BARRON'S

THE TRUSTED NAME IN TEST PREP

PANCE™/ PANRE™ Exam
Premium

Nina Multak, Ph.D., PA-C, DFAAPA

Published by Kaplan North America, LLC, dba Barron's Educational Series
1515 W Cypress Creek Road
Fort Lauderdale, FL 33309
www.barronseduc.com

ISBN: 978-1-5062-6694-7

10 9 8 7 6 5 4 3 2 1

Kaplan North America, LLC, dba Barron's Educational Series print books are available at special quantity discounts to use for sales promotions, employee premiums, or educational purposes. For more information or to purchase books, please call the Simon & Schuster special sales department at 866-506-1949.

About the Author

Nina Multak, PhD, MPAS, PA-C, DFAAPA, is the Associate Dean and Randolph B. Mahoney Director of the University of Florida School of Physician Assistant Studies. She received her doctoral training from the Drexel University College of Computing and Informatics and her master's in Physician Assistant Studies from the University of Nebraska College of Medicine with an emphasis on educational innovation for physician assistant students. She completed her PA training from the Drexel University PA Program (then Hahnemann University). Her clinical experience includes obstetrics and gynecology, ophthalmology, and cardiovascular and thoracic surgery. Dr. Multak has held previous faculty appointments where she also taught PA students, including at Drexel University, NOVA Southeastern University, and the Philadelphia College of Osteopathic Medicine.

Acknowledgments

My sincerest gratitude to the PA and MD faculty from the University of Florida, who provide educational excellence to our PA students and help prepare them for success. Each of you contributes to the development of individuals who dedicate their lives to the pursuit of excellence and providing health care to all citizens, especially those in most need of clinical care.

To my PA colleagues: Your dedication to patient care and to training the next generation of PAs is held in the highest regard. Thanks for all you have done to prepare our students to take the PANCE and prepare them for this important rite of passage as they begin their careers. To those of you using this resource to prepare for your PANRE—good luck! It is a pleasure to call you colleagues and friends.

To all the PA students using this text to prepare to take the PANCE: You are taking the right steps to prepare for a good outcome! Wishing you success on the exam and in your careers.

To the team at Barron's: Thank you for your dedication to providing a resource to help PAs succeed in their initial certification and recertification.

To my family: Alex, Ariel, Ilana, and Ben—your love and support mean the world to me.

Contributors and Reviewers

Roddy J. Bernard, MD, Department of Medicine, University of Florida, Gainesville, FL

Petar Breitinger, MPAS, PA-C, School of PA Studies, College of Medicine, University of Florida, Gainesville, FL

Elizabeth Brownlee, MPAS, PA-C, School of Physician Assistant Studies, College of Medicine, University of Florida, Gainesville, FL

Breann Garbas, DHSc, PA-C, School of Physician Assistant Studies, College of Medicine, University of Florida, Gainesville, FL

Richard Davis, PA-C, University of Florida Health, Gainesville, FL

Paola Gonzalez, MPAS, PA-C, University of Florida Health, Gainesville, FL

Travis Grant, MHS, PA-C, School of PA Studies, College of Medicine, University of Florida, Gainesville, FL

Thao Jinwright, MPAS, PA-C, School of PA Studies, College of Medicine, University of Florida, Gainesville, FL

Amie Ogunsakin, MD, Division of Endocrinology, Diabetes and Metabolism, College of Medicine, University of Florida, Gainsville, FL

Eric S. Papierniak, DO, Division of Pulmonary, Critical Care, and Sleep Medicine, University of Florida, Gainesville, FL

Raju Reddy, MD, University of Florida, Gainesville, FL

Scott Ryals, MD, Division of Pulmonary, Critical Care, and Sleep Medicine, University of Florida, Gainesville, FL

Ashutosh M. Shukla, MD, Director of Advanced CKD and Home Dialysis Services, University of Florida, Gainesville, FL

John Trainer, MD, Community and Family Medicine-Student Health Care Center at Shands, University of Florida, Gainesville, FL

Melissa Turley, PharmD, PA-C, School of Physician Assistant Studies, College of Medicine, University of Florida, Gainesville, FL

Brittany Venegas, MPAS, PA-C, Surgical Critical Care, University of Florida, Gainesville, FL

Whitney Woodmansee, MD, Division of Diabetes, Metabolism and Endocrinology, University of Florida, Gainesville, FL

Yeow Chye Ng, PhD, APRN, AAHWE, CPC, FAAN, Assoc. Prof., University of Alabama, Huntsville, AL

Angela Caires, DNP, CRNP, University of Alabama, Huntsville, AL

Table of Contents

PRACTICE TESTS

How to Use This Book

This book provides comprehensive review and practice for the latest Physician Assistant National Certifying Exam (PANCE™) in alignment with the NCCPA exam blueprint.

Exam Overview

Begin with Chapter 1, the Introduction, which discusses the Physician Assistant National Certifying Exam and the Physician Assistant National Recertifying Exam (also known as PANCE™/ PANRE™). This chapter provides a detailed overview of the exam, including a breakdown of the two main categories (Medical Content Categories and Task Categories) from the most recent blueprint and the percentage of exam content devoted to each topic within each of the categories. Review the directions for scheduling your exam, and learn how the exam is scored.

Preparing for the Exam and Steps for Recertification

Once you're familiar with the exam format, continue reading through Chapter 1 to review expert advice on preparing for test day. Learn how to set up a study plan and how to divvy up the categories and topics into daily and weekly review sessions. Take a look ahead at the beginning of each chapter to see which topics will be covered so you can include them in your study plan. Then, review the details about the exam day experience so you know exactly what to expect. Make sure to also review the requirements for recertification or reinstatement of certification to confirm that you're up-to-date with the latest information.

Review and Practice

Next, study Chapters 2 through 14, which are organized by the two main categories of the PANCE blueprint followed by each topic they explore. Review the Medical Content Categories (including the Cardiovascular, Immune, and Musculoskeletal systems, as well as Infectious Diseases) and the Task Categories (including Using Diagnostics and Labs, Health Maintenance, and Using Pharmaceuticals). These are just a few important topics from the complete list of what you need to know to pass the exam. End-of-chapter practice questions with explanations have also been provided for extra practice of the topics within each chapter.

Practice Tests

There are two full-length practice tests that mirror the actual PANCE in format, content, and level of difficulty. These tests assess your knowledge of the topics within each category, and the percentage of each content area is based on the actual exam structure. Each test is followed by detailed answers and explanations for all questions.

Resources

This book concludes with a list of quick references and resources that can be used for additional studying, as well as an acknowledgment of the contributors who helped put this valuable study guide together.

Online Practice

There is also one additional full-length practice test online. Like the book tests, the online test provides an in-depth review of all tested topics and is structured to mimic the actual exam. You may take this test in practice (untimed) mode or in timed mode. All questions are answered and explained. Refer to the card at the beginning of this book, which provides instructions for accessing this test.

One Final Note

Use this book to supplement your current physician assistant–related knowledge as you prepare for your certification exam. Determine what you know. Make a list of topics that you need to review further as you continue to prepare for your test. Take the practice tests to simulate the conditions you will encounter on test day and to practice what you've learned. Congratulations on your journey to embark on a career as a physician's assistant. Best of luck on your exam!

1

Introduction

Congratulations on selecting a career as a physician assistant (PA)!

The PA profession is a health care innovation that evolved to help fill health care gaps, first in primary care and, today, in all medical and surgical specialties and subspecialties. The tremendous growth and expansion of our profession is reflective of the rapidly changing health care system and is a tribute to thousands of PAs willing to venture into new and different clinical settings and disciplines to provide needed services around the nation and globally.

If you are reading this text, you are likely preparing for the next step in your career—initial certification or recertification. Whether you're preparing to take the Physician Assistant National Certifying Exam (PANCE) or the Physician Assistant National Recertifying Exam (PANRE), this text will help you prepare for success! We'll share with you what to expect on exam day and the days preceding it, how to study, and guidance through the content that should be reviewed. The process to acquire certification is an endurance challenge and your preparation and studying will be like training for a marathon. Just as you planned your path to this point, it is important to set aside time and establish a study plan and schedule to help you achieve success.

The initial certification exam is taken upon graduation from an accredited physician assistant program, and the recertification exam is taken every 10 years after successful completion of the initial certification. The PANCE is composed of 300 multiple-choice questions completed over 5 hours, and the PANRE has 240 multiple-choice questions over a 4-hour time frame. The PANCE consists of 300 multiple-choice questions, which are organized into five blocks of 60 questions each. Exam takers are given 1 hour to complete each block of questions. Although there is no time limit per question, on average a test taker will have 1 minute per question. There is a total of 45 minutes allotted for breaks between blocks, and each exam candidate will be responsible for managing break time. You will have 15 minutes to complete the tutorial prior to beginning the exam.

Becoming a PA

If you are thinking about becoming a PA, but have not yet attended a PA training program, you may be interested in the following information:

- A PA is a nationally certified and state-licensed medical professional.
- PAs practice medicine on health care teams with physicians and other providers.
- PAs practice and prescribe medication in all 50 states, the District of Columbia, the majority of the U.S. territories, the uniformed services, and internationally. Global PA practice is expanding in countries outside the U.S.
- Applicants to physician assistant programs have a bachelor's degree and competitive grades in prerequisite courses like human anatomy and physiology, biology, chemistry, and math. Applicants can also apply to a 5-year, freshman entry-level program.
- Physician assistant training typically occurs in a master's degree program.
- PA programs require applicants to have several hundred hours of experience working or volunteering in health care.

- Most PA programs can be completed in about 2 years to 28 months. Classes may include physiology, pharmacology, and medical ethics. Students are also required to complete clinical rotations at hospitals affiliated with the PA school. During clinical rotations, students work under the supervision of doctors and licensed physician assistants and gain hands-on experience treating patients.
- After completion of an accredited PA training program, the PA will:
    - Become certified by passing the PANCE
    - Get a state license
    - Complete continuing medical education (CME) and recertification/PANRE

Be PANCE Ready with This Book

Exam candidates should review this text as they begin to study for the exam. Study preparation guidance as well as clinical content are included in this resource, which will benefit preparation for the PANCE and PANRE. There will be sections on exam preparation strategies, test-taking strategies, exam content, and general information about medical conditions including pathophysiology, signs and symptoms, diagnostic and lab evaluation, and treatment options. The chapters on study preparation and exam tips should be reviewed first, and after these elements are completed, the practice exam should be taken.

Exam Preparation

Give Yourself Plenty of Time to Prepare

Preparing for the PANCE or PANRE is like preparing for a marathon. It is different from a sprint or short distance run, and there are multiple factors that need to be considered. Exam candidates report allocating at least 6 months of study time to prepare for these exams. Candidates who are taking the PANCE often allocate 3–8 weeks of dedicated time after graduation prior to the scheduled date of the PANCE. Often the hardest part of studying for your PANCE or PANRE is figuring out where to begin.

Begin with the End in Mind

This is a principle important in developing your study plan. When you begin to study for your exam, understand your goals, envision what you want to accomplish, and work backwards from there. In this case, your main goal is to review and understand exam-related information in a specific time period.

Develop a Study Plan

As you get ready for the Physician Assistant National Certification Exam or Recertification Exam, we wanted to share a few tips to help you on your path to success! Like anything in life that is worth a great amount of effort to achieve, it is important to develop a plan and a study strategy to make sure you make the most effective use of your study time leading up to the exam. Having a plan will also reduce your feeling of stress. You should develop your study plan as soon as possible and give yourself plenty of time to prepare. If you do that, you will develop consistent progress and will not feel quite as rushed or anxious about having ample time to study. As you cover each subject area within the exam blueprint, testing your understanding using practice questions is critical to getting the real-time feedback you need to identify your strengths and weaknesses.

Develop a study schedule by starting with a master plan. Your master plan will cover the months you will study and the time you plan to attribute to specific topic review. Your study schedule should list each topic by the month in which it will be completed, as well as the specific days you plan to complete the different subtopics. If possible, study at the same time of day for each session and study consistently. It is much more productive to study in small chunks several times per week than to study for many hours every other week. Decide how long to spend on each topic.

You may be able to plan this through a review of the Physician Assistant Clinical Knowledge Rating and Assessment Tool (PACKRAT) exam you took while enrolled in PA training. Take a look at the results and identify where your strengths and weaknesses lie. Use this information to guide the architecture of your overall study plan and determine exactly how long to take with each topic. While there is no single studying strategy that works best for everyone, you should start by creating a weekly study plan that highlights the category or categories of content you will be reviewing each specific week, and include the right mix of study resources you want to use in addition to this book.

> **NOTE**
>
> The NCCPA also offers practice exams for a fee. Additional information can be found here: *https:// www.nccpa.net/ practiceexams*.

Recertification/PANRE

Taking initial certification exams and recertification exams, the high-stakes exams to verify competency, is a part of the professional journey for every PA. It represents our commitment to lifelong learning. It is required for each PA every 10 years. PAs can recertify during the last 2 years of the certification maintenance cycle. Eligibility for PANRE is available through the National Commission for Certification of Physician Assistants (*https://www.nccpa.net/panre-eligibility*).

Develop Your Plan

In marathon training, you incrementally increase the number of miles you run leading up to the actual race. Building stamina for your PANCE or PANRE is similar. Practicing is key to success. You will spend many hours and hours preparing for your PANCE/PANRE, and you should prepare to focus for long periods of time during the exam. The way to build up stamina in test-taking is very similar to training for a marathon. Once you are two weeks from exam day, set aside time to practice questions without interruption.

Two weeks before exam day: Take a block of 60 questions and give yourself 1 hour to complete it. Limit your break to 5 minutes before starting the second block of 60 questions. Two blocks of 60 questions (about 2 hours of test taking) is your goal. Slowly introduce your body and brain to long periods of focus.

Ten days before exam day: Do the same as above, but now work through three blocks of 60 questions for a total work time of 3 hours.

Seven days before exam day: Simulate the actual exam. Work through five blocks of 60 questions. Limit your breaks to 5–10 minutes between blocks. Take a 20- to 30-minute break. Turn off all notifications on your computer. No food or beverages while you answer your questions. Don't answer the door or phone. You want to simulate the exam experience as closely as possible.

Three days before exam day: Complete three blocks of 60 questions.
You can modify any of the variables above. The most important thing is to expose your mind and body to 5 hours of continuous focus. However, just like in marathon training, you need to provide your brain and body a recovery period. It is suggested that you avoid taking a full-length exam within 24 hours of exam day.

Exam Checklist

Night Before Exam	Day of Exam
☐ Identify how long it is going to take you to get to the testing center.	☐ Eat breakfast.
☐ Locate your car keys or confirm public transportation plan.	☐ Leave your house with enough time to arrive at the testing center (actually in the center, not the parking lot) 30 minutes before your scheduled exam time (factor in parking time).
☐ Confirm you have enough gas in your car to get to the exam and funds for transportation and/or parking.	☐ Check in with registration.
☐ Locate your picture ID and pack it with what you are bringing to the testing center.	☐ Place your belongings in your locker.
☐ Lay out your clothes.	☐ You will be escorted to your testing station. Get comfortable, look around your cubicle, adjust your chair. Adjust clothing layers if necessary.
☐ Pack your lunch or snack.	☐ Before you begin your exam, take a slow deep breath in and slowly exhale.
	☐ Begin exam—you've prepared for success.

Repetition and Review

It's important to reinforce what you've learned in the past. It's natural to forget some concepts as you learn new information. We believe that many students in their quest to get through all the material as quickly as possible simply do not spend enough time reviewing material they've studied a few days, weeks, or months ago. It's important to remember that the key is not to be a quick learner, but to be efficient. Repetition and regular review are key to developing any new skill, and we believe fundamental to succeeding on the PANCE and PANRE.

Find a Good Place to Study

You should identify a place to study. It is up to you to decide what works best for you: home, library, music, silence, etc. The important thing is to be consistent. The more often you study in the same place, the easier it will make the most effective use of your time. You are going to want to pick a place where you are not going to be distracted.

Study location tips and suggestions:

- Avoid areas that friends and family can easily make contact with you.
- Avoid areas where people are continually entering and exiting (this causes you to look up often and breaks concentration).

We know that preparing for the PANCE and PANRE can be a stressful experience, and it is important to prioritize your preparation above everything else. At the same time, don't sacrifice regular physical activity in the process. In the weeks and months ahead, as you work toward entering a career in which you will help countless people live healthy lives, it is important not to sacrifice your own. Be sure to get fresh air and sufficient exercise, and include it as part of your study plan if you have to!

Identify a Study Partner or Group

You may benefit by interspersing individual study with a study partner or small group. Studying with an equally motivated study partner can be a great way to learn. Study partners provide you with accountability to keep you on track and the ability to review areas of comfort or clarify information blind spots you may have.

If you are currently in PA school, or graduated recently, your classmates can be terrific study partners. During your first group meeting, it's a good idea to determine your compatibility by comparing schedules to make sure you won't struggle to find times that work well for both of you. While you are waiting to form a study group, remember to also consider a significant other, sibling, or friend as a study partner even if they are not preparing for the PANCE or PANRE exam themselves. Although they may not be able to explain or clarify PA concepts to you, they can be great sounding boards as you talk through concepts out loud and terrific at quizzing you using this text, flash cards, or a study guide.

Review of Exam Blueprint

Multiple-choice examinations are the most commonly employed method for assessment of cognitive skills in medical education. The practice tests associated with this resource are single best answer multiple-choice questions that are the same format as on the PANCE and PANRE.

Know What to Study

The National Commission for Certification of PAs publishes an exam blueprint on their website: *https://www.nccpa.net/become-certified/pance-blueprint/*. This provides information on the content and topic areas. Focus should include the following for each topic:

- Pathophysiology
- Clinical Presentation
- Symptoms
- Signs
- Diagnostic and Lab Studies
- Differential Diagnosis/Formulating the Most Likely Diagnosis
- Health Maintenance and Patient Education
- Treatment (Pharmaceutical and Clinical Intervention)
- Professional Considerations

NOTE

When one of the list items is not applicable to the condition discussed, it will not appear under the topic. Sometimes symptoms and signs are grouped together depending on the condition being explained.

Medical Content Categories

Category	% of Content
Cardiovascular System	16%
Pulmonary System	12%
Gastrointestinal System/Nutrition	10%
Musculoskeletal System	10%
Eyes, Ears, Nose, and Throat	9%
Reproductive System	8%
Endocrine System	6%
Genitourinary System	6%
Neurologic System	6%
Psychiatry/Behavioral	6%
Dermatologic System	5%
Hematologic System	3%
Infectious Diseases	3%
Total	**100%**

Professional Task Categories

Formulating most likely diagnosis: 18%

Pharmaceutical therapeutics: 18%

History taking & physical exams: 16%

Using laboratory & diagnostic studies: 14%

Clinical intervention: 14%

Health maintenance: 10%

Applying basic science concepts: 10%

2

Cardiovascular Review

Learning Objectives

In this chapter, you will review:

→ Conduction disorders
→ Congenital heart disease
→ Coronary artery disease
→ Heart failure
→ Hypertension
→ Hypotension
→ Lipid disorders
→ Trauma
→ Infectious and inflammatory heart conditions
→ Valvular disorders and vascular disease

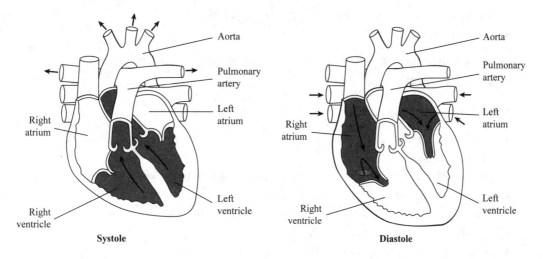

Figure 2.1 Physiology: The cardiac cycle

Cardiomyopathy

Cardiomyopathies are a group of diseases of the myocardium associated with mechanical and/or electrical dysfunction that usually exhibit inappropriate ventricular hypertrophy or dilatation and are due to a variety of causes that frequently are genetic.

Cardiomyopathies are divided into two major groups based on predominant organ involvement. **Primary cardiomyopathies** (genetic, nongenetic, acquired) are those solely or predominantly confined to heart muscle and are relatively few in number. **Secondary cardiomyopathies** show pathological myocardial involvement as part of a large number and variety of multi-organ disorders. The current American Heart Association definition divides cardiomyopathies into primary, which affect the heart alone, and secondary, which are the result of illness affecting other parts of the body.

Types of cardiomyopathy include *hypertrophic* cardiomyopathy, *dilated* cardiomyopathy, *restrictive* cardiomyopathy, *arrhythmogenic right ventricular dysplasia*, and *takotsubo* cardiomyopathy.

All types of cardiomyopathy may be associated with atrioventricular (AV) valve regurgitation, typical and atypical chest pain, atrial and ventricular tachyarrhythmias, and embolic events. The nonspecific term *congestive heart failure* describes only the resulting syndrome of fluid retention, which is common to all three types of cardiomyopathy and also to cardiac structural diseases associated with elevated filling pressures.

Characteristics of cardiomyopathies include:

- Hypertrophic cardiomyopathy: The heart muscle enlarges and thickens.
- Dilated cardiomyopathy: The ventricles enlarge and weaken.
- Restrictive cardiomyopathy: The ventricle stiffens.

Dilated Cardiomyopathy

Pathophysiology

- Dilated cardiomyopathy in adults is most commonly caused by CAD (ischemic cardiomyopathy) and hypertension.
- Characterized by an enlarged left ventricle with reduced systolic function as measured by left ventricular ejection fraction.
- Enlarged and weakened ventricles

Dilated cardiomyopathy can lead to heart failure, heart valve disease, irregular heart rate, and blood clots in the heart.

Clinical Presentation

- Shortness of breath, fatigue, cough, orthopnea, paroxysmal nocturnal dyspnea, edema, syncope, S3 gallop, rales
- Early symptoms often relate to exertional intolerance with breathlessness or fatigue.
- Symptoms may initially be unnoticed or attributed to other causes.
- Harsh murmur heard at left sternal edge that increases with Valsalva maneuver.
- Standing position often heard on auscultation.
- Peripheral edema may be absent despite severe fluid retention.

As fluid retention leads to elevation of resting filling pressures, shortness of breath may occur during routine daily activity, such as dressing, and may manifest as dyspnea or cough when lying down at night.

Diagnostic and Lab Studies

Echocardiography is a key diagnostic modality for patients with suspected cardiomyopathy. In dilated cardiomyopathy, echocardiography typically demonstrates an enlarged ventricular chamber with normal or decreased wall thickness and systolic dysfunction.

- ECG will show left ventricular hypertrophy, as well as a large QRS complex, Q-waves with no history of CAD, and frequent T-wave inversion.
  - In patients with familial idiopathic dilated cardiomyopathy, the American College of Cardiology (ACC)/AHA heart failure guidelines recommend screening asymptomatic

first-degree relatives with echocardiography and ECG, as well as possible referral to a cardiovascular genetics center.

○ ECG typically reveals decreased voltage despite signs of left ventricular hypertrophy.

■ Echocardiography typically reveals global or segmental wall abnormalities with or without wall motion abnormalities. The ECG shows abnormal repolarization and small-amplitude potentials at the end of the QRS complex (epsilon wave). The diagnosis is typically made by evaluating for electrical, functional, and anatomic abnormalities that may have been evaluated previously because of a sudden arrhythmia, syncope, or cardiac arrest.

Differential Diagnosis/Formulating the Most Likely Diagnosis

Dilated cardiomyopathy is also associated with HIV, Chagas disease, rheumatologic disorders, iron overload, sleep apnea, amyloidosis, sarcoidosis, chronic alcohol usage, and end-stage kidney disease.

Health Maintenance and Patient Education

■ Identify behaviors that may predispose patient to the disease or family history.
■ Alcohol use should be discontinued, since there is often marked recovery of cardiac function following a period of abstinence.
■ Endocrine causes should be treated.

Treatment (Pharmaceutical and Clinical Intervention)

Treatment for dilated cardiomyopathy is directed at the underlying disease. Most patients have heart failure; therefore, treatment should follow the ACC/AHA heart failure guidelines. Lifestyle changes should include reduced alcohol consumption, weight loss, exercise, smoking cessation, and a low-sodium diet.

Treatment includes administration of an angiotensin-converting enzyme inhibitor or angiotensin receptor blocker, a loop diuretic, spironolactone (Aldactone) for New York Heart Association (NYHA) class III or IV heart failure, and a beta-blocker. Metoprolol (Lopressor), carvedilol (Coreg), and bisoprolol (Zebeta) are the only beta-blockers with proven benefit in heart failure.

Professional Considerations

■ Monitoring severity of RV dysfunction is critical in long-term prognosis.
■ Patients with new or worsening symptoms of heart failure with dilated cardiomyopathy should be referred to a cardiologist.
■ Patients with continued symptoms of heart failure and reduced LVEF (35% or less) should be referred to a cardiologist for consideration of placement of an ICD.
■ Patients with advanced refractory symptoms should be referred to a cardiologist for consideration of heart transplant or LV assist device.
■ Patients with hypoxia, fluid overload, or pulmonary edema unable to be managed and resolved in an outpatient setting should be admitted to the hospital for stabilization.

Hypertrophic Cardiomyopathy

Pathophysiology

Hypertrophic cardiomyopathy is very common and can affect people of any age. It affects men and women equally, and about 1 out of every 500 people has the disease. Hypertrophic cardiomyopathy happens when the heart muscle enlarges and thickens without an obvious cause. Usually the ventricles, lower chambers of the heart, and septum (the wall that separates the left and right side of the heart) thicken. The thickened areas create narrowing or blockages in the ventricles, making it harder for the heart to pump blood. Hypertrophic cardiomyopathy also can cause stiffness of the ventricles, changes in the mitral valve, and cellular changes in the heart tissue.

Clinical Presentation

- Same as dilated cardiomyopathy—dyspnea, chest pain, syncope; sudden cardiac death
- Arrhythmias, angina, or even asymptomatic PE—sustained PMI, S4 gallop

Diagnostic and Lab Studies

- Endomyocardial bx to determine type of cardiomyopathy may be necessary—amyloidosis, radiation, etc.
- Echocardiogram is diagnostic.
- ECG shows LVH, large QRS complex, Q-waves, and frequent T-wave inversion.
- Echocardiography shows LVH with reduction in ventricular chamber volume.

Differential Diagnosis/Formulating the Most Likely Diagnosis

Distinguish from athletic hypertrophy, which has no diastolic dysfunction, and hypertrophic cardiomyopathy in older adults that is usually associated with hypertension.

Health Maintenance and Patient Education

- Patients with malignant ventricular arrhythmias and/or unexplained syncope in the presence of a positive family history for sudden death, with or without an abnormal BP response to exercise, are best managed with an implantable defibrillator.
- Reasonable to consider an implantable cardioverter-defibrillator (ICD) for patients with hypertrophic cardiomyopathy and maximum wall thickness of at least 30 mm, sudden cardiac death in a first-degree relative, and/or unexplained syncope in the last 6 months.

Treatment (Pharmaceutical and Clinical Intervention)

- Beta-blockers should be the initial medication in symptomatic individuals.
  - The resulting slower heart rates assist with diastolic filling of the stiff LV. Dyspnea, angina, and arrhythmias respond in about 50% of patients.
- Calcium channel blockers, especially verapamil, have also been effective in symptomatic patients. Verapamil is preferred due to its more potent effects on the myocardium. Their effect is due primarily to improved diastolic function; however, their vasodilating actions can also increase outflow obstruction and cause hypotension.
- Septal myomectomy (only in patients with obstructive hypertrophic cardiomyopathy), biventricular pacing, implantable cardioverter-defibrillator

Professional Considerations

- Increased risk of sudden death
- Genetic testing is recommended if first-degree relatives are available to participate. Some patients remain asymptomatic for many years or for life.

- The highest risk patients are those with a personal history of ventricular arrhythmias, a family history of sudden death, unexplained syncope, or documented ventricular tachycardia.
- Patients should be referred to a cardiologist when symptoms are difficult to control, syncope has occurred, or there are any of the high-risk features present.

Restrictive Cardiomyopathy

Pathophysiology

Restrictive cardiomyopathies (RCM) are characterized by small, stiff ventricles with progressive impairment of diastolic filling, leading to the hemodynamic flow preload but high filling pressures. This pattern of diastolic dysfunction leads to dilated atria and elevated mean atrial pressures, resulting clinically in biventricular "backward failure" manifest as pulmonary venous congestion (dyspnea), as well as systemic venous pressure elevation (peripheral edema).

Clinical Presentation

- Pedal edema, abdominal swelling, and loss of appetite
- Physical exam reveals elevated jugular venous pressure often with Kussmaul sign, peripheral edema, and ascites.
- Patients typically are limited by dyspnea on exertion attributable to left heart diastolic dysfunction.

Diagnostic and Lab Studies

- Echocardiography: small stiff ventricles, preserved systolic function (until late stages), dilated atria, and diastolic dysfunction by Doppler
- Cardiac magnetic resonance imaging is powerful: delineates myocardial infiltration, inflammation, and fibrosis and assesses pericardium.

Differential Diagnosis/Formulating the Most Likely Diagnosis

- Constrictive pericarditis
- Hypertrophic obstructive cardiomyopathy (HOCM)
- Hypertensive heart disease
- Ischemic heart disease
- Dilated cardiomyopathy

Health Maintenance and Patient Education

In the early stages of disease, systolic function is typically preserved, although deterioration in contractility may be observed as the disease progresses.

Treatment (Pharmaceutical and Clinical Intervention)

- Disease etiologies are often untreatable.
- Management is based on diuretics to reduce systemic and pulmonary venous congestions.

Professional Considerations

A tissue biopsy may be necessary for a definitive diagnosis.

Conduction Disorders/Dysrhythmias

Atrial Fibrillation/Flutter

Pathophysiology

Atrial fibrillation is an arrhythmia characterized by rapid, irregular, disorganized atrial activation with an irregular ventricular response. The ventricular response is usually between 120–160 beats/minute, but occasionally can be seen with high rates of 200 beats/minute or a slow ventricular rate in patients with high vagal tone or atrioventricular (AV) nodal conduction disease. An electrocardiogram (ECG) may depict absence of distinct P-waves with an irregularly irregular ventricular response.

- This arrhythmia is caused by triggering foci. Paroxysmal atrial fibrillation may be associated with hypoxia, anemia, thyroid disease, acute alcohol intoxication (also known as holiday heart), electrolyte imbalances, postsurgical patients, or an acute illness. Development of atrial arrhythmias occur more often in patients with hypertension, heart failure, and rheumatic heart disease.
- Atrial flutter is largely due to a reentry circuit, associated with a circuit that revolves around the tricuspid valve annulus. This produces a characteristic saw tooth flutter wave on ECG.
- The atrial rate of flutter is around 240–300 beats/minute. It often conducts with a 2:1 response to the ventricles, creating a "regular" appearing tachycardia at the rate of 150 beats/minute, with difficult P-wave visualization.

Clinical Presentation

A patient may present with a variety of symptoms that can be nonspecific to their diagnosis. In addition, atrial fibrillation can be concurrent with both cardiac and noncardiac conditions, or it can be identified after an initial presentation of stroke, heart failure, or thromboembolic disease. Patients can also be asymptomatic at time of presentation.

Risk factors such as hypertension, heart failure, sleep apnea, and diabetes may identify patients who may be evaluated for an arrhythmia such as atrial fibrillation.

- Incidence of atrial fibrillation increases with age.
- Atrial fibrillation may also be seen in the context of cardiothoracic and noncardiac surgery, pericarditis, myocarditis, electrocution, pneumonia, and pulmonary embolisms.

Symptoms
- Palpitations
- Syncope
- Dizziness
- Dyspnea
- Breathlessness
- Chest discomfort
- Stroke/TIA (transient ischemic attack) with no other explanatory cause
- It may also occur with hypotension, heart failure, or fatigue.

Signs
- A prudent physical exam should identify patients who have a palpable irregular pulse or audible irregular heartbeat. An irregular pulse on a physical exam is found to be sensitive to the presence of atrial fibrillation.

- The pulse has a loss of *a*-waves when palpating the jugular venous pulse. There may also be a pulse deficit, where the left ventricle may not be able to produce a peripheral pressure wave when faced with tachycardia, and physical exam may find that the apical ventricular rate is faster than the rate palpated at the wrist.
    - Variations on the intensity of the first heart sound or the absence of a fourth heart sound may be discovered.
    - The pulse in atrial flutter may be rapid and regular. Jugular venous pulse oscillations may be visible.

Diagnostic and Lab Studies

- All patients should obtain an electrocardiogram if atrial fibrillation is expected. In patients that have suspected paroxysmal timing, a 24-hour ambulatory ECG monitor may be utilized with symptoms occurring less than 24 hours apart or an event recorder ECG in those with symptoms occurring greater than 24 hours apart.
- Atrial fibrillation appears on ECG with the absence of P-waves and presence of fibrillatory waves between the QRS complexes at a rate of 300/minute. They are irregular in timing and morphology and appear with irregularly irregular R-R intervals.
- Atrial flutter produces a characteristic sawtooth flutter wave on ECG. The atrial rate of flutter is around 240–300 beats/minute. It often conducts with a 2:1 response to the ventricles, creating a "regular" appearing tachycardia at the rate of 150 beats/minute, with difficult P-wave visualization.

Transthoracic echocardiography (TTE) will be performed in patients with atrial fibrillation for whom a baseline TTE is important in their long-term management, for whom a possible cardioversion is being considered, for whom there is high risk or a question of underlying structural/functional heart disease, such as heart failure or a murmur, or for whom clinical risk stratification is needed for choosing antithrombotic therapy. TTE should not be performed routinely in those whom the provider and the patient have already decided on the initiation of anticoagulation therapy with the appropriate criteria. Transesophageal echocardiography (TEE) can be utilized when patients with atrial fibrillation have an abnormality on the TTE that needs more clarification, such as valvular abnormalities, if a TTE is technically difficult, or in patients for whom a TEE-guided cardioversion is being offered.

Differential Diagnosis/Formulating the Most Likely Diagnosis

Defining the timing of atrial fibrillation may clarify a treatment strategy for providers. Paroxysmal atrial fibrillation is defined by arrhythmias that start and stop spontaneously within 7 days of onset. Persistent atrial fibrillation is longer than 7 days or requires an intervention to terminate the rhythm. Long-standing persistent atrial fibrillation lasts over 1 year but still has the opportunity to convert into sinus rhythm. Permanent atrial fibrillation is defined when cardioversion is failed or not attempted, whether in patients for whom a decision has been made to not attempt cardioversion or those who have greater risks than benefits of chemical or electrical cardioversion.

Health Maintenance and Patient Education

Patients with atrial fibrillation require personalized care and education. Since care of atrial fibrillation is now increasingly patient-centered and symptom-directed, this education should include items such as arrhythmia causes and effects, possible complications of atrial fibrillation, stroke awareness and mechanisms to prevent stroke occurrences, rate and rhythm control with symptom recognition, anticoagulation therapy, and support networks. Some patients may be referred to cardiology, electrophysiologists, psychological support, and other networks for atrial fibrillation advice.

Treatment (Pharmaceutical and Clinical Intervention)

In any patient with life-threatening hemodynamic instability, an emergent electrical cardioversion should be performed without delay for anticoagulation. In patients who present with new-onset atrial fibrillation, and the atrial fibrillation is thought to be the primary problem for their presentation, a rhythm control strategy can be taken. A patient's duration of atrial fibrillation and their thromboembolic risk are important factors in the decision for rhythm control over rate control. A restoration of sinus rhythm in this population can be performed with pharmacological and/or electrical cardioversion. Other rhythm control medications are available but will not be discussed in this context.

As a first-line strategy, rate control should be offered for patients, except for those who have a reversible cause of atrial fibrillation, those who have heart failure thought to be caused by atrial fibrillation, new-onset arrhythmia, those with atrial flutter who are suitable for an ablation to restore sinus rhythm, or those for whom rhythm control would be more suitable, based on the clinical judgement of the provider. In patients who still experience symptoms with adequate trial of drug therapy, a left atrial ablation may be offered for patients with paroxysmal atrial fibrillation, or a left atrial catheter or surgical ablation for patients with persistent atrial fibrillation. Rate control medications may include a standard beta-blocker or a rate-limiting calcium channel blocker as initial monotherapy. Digoxin monotherapy may be offered for patients who have non-paroxysmal atrial fibrillation only if they have a sedentary lifestyle. A combination drug therapy may be chosen if escalating monotherapy does not control symptoms or if rate control is poor. Amiodarone should not be offered for long-term rate control.

If a patient still remains symptomatic after optimal heart rate-control, a pharmacological or electrical rhythm control can be offered, understanding that in patients with atrial fibrillation lasting longer than 48 hours, an electrical cardioversion should be indicated. If possible, delay the electrical cardioversion until optimal anticoagulation has been achieved at a minimum of 3 weeks, or consider TEE for evaluation of a thrombus prior to cardioversion. If patients have symptoms that are caused by known precipitants (e.g., alcohol, caffeine, etc.), or with other infrequent occasions of arrhythmia, a "no drug treatment" or "pill-in-the-pocket" strategies may be considered. The criteria for these strategies include patients who are reliable to understand how to and when to take the medication, have an adequate blood pressure and heart rate at baseline, have infrequent symptomatic episodes of paroxysmal atrial fibrillation, and have no history of ischemic heart disease, valvular heart disease, or history of left ventricular function.

- Stroke risk should be assessed for patients with atrial fibrillation utilizing the CHA2DS2-VASc stroke risk score if the patients have atrial flutter, either symptomatic or asymptomatic paroxysmal, persistent or permanent atrial fibrillation, or a risk of recurrence of atrial fibrillation after cardioversion back into sinus rhythm.
- Bleeding risk also should be calculated in patients to assess the risk of bleeding in those who have or are starting anticoagulation, utilizing the HAS-BLED score.

Several risk factors should also be modified, including uncontrolled hypertension, harmful alcohol consumption, poor control of international normalized ratio (INR), and evaluation of other interacting medications, such as NSAID or aspirin. Aspirin should not be offered as monotherapy for the sole prevention of strokes with atrial fibrillation.

- Anticoagulation should be considered in men with CHA2DS2-VASc score over 1, or with patients with CHA2DS2-VASc over 2, while taking bleeding risk into account. Do not offer stroke prevention therapy to patients under age 65 with no other risk factors other than their sex.
- A time in therapeutic range (TTR) may be a helpful tool in measuring a patient's anticoagulation control with vitamin K antagonists. In order to calculate a TTR, utilize a maintenance period of at least 6 months, while excluding the first 6 weeks of treatment with anticoagulation.
  - Use a validated method, such as computer-assisted dosing, the Rosendaal method, or a proportion of tests in range for manual dosing, to assess a patient's appropriate response to their anticoagulation control.
  - If the anticoagulation control is poor and cannot be improved, the risks and benefits of continuing or stopping anticoagulation control with education of alternative stroke prevention strategies must be discussed with the patient, and a decision made conjointly.
- Treatment of atrial flutter is very similar to atrial fibrillation. If a patient is hemodynamically compromised, a cardioversion is recommended. Rate control strategy and anticoagulation therapy is recommended with guidelines similar to those with atrial fibrillation. Ablation can also be offered by an electrophysiologist in patients with recurrent atrial flutter.

Professional Considerations

When discussing the risks and benefits of anticoagulation, it should be explained that for most patients, the benefit of anticoagulation outweighs the risk of bleeding. Also, for patients with an increased HAS-BLED risk of bleeding, the benefit of anticoagulation may not always outweigh the bleeding risk. Thus, careful decision making and monitoring of the choice of anticoagulation is important. In addition, review the need and quality of anticoagulation annually, or more frequently if a clinical event occurs.

Atrial fibrillation, due to the loss of atrial contraction, can lower the cardiac output by about 10%, compared to a patient's sinus rhythm. This decrease is usually tolerated well, except in cases where a patient's heart rate is fast or when patients already have a lower cardiac output at baseline. This effect to cardiac output should be weighed heavily when discussion regarding rate or rhythm control is had. Some patients, when left in atrial fibrillation, may develop heart failure.

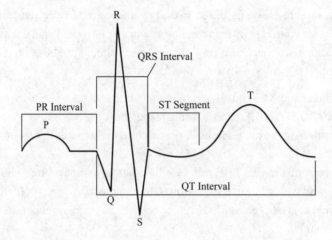

Figure 2.2 Cardiac output/ECG intervals

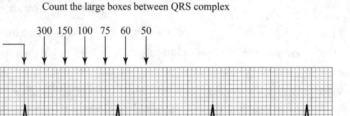

Figure 2.3 EKG sample

Atrioventricular Block

Pathophysiology

An atrioventricular (AV) block is an arrhythmia in which the electrical passage from the atria to the ventricles is either delayed or stopped. This may be due to an anatomical defect or a functional impairment with the conduction system. The most common causes of AV block are idiopathic fibrosis and sclerosis of the conduction system and ischemic heart disease.

Other causes are drugs (such as beta-blockers, calcium channel blockers, digoxin, and amiodarone), increased vagal tone, valvulopathy, congenital heart, genetic, cardiomyopathies, infections, cardiac surgery, or other causes.

Clinical Presentation

- A first-degree AV block and a second-degree type I block may occur in younger patients who have a higher vagal tone, as well as in well-trained athletes. There may be no physical exam findings.
  - First-degree AV block is usually asymptomatic.

- Second- and third-degree AV blocks may occur with a slow palpable pulse that may or may not be irregular due to dropped beats in second-degree AV block or slow ventricular escape rhythm in third-degree AV block.
  - Second-degree AV block may occur with light-headedness, presyncope and syncope, or as an asymptomatic arrhythmia. Depending on the rate and quality of the ventricular rhythm, systemic perfusion may not be reliably maintained, and thus more symptoms may present.
- Third-degree block may also have physical exam findings of cannon *a*-waves, changes in the loudness of S1, or blood pressure fluctuations.
  - Third-degree heart block may occur with effort intolerance, postural light-headedness, fatigue, weakness, and bradycardia.

Diagnostic and Lab Studies

- First-degree AV block is defined by a fixed P-R interval of greater than 200 milliseconds (five small squares on the ECG). Each P-wave is followed by a QRS complex.
- A second-degree AV block is separated into two types: type I (Mobitz I or Wenckebach) and type II (Mobitz II). Second-degree type I shows a pattern of gradual, repeated prolongation of the P-R interval, which eventually cycles after a failure of conduction of an atrial beat.
  - A second-degree type II AV block occurs during a rhythm in which most beats have a constant P-R interval, but on occasion, an atrial depolarization is not followed by a ventricular depolarization. This block is usually in a repeating cycle of every third (3:1 block) or fourth (4:1 block) P-wave. The P-P interval is constant, and the R-R interval will be constant until the dropped beat occurs.
- A third-degree heart block, or complete heart block, is shown when there is complete dissociation of QRS complexes from their respective P-waves.
  - The P-P and R-R intervals remain constant but are independent of each other. The atrial rate is usually faster than the ventricular rate. Usually, ventricular escape complexes occur at a rate of 30–40 bpm and are wide.

Differential Diagnosis/Formulating the Most Likely Diagnosis

Differentiating between the AV blocks may be determined by reviewing an ECG, or a rhythm strip, to determine intervals of the PR, QRS, and frequency of dropped beats.

Health Maintenance and Patient Education

- A first-degree AV block and a second-degree type I AV block can occur in normal, healthy individuals with likely no progression to further blocks.
- A second-degree type II AV block and third-degree AV block can progress due to the disease within the conduction system, and a pacemaker is usually indicated.

Treatment (Pharmaceutical and Clinical Intervention)

- For a first-degree block and second-degree type I block, no specific therapy is required, yet this rhythm may be a marker of an underlying problem, such as MI, myocarditis, degenerative diseases, or a drug effect (e.g., tricyclic antidepressants).
- In a second-degree type II block, usually treatment is pacing, whether temporary or permanent pacing, even in those who present with no symptoms. When this block presents, it indicates a disease of the conduction system distal to the AV node and can lead to further AV blocks.

- Third-degree heart blocks require permanent pacing, regardless of symptoms. Emergent temporary pacing may be necessary if there is hemodynamic instability.

Professional Considerations

All reversible causes of heart block should be taken into consideration when approaching a patient with a newly diagnosed AV block. Functional causes of AV block (autonomic, metabolic/endocrine, and drug-related) tend to be reversible.

- Pharmacologic treatment: atropine; treat reversible causes—hyperkalemia, endocarditis, myocarditis
- Medications that prolong intervals (inotropes and vasopressors), electrical imbalances, trauma, surgery, or infection may contribute to the AV block. The workup of these items may prevent the patient from potentiating further into more severe blocks or arrhythmias.

Bundle Branch Block

Pathophysiology

A bundle branch block occurs when there is a dysfunction in the bundle of His, leading to a block of the electrical passage either into the left or right bundle of His. This kind of block may occur due to other heart disorders, including intrinsic degeneration. A right bundle branch block (RBBB) occurs when conduction is delayed through the right bundle, but the depolarization through the left bundle occurs normally. Because of this, a secondary R-wave will occur. A left bundle branch block (LBBB) occurs when conduction through the left bundle is delayed and electrical activity through the right bundle occurs normally. This will produce tall R-waves in the lateral leads and deep S-waves in the right precordial leads.

Clinical Presentation

- RBBB will increase prevalence with age. Because the anatomy of the right bundle branch tracks near the sub-endocardial surface, it can be compromised by stretch and trauma. It is more likely to be seen in patients with increased right ventricular pressure, such as RV hypertrophy, pulmonary embolism, myocardial inflammation, ischemia, or infarction, and certain procedures or interventions.
- LBBB can occur in patients with underlying heart disease, as the conduction system can be injured with ischemia and infarction of tissue. LBBB can also present in patients with a structurally normal heart and without symptoms. As with RBBB, LBBB increases prevalence with age, and it can be caused by slowly progressing cardiac disease.

Patients with bundle branch blocks are generally asymptomatic unless they occur with another specific disease that may be causing symptoms, such as chest pain or shortness of breath. Symptoms that can present are fatigue, dyspnea, palpitations, exercise intolerance, and syncope.

Diseases such as pulmonary hypertension, obstructive sleep apnea, pulmonary embolism, myocardial infarction, endocarditis, or syncope may present with symptoms that can be associated with bundle branch blocks.

Diagnostic and Lab Studies

On ECG, the QRS will appear wide, usually without any problem with AV conduction (i.e., they usually are in normal sinus rhythm). In a left bundle branch block (LBBB), there will be an "M" appearance in V6 and a "W" pattern in V1. With the right bundle branch block (RBBB), there is an RSR complex in V1, and a QRS complex in V6. There will also be ST depression and T-wave inversion in R precordial leads and a slurred S-wave in the lateral leads. Additional testing includes an echocardiogram to evaluate heart function and for valvular disorders or stress testing or imaging to evaluate for ischemia or infarction.

Differential Diagnosis/Formulating the Most Likely Diagnosis

- Ventricular tachycardia and other ventricle-initiated rhythms may appear similar to bundle branch blocks. If a ventricular rhythm originates in the ventricle, the QRS will appear widened and can look like bundle branch blocks. However, the ventricular rhythms will have AV dissociation, which will separate the diagnoses.
- Ventricular pacing may also appear to have a wide QRS, such as bundle branch blocks, but the presence of pacemaker spikes prior to the QRS complex on an ECG will differentiate the two rhythms.

Health Maintenance and Patient Education

The presence of a bundle branch block with an acute myocardial infarction and in heart failure is associated with a significant increase in mortality. LBBB and RBBB are also an independent predictor of all-cause mortality in patients with cardiovascular disease. Therefore, evaluation for hypertension, coronary disease, myocarditis, valvular heart disease, and cardiomyopathies should occur. Close follow-up is indicated.

Treatment (Pharmaceutical and Clinical Intervention)

Bundle branch blocks are found commonly in the population. Neither by itself is an indication for pacing, but they both may indicate an increased risk of cardiovascular disease. If the LBBB is determined to be new, it may be a cause of concern. If it coexists with symptoms of angina, it may indicate an MI. A new RBBB may occur with no evidence of heart disease, but also with anterior myocardial infarction or after a pulmonary embolism. Even without structural heart disease, an LBBB is associated with dyssynchronous left ventricular activation, which in turn will reduce the quality of left ventricular contraction. This may cause a lower left ventricular ejection fraction and cardiac output, which may cause hypotension and worsening heart failure symptoms. Consults to cardiology and electrophysiology may be needed for further diagnosis, heart failure treatment optimization, and even implantation of a pacemaker for resynchronization with biventricular pacing.

Professional Considerations

A STEMI is a difficult diagnosis to make with an LBBB. ST elevation, ST depression, and T-wave inversions may be present in both diagnoses. The Sgarbossa criteria is used to help diagnose a STEMI in the presence of LBBB.

Paroxysmal Supraventricular Tachycardia

Pathophysiology

Paroxysmal supraventricular tachycardia (PSVT) denotes a tachyarrhythmia that arises above the His bundle bifurcation. This arrhythmia occurs mostly as a reentrant mechanism but may also occur due to increased automaticity. The most common form of PSVT is atrioventricular nodal reentrant tachycardia (AVNRT). It has a sudden onset and end, with heart rates usually between 180–200 beats/min. Due to this arrhythmia's reentrant mechanism location within the AV node, the atria and ventricles can be simultaneously stimulated, causing concurrent P-waves within the QRS complexes. The second most common form of PSVT is atrioventricular reciprocating tachycardia (AVRT). This occurs when electrical activity travels from the AV node to a retrograde accessory bypass tract. The QRS morphology is normal appearing because the ventricular activation occurs through standard pathways; thus, the accessory pathway is concealed. ECG findings include a heart rate faster than 200 beats/min or P-waves seen following the QRS complex. Other less common PSVT forms include sinus node reentry, intra-atrial reentry, and automatic atrial tachycardia. These tachyarrhythmias are more often seen in patients with cardiac disease.

Clinical Presentation

Typically, patients with AVNRT present in the third and fourth decade of life, and 70% of the patients are female. Majority of patients with AVNRT do not have cardiac disease. The less common forms of PSVT can be seen in patients with underlying cardiac disease.

Patients may present with symptoms such as palpitations, light-headedness, diaphoresis, or syncope.

- Rapid heart rates may also present with angina, hypotension, and symptoms of pulmonary edema, such as leg swelling and shortness of breath. The rapid heart rate is usually abrupt in onset.
- A physical exam may show a rapid pulse and a cardiac auscultation of a rapid heartbeat.

Diagnostic and Lab Studies

An ECG will show a narrow complex tachycardia, with a rate greater than 100 beats per minute and QRS less than 120 milliseconds.

Many patients with this arrhythmia should be referred for an echocardiogram to evaluate for any evidence of structural heart disease. In addition, further testing may be considered, such as ambulatory ECG monitoring or stress testing.

Differential Diagnosis/Formulating the Most Likely Diagnosis

In order to differentiate common forms of tachycardias, initial management may be to increase vagal tone, utilizing carotid sinus massage, Valsalva maneuver, or the diving reflex, in order to slow down the pathway. In a number of patients, the tachycardia will terminate spontaneously with the maneuvers. If it does not, an adenosine challenge may be performed to produce a temporary AV block, interrupting reentry, and it can diagnose an underlying atrial rhythm of AVNRT. In addition, a short-acting beta-blocker, a calcium channel blocker, or verapamil may be helpful in diagnosing or converting a patient in AVNRT.

Health Maintenance and Patient Education

- AVNRT is commonly triggered by alcohol, caffeine, and sympathomimetic amines.
- On occasion, when AVNRT has multiple recurrences, education regarding avoidance of these substances is necessary.

Treatment (Pharmaceutical and Clinical Intervention)

Any hemodynamically unstable PSVT rhythm requires immediate synchronized direct-current cardioversion, starting with 50–100 J, then to increase the dose in increments of 50 J until sinus rhythm is achieved.

- If unable to perform immediate cardioversion, vagal stimulation in the form of physical maneuvers may be trialed.

Stimulation of the vagal nerve may be performed by the Valsalva or modified Valsalva maneuver, cold-water facial immersion, or carotid sinus massage.

As AVNRT and AVRT are nodal-dependent rhythms, treatment focuses on pharmacologics that reduce conduction through the AV node.

- Medications such as adenosine, beta-blockers, or calcium channel blockers may be administered. Adenosine is 90% successful in terminating PSVTs due to AV nodal reentry mechanisms. It may possibly be effective in sinus node reentry tachycardia but is often ineffective in treating automatic atrial tachycardia.
- Care needs to be given to patients with a history of reactive airway disease as it may provoke vasospasms.

In addition, adenosine is preferential in patients who are being treated with beta-blockers or with impaired cardiac function or hypotension.

- Beta-blockers and calcium channel blockers are often effective at slowing conduction through the AV node and ceasing impulse conditions.
- These medications should be given with caution to patients with CHF or COPD. Medications such as digoxin and amiodarone may be effective, but their initial slow onset of action may be undesirable.

A hemodynamically stable patient with PSVT usually tolerates the arrhythmia well, unless they have underlying cardiac disease or left ventricular dysfunction.

Professional Considerations

If serious signs and symptoms arise with PSVT, hospitalization should be considered. If the patient requires emergency cardioversion, or if they have arrhythmias refractory to treatment, they may also be considered for hospitalization. If a patient is seen in the emergency department with transient PSVT, outpatient follow-up care should be provided.

Premature Beats

Pathophysiology

Premature beats include premature atrial contraction (PAC), premature junctional contraction (PJC), and premature ventricular contraction (PVC). These are beats that arise from a premature activation of a site that is not the sinus node.

Clinical Presentation

PAC are common and may occur in normal hearts with or without risk factors. They may occur with ingestion of triggering substances, such as coffee, tea, alcohol, or pseudoephedrine, or they may be a sign of heart disease. They are also common in patients with chronic obstructive pulmonary disease (COPD). PACs also occur frequently in those patients with mitral valve disease and with left ventricular dysfunction. They also can occur at a higher incidence with patients who are soon to delve into atrial fibrillation.

- PJCs are less common than PACs and PVCs.
- They may occur alongside other types of diagnoses, such as hypokalemia, lung disease, myocardial infarction, caffeine, nicotine or alcohol use, amphetamine use, stress, digitalis use, thyroid disease, pericarditis, heart failure, or valvular heart disease.
- PVCs occur more frequently in the older population and in those with known heart disease and hypertension. They also occur commonly in the "healthy" population.

Symptoms

- Generally, premature beats can cause palpitations. This is true of all premature beats regardless of their origin. Patients may also feel like their heart is "skipping a beat."

Signs

- A palpation of the peripheral pulse may reveal a premature pulse wave or a pause during the compensation period. When heart sounds are auscultated, the same premature sound or a pause may be discovered if the timing allows.

Diagnostic and Lab Studies

Diagnosis occurs with an ECG. PAC appears to be a P-wave followed by a regular interval, narrow QRS followed by a T-wave that does not occur in a regular fashion after the patient's rhythm. They are usually followed by a compensatory pause before the next regular beat. A PJC may be observed when there is a normal QRS complex with no P-wave, or a P-wave that is at the end of the QRS complex near the ST segment, or even on the T-wave. A PVC occurs when a QRS is greater than 120 milliseconds and the QRS morphology is different from the usual appearance of other QRS complexes on the ECG. The T-wave may also be in the opposite direction. In addition, there may be a compensatory pause after the PVC.

Differential Diagnosis/Formulating the Most Likely Diagnosis

At times, a 24-hour Holter monitor or an ambulatory ECG monitor may be ordered to help determine the frequency of premature beats. This evaluation may also determine if the beats are mono- or multi-morphic, which can help determine the location of the ectopy. An echocardiogram may also be ordered to evaluate for structural or functional changes.

Other laboratory tests may be helpful, such as thyroid function tests, CBC, BNP, digoxin level, drug screen, or electrolyte levels.

Health Maintenance and Patient Education

If a patient is found to be symptomatic with premature beats, it may be advisable to council to avoid alcohol, caffeine, or nicotine use. In addition, careful questioning regarding medications or other comorbid conditions may be wise. PACs are not life-threatening by themselves, and a patient should be advised so. Nevertheless, PACs may initiate other arrhythmias, such as supraventricular or ventricular arrhythmias, as well as atrial fibrillation, and those rhythms should be carefully observed for an occurrence.

- PVCs may occur with other cardiac and noncardiac conditions. These comorbidities may include hypertension, left ventricular hypertrophy, myocardial infarction, heart failure, myocarditis, cardiomyopathies, and congenital heart disease.
- In addition, noncardiac conditions in which PVCs may frequently occur include sleep apnea, pulmonary hypertension, COPD, thyroid, adrenal, or gonadal conditions, or other medications or substances that may cause ectopy.

Treatment (Pharmaceutical and Clinical Intervention)

Occasional premature beats may require no intervention, especially if the patient is asymptomatic. Although if the ectopy is frequent, further evaluation may be warranted to identify structural heart disease. Many patients may be counseled to avoid triggering substances, such as smoking, alcohol, caffeine, or stressful situations. If a patient has frequent, symptomatic occurrences, medical therapy with a beta-blocker or another antiarrhythmic medication or a catheter ablation may be offered.

Professional Considerations

A personal or family history of cardiac disease, symptoms of any angina, syncope, or heart failure, a new cardiac murmur, multifocal PVCs, or other ECG abnormalities may indicate the need for additional testing.

Sick Sinus Syndrome

Pathophysiology

Sick sinus syndrome (sinus node dysfunction) is an arrhythmia that causes inappropriate atrial rates. This may include dysfunctions such as:

- Inappropriate sinus bradycardia
- Tachycardia-bradycardia syndrome
- Sinus pause or arrest
- Sinoatrial (SA) exit block

This may occur due to:

- Idiopathic sinus node fibrosis, commonly due to collagen vascular disease, surgery, or cancer
- Degeneration of the conduction system
- Recreational drugs
- Increased vagal tone and other disorders, such as:
  - Ischemic
  - Inflammatory
  - Infiltrative

Medications may also cause sinus node dysfunction, such as beta-blockers, calcium channel blockers, digoxin, antiarrhythmic medications, or acetylcholinesterase inhibitors.

Clinical Presentation

This arrhythmia more commonly occurs in older patients, especially those who have another cardiac disorder or diabetes.

Symptoms
- Dizziness
- Palpitations
- Syncope
- Effort intolerance
- Fatigue or weakness

Sick sinus syndrome may also occur with minimal symptoms or be asymptomatic if the heart rate is adequate for perfusion.

Diagnostic and Lab Studies

Sick sinus syndrome may present in numerous ways on an ECG. Sinus node dysfunction is always present and may occur with abnormalities such as sinus bradycardia, sinus pauses, sinus arrest,

SA nodal exit block, or inadequate heart rate response to physical activity. In addition, sick sinus syndrome may occur with atrial fibrillation, atrial flutter, and atrial tachycardia. The combination of these two arrhythmias will create the tachycardia-bradycardia syndrome.

Differential Diagnosis/Formulating the Most Likely Diagnosis

A sinus pause occurs when the sinus node activity ceases temporarily, as seen with disappearing P-waves for a duration of seconds to minutes. In SA exit block, the conduction of SA node impulses to atrial tissue is impaired. An ECG should be performed, as well as evaluating previous ECGs to identify a pattern of sinus node dysfunction. It may also be helpful to perform an exercise stress test to evaluate the sinus node's response to exercise, to identify the inability to obtain a faster heart rate in response to testing.

Treatment (Pharmaceutical and Clinical Intervention)

Pacing may be indicated when an evaluation of other causes for sinus node dysfunction should occur. This may be due to medication use, myocardial ischemia, hypothyroidism, or autonomic imbalances.

Professional Considerations

Invasive electrophysiologic studies are rarely used for the evaluation of sick sinus syndrome. However, EPS may be helpful in identifying patients with certain tachycardias that may be potentially curable with ablation. In addition, EPS may prescribe an implantable cardiac monitor that may evaluate a patient's rhythm for up to three years to identify ambulatory and nonambulatory sinus node dysfunctions that may be difficult to discover on a typical Holter monitor or 24-hour monitoring. Referral to an electrophysiologist may be needed.

Sinus Arrhythmia

Pathophysiology

Sinus arrhythmia is a variation in the rate of the sinus node. Can be caused by occasions such as normal respiratory variation, sympathetic mechanisms such as arterial elevations in carbon dioxide, or drug-induced increases on a patient's vagal tone. During inspiration, vagal tone will be inhibited, thereby increasing a sinus rate; with expiration, vagal tone will increase again to the natural state, thus the sinus rhythm rate will decline.

Clinical Presentation

Sinus arrhythmia occurrences will increase with a patient's age. It has also been associated with diabetes mellitus, obesity, and hypertension. Drugs that may cause an increased vagal tone may be morphine or digitalis. Patients who present with an increased arterial PCO_2 may also have more pronounced sinus arrhythmia. Typically, sinus arrhythmia does not present with symptoms.

Diagnostic and Lab Studies

On ECG, the clinician will find that the sinus rhythm will vary in the rate. There will be an irregularity in the P-P interval as much as 120 milliseconds, but the atrial electrical activity will still be originating at the sinus node. A patient that has respiratory sinus arrhythmia will cease to have this arrhythmia during a breath hold.

Differential Diagnosis/Formulating the Most Likely Diagnosis

Differential diagnosis may include third-degree heart block or premature beats with a compensatory pause. Neither of these have a sinus node origin nor regularity of sinus beats, which is prominent in sinus arrhythmia.

Health Maintenance and Patient Education

Respiratory variations causing sinus arrhythmia are common and benign. A patient can be educated that this is related to changes in cardiac filling during breathing.

Treatment (Pharmaceutical and Clinical Intervention)

There is no specific treatment for sinus arrhythmia as it is usually asymptomatic and benign.

Professional Considerations

Evaluation for other causes of sinus arrhythmia may be searched, including those diagnoses commonly associated with this arrhythmia, including obesity, hypertension, or diabetes mellitus.

Also, any causation drugs may be evaluated and changed if the arrhythmia is significant. These evaluations should be performed on an individual basis if the patient's history and physical elude to other diagnoses.

Torsades de Pointes

Pathophysiology

Torsades de pointes is a form of ventricular tachycardia that occurs in patients with long QT intervals. The long QT interval can have a drug-induced or congenital cause.

A long QT will predispose a patient to this arrhythmia by prolonging repolarization, thus causing early after-depolarizations and the dispersion of the refractory period. An R on T phenomenon may result in torsades de pointes, where an ectopic beat is generated during the prolonged repolarization phase.

Clinical Presentation

- Patients in torsades de pointes will most likely be hemodynamically compromised with rapid or absent pulse and very low or undetectable blood pressure. They may have loss of consciousness at the time of presentation.
- Patients that are at higher risk for torsades de pointes are those with older age; female gender; low potassium, magnesium, or calcium levels; underlying bradycardia; heart disease; or who take diuretic medications.
- A patient may experience palpitations, syncope, presyncope, shortness of breath, feelings of doom, or be unresponsive at the time of this rhythm.

Diagnostic and Lab Studies

An ECG will show rapid and irregular QRS complexes that appear to be "twisting" around a baseline. They have been described to look like a ribbon or streamer. The QRS rate will be around 200–250 beats per minute, and a QTc will be greater than 450 milliseconds. A QTc greater than 500 milliseconds has been associated with an increased risk for torsades de pointes. The rhythm may terminate spontaneously, or it may transfer into ventricular fibrillation.

Studies should focus around the cause of the patient's arrhythmia. Common causes for torsades de pointes can be medications (e.g., antiarrhythmics, tricyclic antidepressants, phenothiazines, and certain antifungals and antivirals) or another diagnosis such as congenital long QT syndrome.

Differential Diagnosis/Formulating the Most Likely Diagnosis

Torsades de pointes differs from ventricular fibrillation in that it can spontaneously resolve; however, if left untreated, it can progress into ventricular fibrillation.

Health Maintenance and Patient Education

The prevention of torsades de pointes may be the most important treatment. Correcting electrolyte levels, especially potassium, magnesium, and calcium, and discontinuing any QT prolonging medications may gain the biggest prophylactic benefit for patients.

Treatment (Pharmaceutical and Clinical Intervention)

Torsades de pointes, if pulseless, should be treated with unsynchronized direct-current cardioversion. In addition, correction of electrolytes is key, especially potassium and magnesium. Intravenous magnesium is the first-line pharmacologic therapy. Lidocaine may also be utilized because it shortens the QTC interval. Avoid using antiarrhythmic medications such as class Ia, Ic, and III.

Professional Considerations

Patient stability should be the number one focus with a patient presenting with torsades de pointes. Emphasis should be placed on converting the patient out of this rhythm and obtaining hemodynamic stability. Once this is achieved, the underlying cause of this rhythm should be determined.

Ventricular Fibrillation

Pathophysiology

Ventricular fibrillation (VF) is caused by multiple uncoordinated quivers of the ventricle, with no useful contractions. This electrical activity is irregular in morphology and timing. It is a wide complex tachycardia with a ventricular rate greater than 300 beats per minute, with a varying morphology of the QRS. There are no identifiable P-waves, QRS complexes, or T-waves.

Clinical Presentation

VF is commonly seen as the presenting rhythm in cardiac arrest patients. Ventricular contraction is abnormal, and thus cardiac output is very low. It can be exacerbated by electrolyte abnormalities, acidosis, hypoxemia, or ischemia. In addition, conditions such as hypothermia, cardiomyopathies, family history of sudden cardiac death, congenital QT abnormalities, Brugada syndrome, or alcohol use may be associated with ventricular fibrillation.

Patients typically present with a sudden collapse from cardiac arrest, with symptoms of unconsciousness, unresponsiveness, or pulselessness. They may present with symptoms such as chest pain, nausea, vomiting, or shortness of breath.

Diagnostic and Lab Studies

Lab studies that may help the provider correct reversible causes of this arrhythmia include serum electrolytes, cardiac enzymes, medication levels, toxicology screen, complete blood count, arterial blood gas, or BNP levels. An ECG can be performed to evaluate for certain rhythms, such as an acute myocardial infarction, Brugada syndrome, WPW, digitalis toxicity, or QT interval prolongation. An echocardiogram may reveal wall motion abnormalities or any valvular problems, as well as any pericardial effusion that may be present.

Differential Diagnosis/Formulating the Most Likely Diagnosis

Differential diagnosis may include rhythms such as asystole, pulseless electrical activity (PEA), polymorphic ventricular tachycardia, torsades de pointes, SVT with aberrancy, or accelerated idioventricular rhythm. Careful ECG interpretation should be performed to distinguish between these rhythms.

Health Maintenance and Patient Education

Complications of this rhythm may be anoxic brain injury, other arrhythmias, injuries related to CPR, myocardial injury, long-term disability, and death. Mortality of this rhythm remains high, thus family involvement and education about the patient's condition is important.

Treatment (Pharmaceutical and Clinical Intervention)

Nearly 70% of cardiac arrest patients have been identified to have ventricular fibrillation as a rhythm. Without quick treatment, this rhythm will lead to death within minutes. Advanced Cardiac Life Support protocol should be followed.

- Ventricular fibrillation should be defibrillated immediately. Patients with prompt defibrillation have been shown to have improved survival compared to those in whom defibrillation was delayed by 2 minutes or more. Medications such as epinephrine and amiodarone as per the ACLS protocol should be administered.
- Most patients in VF have an underlying heart disorder, such as ischemic, hypertrophic, or dilated cardiomyopathy. After return of spontaneous circulation (ROSC) is obtained, the focus should be shifted into evaluating and identifying these conditions that caused VF.

Professional Considerations

If a patient has a significant risk to this arrhythmia, preventative therapies may be considered. This preventative management includes medication therapy or the implantation of an ICD.

- Primary prevention includes inserting an ICD in patients who are at high risk of ventricular fibrillation or ventricular tachycardia.
- Secondary prevention recommends inserting an ICD in patients with prior episodes of ventricular fibrillation and sustained ventricular tachycardia.

Ventricular Tachycardia

Pathophysiology

Ventricular tachycardia (VT) occurs from a stable focus or reentry circuit in the ventricle. In a patient with structural heart disease, there may be an infarcted patch of tissue or inflammation that can create reentry pathways leading to VT. This rhythm may also be related to reentry or automaticity in a diseased Purkinje system. It is also possible for no structural disease to be present, and VT may occur due to a focal region of automaticity.

Clinical Presentation

A patient may present in various ways, depending on the rate of the VT, underlying heart function, and the patient's autonomic adaptation to the arrhythmia. Hypotension or syncope may be the initial symptom if the arrhythmia is over 200 beats/min. A patient may tolerate VT if at a slower rate around 150 beats/min.

Symptoms
- Diaphoresis and chest pain
- Palpitations
- Light-headedness
- Syncope
- Unresponsiveness

Diagnostic and Lab Studies

Ventricular tachycardia occurs with a broad QRS of greater than 0.14 seconds, AV dissociation, concordance of all QRS complexes in V1 through V6 being either positive or negative, fusion beats, and capture beats. In addition, cardiac biomarkers for evaluation of ischemic disease, electrolyte levels, and certain drug levels may be drawn for evaluation.

Differential Diagnosis/Formulating the Most Likely Diagnosis

Monomorphic VT may need to be distinguished from other wide-complex tachycardias, such as bundle branch blocks with aberrant conditions, SVT, or rapid cardiac pacing. An adenosine challenge will differentiate between SVT and VT. When given adenosine, SVT will be interrupted, whereas VT will not be affected. In times where it can be difficult to distinguish between VT and SVT with aberrancy, treat it as VT. At times, an electrophysiological study may be needed for definitive diagnosis.

Health Maintenance and Patient Education

In patients who have VT, implantation of an implantable cardioverter defibrillator (ICD) may be discussed if there is an expectation of survival with reasonable functional status for the next 1 year. A patient should be educated regarding the risks, benefits, and alternatives of ICD placement. Chronic medication therapy, such as amiodorone, may also be used. Some patients may be offered catheter ablation if they have frequent symptomatic recurrences.

Treatment (Pharmaceutical and Clinical Intervention)

If VT is clear or if a patient is hemodynamically unstable, an immediate cardioversion is required. If a patient is not hemodynamically unstable, IV amiodarone, IV magnesium, IV lidocaine, or overdrive pacing may be utilized.

Chronic VT may be controlled with medications such as sotalol, flecainide, amiodarone, propafenone, and disopyramide. In addition, ablation of the right ventricular outflow tract (RVOT) can be helpful at the cessation of VT. An automatic implantable cardioverter defibrillator (AICD) may also be implanted for internal defibrillation of this dysrhythmia.

Professional Considerations

Management and investigation of VT causes should be carried out by a cardiologist or an electrophysiologist. There may be a precipitating event, such as an MI or ischemic heart disease, both of which will require heart catheterization. In other cases, invasive electrophysiological testing may be desired to identify root causes of VT. To identify scar tissue causing VT, a TTE, nuclear imaging, or MR imaging may be needed. Patient stability should be the number one focus in a patient presenting with torsades de pointes. Emphasis should be placed on converting the patient out of this rhythm and obtaining hemodynamic stability. Once this is achieved, the underlying cause of this rhythm should be determined.

Congenital Heart Disease

Atrial Septal Defect

Pathophysiology

Females > Males (2:1)
Shunting of blood flow from left to right is most likely in an acyanotic person with an ASD.

- The increased flow leads to right sided and pulmonary artery dilatation and the pulmonary vasculature increases due to volume overload, which can be tolerated very well for years.
- The size of the shunt determines the degree of cardiac enlargement.
- Development of pulmonary hypertension (Eisenmenger syndrome)
- ASDs are classified by the area they form in:

    1. Primum: forming when the septal primum tissue does not adhere to the endocardial cushions and creates an opening at the base of the interatrial septum
    2. Secundum: most common ASD location, located in the fossa ovalis
    3. Sinus venosus: opening occurring either where the superior or inferior vena cava meet the atrial septum. Can be associated with a partial anomalous pulmonary connection of the right pulmonary vein (PAPVR).
    4. Coronary Sinus: This rare defect unroofs the coronary sinus creating an opening to the left atrium. PFO (patent foramen ovale) is not an ASD, but the natural communication between the atria formed as the anterior and posterior atrial septums come together.

Clinical Presentation

Symptoms
- Most small ASDs do not cause symptoms in infancy or childhood, but if symptoms appear they will present as recurrent respiratory infections, easy fatigability, and exertional dyspnea.
- Large defects may present with symptoms of heart failure, respiratory infections, or failure to thrive.

Signs
- Wide, fixed split S2 due to increased RV volume resulting in delaying PV opening
- II-III/VI mid-systolic ejection murmur (SEM) at left upper sternal border (LUSB) due to increased flow across pulmonary valve
- Early mid-diastolic murmur along LLSB (left lower sternal border) due to increased volume of blood shunted across a relative tricuspid stenosis

Heart Failure Signs
- Failure to thrive
- Tachypnea
- Rales
- Hepatomegaly

Diagnostic and Lab Studies

- ECG: small ASD → normal; if hemodynamically significant → right axis deviation (RAD) and mild RVH or RBBB
- CXR: normal with a small PDA; significant shunt may see cardiomegaly, prominent pulm artery, and increased pulmonary vascular markings.
- Echocardiogram is study of choice to be able to differentiate ASDs and estimate shunt volume and pulmonary artery pressures.
- TEE (transesophageal echocardiogram) is best to determine margin size prior to catheter closure.
- MRI helpful if other defects noted like PAPVR to determine volumes and pulmonary/systemic flow.

Differential Diagnosis/Formulating the Most Likely Diagnosis

- Mitral stenosis
- Pulmonic stenosis
- Ventricular septal defect (VSD)
- Innocent murmur
- Patent ductus arteriosus (PDA)

Health Maintenance and Patient Education

Long-term follow-up care is required if surgical or percutaneous ASD closure or other associated cardiac lesions. Antibiotic prophylaxis is not required with an isolated ASD except if repaired with a device or prosthetic material during the first 6 months after repair or if there is a residual defect at site of repair.

- No exercise restrictions in children with uncomplicated ASD repair.
- Monitor growth parameters for failure to thrive.

Treatment (Pharmaceutical and Clinical Intervention)

- Most small ASDs (< 3 mm) will spontaneously close, otherwise closure is delayed until the child is 2–5 years old depending on symptomatology.
- Percutaneous transcatheter device closure for small to moderate sized secundum ASDs followed by anticoagulation (ASA, clopidogrel) for 6 months.

Indications for surgical closure:
- Sinus venosus, primum, coronary sinus ASDs, and/or with complex cardiac lesions
- CHF unresponsive to medicine
- L to R shunt with increased pulm to systemic blood flow (pulmonary hypertension contraindication)
- Bronchopulmonary dysplasia
- Surgical closure uses either a Dacron or pericardial patch.

Professional Considerations

Referral to pediatric cardiology.

Coarcatation of Aorta

Pathophysiology

Coarctation of the aorta (COA) is defined as a descending aorta narrowing located at the insertion of the ductus arteriosus distal to the left subclavian artery. As the patent ductus arteriosus and foramen ovale close in the neonatal period, the cardiac output begins to increase. Due to the narrowing of the aorta, hypertension and heart failure occur. Left ventricular afterload increases due to the obstruction, which increases the systolic pressure gradient. Development of left ventricular hypertrophy and collateral blood flow becomes a compensatory mechanism over time. If severe enough obstruction, heart failure develops in the neonates.

COA can have a genetic predisposition and may be accompanied by other cardiac lesions, such as bicuspid aortic valve, ventricular septal defects, patent ductus arteriosus.

Clinical Presentation

Symptoms

- Infancy CHF (LV failure)
- Diaphoresis
- Poor feeding
- Poor weight gain
- Circulatory shock
- Severe acidemia
- Respiratory distress between 2–3 weeks of life after ductus closes

Late Presentation—Child/Adolescent Claudication

- Weakness or pain in the legs with exercise
- HTN
- Murmur
- Headaches
- Chest pain
- Fatigue
- Epistaxis (adults)

Signs

- II-III/VI SEM at LUSB, radiation throughout the precordium/back and may be heard in L interscapular region.
- Summation gallop (S3/tachycardia) if failure
- If bicuspid aortic valve, ejection click at apex
- BP in upper limbs > BP in lower limbs; measured R arm/leg > 15–20 mmHg difference
- Delayed pulses upper extremity to lower extremity
- Absent femoral pulses in severe COA
- Hepatomegaly in neonate with heart failure
- SpO_2 difference > 5% between upper limb and lower limb suggests coarctation.

Diagnostic and Lab Studies

Genetic testing for Turners syndrome should be done on all females with COA.
Echocardiography can be confirmatory.

ECG

- Infancy: rightward axis, RVH or RBBB
- Children: leftward axis, LVH

CXR

- Cardiomegaly
- Pulmonary venous congestion
- Rib notching after age 5 from collateral circulation development
- Figure 3 sign—aorta "pinching" pre and post-coarctation

Cardiovascular MRI or CTA can help define the location of the COA, as well as identify collateral vessels. MRI preferred due to lifetime radiation risk from CTA.

Differential Diagnosis/Formulating the Most Likely Diagnosis

- Congenital adrenal hyperplasia
- Dilated cardiomyopathy
- Hypertension
- Hypertrophic cardiomyopathy
- Pediatric adrenal insufficiency (Addison disease)
- Pediatric hypoplastic left heart syndrome
- Pediatric sepsis
- Pediatric valvar aortic stenosis
- Pediatric viral myocarditis
- Trauma with aortic dissection

Health Maintenance and Patient Education

- Lifelong follow-up care is required of all COA patients with particular focus of monitoring for postoperative complications later in life.
- Antibiotic prophylaxis is not required except if repaired with a conduit; stent during the first 6 months after repair or if there is a history of endocarditis.
- Adolescents should be familiarized with the importance of transitioning of care and the need for lifelong follow-up.
- Women with COA of child-bearing age should be counseled about risks and have a thorough evaluation from an adult congenital cardiac specialist if deciding on becoming pregnant.
- Exercise and sports participation consistent with 2015 AHA/ACC guidelines

Treatment (Pharmaceutical and Clinical Intervention)

- Medical management
  - Neonates with severe COA and risk of heart failure IV prostaglandin E1 (alprostadil) to keep the duct open
  - If heart failure, inotropic support (dopamine, dobutamine) to preserve left ventricular contractility
  - Treatment of hypertension with a beta-blocker, ACE inhibitor, or ARB
- Surgical and catheter intervention
  - Infants less than 4 months, surgical repair is preferred by either:
    - Resection with end-to-end anastomosis

- ▪ Subclavian flap aortoplasty
    - ▪ Bypass graft
  - ○ Infants greater than 4 months may benefit from either surgical or catheter-based interventions such as balloon angioplasty.

Stenting in children and adults is the preferred intervention, although surgery is considered on a case-by-case basis.

Professional Consideration

Referral to Pediatric Cardiology includes:
- ▪ Long-term complications that patients should be educated about, which may include:
  - ○ Berry aneurysms involving circle of Willis (5–10%)
  - ○ Aortic aneurysm formation/dissection
  - ○ Hypertension
  - ○ Need for aortic valve replacement

Patent Ductus Arteriosus

Pathophysiology

Persistent patency of the duct between the left pulmonary artery (LPA) and descending aorta in newborns or preemies. The duct is normally kept open due to low arterial oxygen and prostaglandin E2 (PGE2). At birth, rising arterial oxygen tension and decreasing PGE2 facilitates ductal closure.

Also, large PDAs can cause left ventricular volume overload.

Clinical Presentation

Symptoms
- ▪ Symptoms determined by size of duct, degree of left-to-right shunting, differences of pulmonary and systemic vascular resistances.
- ▪ Small PDAs are asymptomatic and detected by exam.
- ▪ Tachycardia/tachypnea in infants with CHF due to moderate to large PDA.
- ▪ Older children may present with shortness of breath or easy fatigability.

Signs
- ▪ I-IV/VI continuous "machinery-like" murmur loudest at LUSB or left infraclavicular area
- ▪ Bounding peripheral pulses/wide pulse pressure in moderate to large PDAs
- ▪ Hyperactive precordium
- ▪ Exercise intolerance with moderate to large PDA
- ▪ Failure to thrive
- ▪ Poor feeding patterns

Diagnostic and Lab Studies

ECG
Small to moderate PDA → normal or large PDA → biventricular hypertrophy

CXR
Possible cardiomegaly with increased pulmonary vascular markings

Echocardiogram

Confirmatory diagnostic study of choice with the use of Doppler color flow and Doppler to estimate the degree of left-to-right shunting and pulmonary artery pressure.

Differential Diagnosis/Formulating the Most Likely Diagnosis

- Venous hum—located on right and changes with position or compression
- Coronary artery fistula
- Aortic stenosis and aortic regurgitation
- Heart failure

Health Maintenance and Patient Education

- Monitor growth parameters
- Nutritional support/failure to thrive
- Complications include:
  - Heart failure
  - Infective endocarditis—rare
  - Pulmonary hypertension

Treatment (Pharmaceutical and Clinical Intervention)

Management is determined by the degree of left-to-right shunting, age, and size of patient and includes either observation or elective ductal closure. If deferring elective closure, observation with regular monitoring for symptoms of heart failure, increased cardiac workload, or pulmonary vascular changes.

Percutaneous PDA closure includes:

- Coil occlusion with an MRI compatible coil
- Ductal occluders, also MRI compatible
- Treatment of choice in infants, children > 6 kg and adults
- [STAR] Surgical closure
- Preferred approach in infants < 6 kg

Preterm infant's pharmacologic management is with prostaglandin synthesis inhibitors using either indomethacin or ibuprofen to close the duct. Prostaglandin inhibitors are not effective with neonates or older children. PDA closure is not indicated in patients with severe or irreversible pulmonary arterial hypertension.

Professional Considerations

Referral to pediatric cardiology.

Tetralogy of Fallot

Pathophysiology

Tetralogy of Fallot, the most common cyanotic heart disease, is characterized by four major features:

- Ventricular septal defect located in the perimembranous region of the septum
- Right ventricular outflow obstruction (RVOT), which can include:
  - Hypertrophy of RV muscular bands
  - Hypoplastic pulmonary valve annulus

- ◦ Infundibular septal deviation
- ◦ Bicuspid or stenotic pulmonic valve
- ▪ Overriding aorta where the aorta is displaced over the septum accepting blood flow from both ventricles
- ▪ Right ventricular hypertrophy

Other associated cardiac abnormalities may include:
- ▪ Right aortic arch in 25% of patients
- ▪ Coronary artery abnormalities
- ▪ Aorticopulmonary collateral vessels
- ▪ Patent ductus arteriosus

Fifteen percent of patients with TOF may have associated genetic abnormalities such as Down syndrome (trisomy 21), Alagille syndrome (Jag1 mutation), and DiGeorge syndrome (Chromosome 22q11 deletion). The physiological effects are dependent on the degree of right ventricular outflow obstruction and the equalization of pressures between the right ventricle and left ventricle due to the flow across the VSD, not the VSD size. If blood flow across the RVOT obstruction is less than the resistance to flow across the aorta, shunting will be from LV to RV, resulting in the patient being acyanotic. As RVOT obstruction increases, pulmonary blood flow resistance also increases and the shunting is from RV to LV, resulting in the patient being cyanotic.

Hypercyanotic spells (tet spells) is due to transient near occlusion of the RVOT, such as a drop in systemic vascular resistance increasing the right-to-left shunt. It causes hyperventilation, cyanosis, and possibly loss of consciousness or cardiac arrest. Spells can be brought on by crying, after bowel movements, or with increased physical activity. Children may squat, which helps to relieve symptoms by increasing SVR and systemic arterial oxygen saturation.

Clinical Presentation

Symptoms
- ▪ With severe RVOT obstruction, newborns will present with cyanosis.
- ▪ Mild-to-moderate obstruction in infants with balanced pulmonary and systemic flow may be asymptomatic ("pink tets").
- ▪ Minimal obstruction can be asymptomatic initially but may develop signs of heart failure and pulmonary overcirculation within the first 4 to 6 weeks of life.

Signs
- ▪ Cyanosis may be present in the nail beds and lips as well as tongue.
- ▪ Prominent RV impulse
- ▪ Loud III-V/VI systolic ejection murmur along LSB with a single S2 and radiation to the back

Diagnostic and Lab Studies

ECG
- ▪ Right axis deviation and right ventricular hypertrophy
- ▪ "Boot-shaped heart"
  - ◦ Normal size
  - ◦ +/– Increased pulmonary vascular markings depending on pulmonary blood flow (degree of RVOT)

Fetal Echocardiography (if suspected or family history of congenital heart disease)
- ▪ Echocardiography to evaluate hemodynamics, VSD, RVOT obstruction, pulmonary arteries, coronary arteries, aortic arch, and other associated anomalies

- Cardiac catheterization to further evaluate anatomy and hemodynamics, as well as interventions

Differential Diagnosis/Formulating the Most Likely Diagnosis

- Differentiate from other cyanosis-causing disorders
- Total anomalous pulmonary venous connection
  - Tricuspid atresia
  - Transposition of the great vessels
  - Truncus arteriosus

Health Maintenance and Patient Education

- Lifelong follow-up care is required of all TOF patients with particular focus on monitoring for postoperative complications later in life.
- Antibiotic prophylaxis is required if repaired with a device or prosthetic material during the first 6 months after repair or if there is a residual defect at site of repair. Antibiotic prophylaxis is also recommended in patients who have prosthetic heart valves.
- Adolescents should be familiarized with the importance of transitioning of care and the need for lifelong follow-up.
- Pregnancy is not recommended in patients with unrepaired TOF. With corrective surgery and no hemodynamic abnormalities, patients may get pregnant after a thorough evaluation from an adult congenital cardiac specialist.
- Exercise

Treatment (Pharmaceutical and Clinical Intervention)

Medical Management

- Neonates with severe obstruction: IV prostaglandin therapy (alprostadil) to keep the duct patent to maintain some pulmonary flow before surgical intervention
- Heart failure symptoms may be treated with digoxin and a loop diuretic (furosemide).
- Tet spells are treated in a stepwise fashion beginning with placing the patient in a knee-to-chest position, oxygen, IV morphine, and IV fluid bolus.
- Other measures include IV beta-blockers (propranolol) and IV phenylephrine.

Surgical Repair

- Primary surgical repair occurs at age 3 to 6 months consisting of VSD patch closure and enlargement of the RVOT

Long-Term Complications of Surgery

- Arrhythmias
- Aortic root dilation and aortic regurgitation
- Pulmonary regurgitation causing RV enlargement
- Residual RVOT obstruction with RV dysfunction
- Catheterization intervention

Professional Considerations

Referral to pediatric cardiology.

Ventricular Septal Defect

Pathophysiology

Most common defect of acyanotic congenital heart disease:

- Shunting of blood flow from left to right is most likely in an acyanotic person with a VSD.
  - The size of the shunt and physiologic effects are determined by the size of the defect and degree of pulmonary vascular resistance (PVR).
- Infundibular stenosis (sub-aortic membrane) may develop in large shunts, particularly with membranous VSDs.
- Development of pulmonary hypertension (Eisenmenger syndrome) can result in a right-to-left shunt later in life.
- VSDs are classified by the area in which the defect forms:
  - Membranous—beneath the aortic valve and the septal tricuspid leaflet
  - Muscular—located in the muscular septum
  - Subpulmonic (outlet)—located within the conal septum formed by the pulmonic and aortic annulus
  - AV canal (inlet)—located beneath the septal leaflet of the tricuspid valve

Clinical Presentation

Symptoms
- Small VSDs, asymptomatic, normal growth/development
- Large VSDs, delayed growth/development, decreased exercise tolerance, pulmonary infections, CHF

Signs
- II-V/VI holosystolic murmur loudest at left lower sternal border (LLSB)
- Possible thrill at LLSB, P2 may be loud and single (pulmonary HTN), hyperdynamic precordium

Diagnostic and Lab Studies

ECG
- Small VSD → normal
- Med VSD → LVH +/− left atrial enlargement (LAE)
- Large VSD → biventricular hypertrophy +/− LAE

CXR
- Increased pulmonary vasculature, LA and LV enlargement (depends on the degree of L > R shunting)
- Possible RV enlargement as PVR increases
- Echocardiogram
  - Echocardiogram is study of choice to be able to differentiate VSDs, estimating size of shunt volume and pulmonary artery pressures.

Differential Diagnosis/Formulating the Most Likely Diagnosis

- Tricuspid regurgitation
  - Mitral regurgitation

Health Maintenance and Patient Education

Complications include:

- Pulmonary hypertension
- Endocarditis
- Aortic regurgitation due to aortic valve prolapse
- Subaortic stenosis
- RV obstruction
- LV to RA shunting
- Immunizations to include influenza, pneumococcal and RSV
- Guidance on nutritional support if failure to thrive
- Monitor growth parameters
- Exercise

Long-term follow-up care is required if there is surgical or percutaneous VSD closure or other associated cardiac lesions. Antibiotic prophylaxis is not required with an isolated VSD, except if repaired with a device or prosthetic material during the first 6 months after repair or if there is a residual defect at site of repair.

Treatment (Pharmaceutical and Clinical Intervention)

- Small defects (< 4 mm) in asymptomatic infants/children, intervention is not required. Follow up at 6-month intervals.
- Moderate to large VSDs during the first months of life become symptomatic with symptoms due to decrease of PVR. Treat signs of heart failure with diuretic therapy (furosemide, spironolactone) and nutritional support.
- Indications for primary patch closure, the preferred procedure of choice

Professional Considerations

Referral to pediatric cardiology.

Coronary Artery Disease

Acute Myocardial Infarction

Pathophysiology

Inadequate supply of blood and oxygen to a portion of the myocardium; it typically occurs when there is an imbalance between myocardial oxygen supply and demand. The most common cause of myocardial ischemia is atherosclerotic disease of an epicardial coronary artery (or arteries) causing decreased blood flow and inadequate perfusion of the myocardium supplied by the involved coronary artery.

Clinical Presentation

The major risk factors for atherosclerosis:

- High levels of plasma low-density lipoprotein (LDL)
- Low plasma high-density lipoprotein (HDL)
- Cigarette smoking
- Hypertension

- Diabetes mellitus varies in its relative impact on disturbing the normal functions of the vascular endothelium.

Symptoms include chest discomfort due to either angina pectoris or acute myocardial infarction. Can be asymptomatic in mild or less severe disease.

Diagnostic and Lab Studies

- **ECG:** Ischemia also causes characteristic changes such as repolarization abnormalities, as evidenced by inversion of T-waves and, when more severe, displacement of ST segments. T-wave inversion probably reflects non-transmural, intra-myocardial ischemia; transient ST-segment depression often reflects patchy subendocardial ischemia; and ST-segment elevation is thought to be caused by more severe transmural ischemia.
- **Exercise stress tests:** In asymptomatic persons, there may be evidence of silent myocardial ischemia.
- **Echocardiography:** reduced ejection fraction
- **Lab:** blood glucose, creatinine, cholesterol, albumin, CRP
- **Chest X-ray:** signs of cardiac enlargement

Differential Diagnosis/Formulating the Most Likely Diagnosis

- Cardiomegaly
- Heart failure

Health Maintenance and Patient Education

Management of cholesterol, diabetes, hypertension. Management of patients with cholesterol and hyperlipidemia emphasizes reduction of cardiovascular risk factors and maintaining hemoglobin A1C < 5.6%.

Treatment (Pharmaceutical and Clinical Intervention)

The treatment of risk factors, particularly lipid lowering and blood pressure control as described above, and the use of aspirin, statins, and beta-blockers after infarction have been shown to reduce events and improve outcomes in asymptomatic as well as symptomatic patients with ischemia and proven CAD.

Professional Considerations

Frequent episodes of ischemia (symptomatic and asymptomatic) appear to be associated with an increased likelihood of adverse coronary events, and management of risk factors is recommended.

Heart Failure

Pathophysiology

Fluid and sodium retention resulting from changes in myocardial contractility, preload or afterload, heart rate and/or valvular structural integrity; impacts left atrial pressure and cardiac output.

Clinical Presentation

- Common: dyspnea, edema, nocturia
- Left-sided failure:
  - Exertional dyspnea
  - Fatigue
  - Orthopnea
  - Paroxysmal nocturnal dyspnea
  - Basilar rales
  - S3 gallop
- Right-sided failure:
  - JVD/distended neck veins
  - Hepatic congestion
  - Decreased appetite
  - Putting edema
  - Nausea
  - Ascites
  - Weight loss
  - Nocturia

Diagnostic and Lab Studies

- **Lab:** hyperkalemia, hypernatremia, elevated liver enzymes, anemia, and renal insufficiency
- **ECG:** nonspecific changes, underlying arrhythmia, intraventricular conduction defects, left ventricular hypertrophy, and new or previous MI
- **Chest X-ray:** cardiomegaly, bilateral or right-sided pulmonary effusions, interstitial or peri-vascular edema (Kerley B lines), venous dilation, and alveolar fluid
- **Echocardiography:** assesses size and function of chambers, valves, pericardial effusion, and wall abnormalities

Differential Diagnosis/Formulating the Most Likely Diagnosis

- CHF may result from multiple conditions.
- It is important to assess classes of heart failure by limitations of daily activity (New York Heart Association Functional Classification).

Health Maintenance and Patient Education

- Management of reversible causes of CHF
- Recommend exercise, low sodium diet, tobacco cessation, alcohol cessation, and stress reduction.

Treatment (Pharmaceutical and Clinical Intervention)

- Oxygen
- Ace inhibitors or angiotensin II receptor blockers
- Beta-blockers
- Aldosterone receptor antagonists
- Thiazide or loop diuretic needed in patients with right-sided heart failure
- Calcium channel blockers needed if patient also has HTN or angina.
- Consider antiplatelet therapy.

- Implantable cardioverter defibrillators with extremely low ejection fraction
- Severe cases:
  - Consider coronary revascularization or ventricular assistive device; pacer if EF < 35.

Professional Considerations

Echocardiography reveals details about the ejection fraction and is an important prognostic indicator in congestive heart failure.

Hypertension

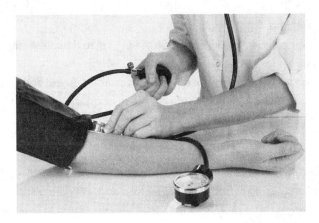

Figure 2.4 Patient's vitals being taken

Essential Hypertension

Pathophysiology

- Essential hypertension-genetic predisposition; increased incidence with age and Black patients
- Environmental factors are contributory: dietary sodium, obesity.
- Excessive use of alcohol, tobacco use, and sedentary lifestyle are exacerbating factors.
- Secondary causes of HTN include:
  - Renal disease
  - Coarctation of the aorta
  - Pheochromocytoma
  - Cushing's syndrome
  - Hyperthyroidism
  - Primary hyperaldosteronism
  - Chronic steroid therapy
  - Hyperthyroid
  - Estrogen use
  - NSAID use

Blood moves through the systemic circulation due to the contraction of the left ventricle. Systole is the pressure measured during contraction, and diastole is the pressure during relaxation. The elastic recoil of the arterial wall is responsible for continuing the forward motion of the blood between contractions. The kidneys are responsible for detecting and responding to signals of intravascular volume. Renal feedback on blood pressure (BP) is made via the renin/angiotensin system.

Baroreceptors in the aortic arch and the carotid sinuses also detect blood pressure and make regulatory adjustments via feedback pathways from the medulla to the autonomic nervous system. Dysfunction in one or more of these systems contributes to the rise in measured BP, and sustained elevations of BP across multiple readings on multiple days is referred to as hypertension.

Clinical Presentation

Most patients with mild-to-moderate hypertension will present with no symptoms at all. Some patients will present with a headache. Further presentations:

- Diagnosed when a patient has an elevated BP reading of greater than 140 mmHg systolic and or 90 mmHg diastolic on at least two visits: usually 1–4 weeks apart OR single reading of > 160/100 and end-organ damage.
- Important to screen for signs and symptoms of end-organ damage at the time of diagnosis of hypertension.
- Sustained elevations of BP can cause damage to any artery in the body and disease to any given artery can lead to damage in the organ it serves, ranging from the retina to the myocardium.

Current diagnostic criteria have been in use for several years at the time of this writing.

- Normal BP is defined < 120/80 mmHg.
- Elevated blood pressures are from 120–129 systolic and less than 80 diastolic.
- Stage 1 hypertension (HTN) is 130–139/80–89.
- Stage 2 HTN is 140/90 or higher.
- A hypertensive crisis is defined as BP greater than 180 or greater than 120.

Diagnostic and Lab Studies

- Optimal accuracy in BP readings is obtained with an appropriately sized cuff.
- ECG: Left ventricular hypertrophy, strain pattern is associated with advanced disease.
- Chest X-ray: May show ventricular hypertrophy.

At the diagnosis of hypertension, obtain a *comprehensive metabolic panel* and *lipid profile* to assess renal function, and also calculate the 10-year risk of cardiovascular (CV) disease. Automated calculators of CV risk are available online and as apps for Google and iOS platforms. Some authors also obtain *urine for microalbumin* to further assess renal health and an *ECG* to assess cardiac status.

Differential Diagnosis/Formulating the Most Likely Diagnosis

Hypertension is reasonably straightforward to diagnose, and consideration should be given to secondary causes. However, 85% of hypertension has no identifiable secondary cause and is simply referred to as primary hypertension. Be more concerned about secondary hypertension in young patients with no lifestyle risk factors or adult patients who do not respond to therapy with a second or third agent. Family history of secondary hypertension increases the likelihood of secondary hypertension in the immediate family.

Health Maintenance and Patient Education

Tobacco cessation

- Patients with HTN should be counseled to cease tobacco use if applicable. Nicotine is a vasoconstrictor and independently can raise BP.

- Inhaled byproducts of combustion also contribute to damage to the endothelium and are a separate risk factor for arterial disease.

Diet
- The DASH diet is shown to be effective in reducing CV disease morbidity and mortality.
- Additional peer-reviewed literature supports the Mediterranean diet and/or a completely plant-based diet as helpful in lowering **CVD risk**.

Obesity is a commonly cited risk factor for HTN. That said, obstructive sleep apnea (OSA) is a common cause of secondary HTN. Obesity contributes to OSA. Screen patients for OSA as indicated. But also note that body mass index (BMI) is a poorly supported tool to assess the health of individuals. Repeated studies have confirmed that regular exercise is more protective against CV morbidity and mortality than ideal body weight. This author encourages patients to eat a healthy diet but no longer emphasizes a goal of normalizing the BMI.

It is commonly held that reducing salt intake should be recommended in addition to other dietary interventions. In the United States, salt consumption is closer to 3,000 mg for women and 4,000 mg for men. Some authors advise a 2,000 mg daily salt limit.

Exercise
Regular cardiovascular exercise is considered beneficial in the control of HTN. Evidence supports 30 minutes of exercise 5 days per week can be helpful.

Patients should be screened for exertional symptoms of coronary insufficiency and evaluated appropriately prior to recommending a formal exercise program.

Treatment (Pharmaceutical and Clinical Intervention)

Treatment goals include lowering systolic by 20 mmHg and diastolic by 10 mmHg. This change is associated with a 50% reduction in CV risk. Ideally, the goal is BP readings below 140/90. Aim for control of BP within 3 months of diagnosis. The 2020 guidelines from the American Heart Association (AHA) call this "essential."
- In persons under age 65, the "optimal" treatment goal is less than 130/80 but higher than 120/70 per the AHA in 2020.
- In persons 65 and older, the optimal treatment goal remains < 140/90, but they add that individual treatment decisions should be made based upon factors such as frailty, independence, fall risk, and tolerability.

This author has found that many patients over age 65 tolerate BP goals that mirror younger patients. If a given patient is deemed not frail or has greater than average life expectancy, then lower goals may be approached as shared decision making. Current guidelines recommend initial therapy with an ACE-inhibitor (ACE-I) or calcium channel blocker (CCB). Beta-blockers were once recommended as preferred in African American patients, but that guideline is no longer supported by national guidelines. Instead, the beta-blocker class is de-emphasized due to common side effects such as erectile dysfunction and decreased exercise tolerance.

- If the patient presents at stage 1, lifestyle modifications can be undertaken as first-line therapy.
- If the patient presents at stage 2, treatment should begin at once. The two most recent revisions of HTN guidelines acknowledge that many patients will tolerate the initiation of two agents at once, and for stage 2 HTN, this is reasonable though not compulsory.

ACE-inhibitors affect BP by reducing the potency of the renal feedback mechanism. They also have well-documented tissue benefits on the lining of the arteries called the endothelium. Diabetic patients should receive an ACE inhibitor for these benefits and their protective effect on the kidneys unless contraindicated. Side effects include cough due to the accumulation of brady-kinin in the pulmonary tissue. This is harmless, but if severe can be a barrier to patient adherence to therapy. Some patients will experience a dramatic adverse reaction called angioedema. This is a permanent contraindication to ACE-I therapy. The overall incidence of ACE-I mediated angio-edema is estimated to be 0.1–0.7 %, but it represents the cause of 40% of ER visits.

- *Angiotensin receptor blocker* (ARB) works "further down" the cascade of renal feedback. It bypasses the production of bradykinin, and thus it does not commonly cause a cough. It is also shown to have tissue benefits in the endothelium and is appropriate instead of ACE-I therapy in a diabetic. There is very little good literature to inform the decision to use ARBs after ACE-I mediated angioedema. But it appears to be uncommon for ARBs to cause angioedema in the general population.
- *Calcium channel blockers* (CCB) work to lower blood pressure by reducing the action of calcium channels in the musculature of the arterial walls. Decreased tension in the vessel wall contributes to lower BP readings.

Additional benefits of the dihydropyridine class of CCBs include a long pharmacologic half-life, which reduces the risk of BP excursions when a patient forgets a dose. In patients with angina, CCBs also have an antianginal effect.

- *Diuretics* appear to exert their antihypertensive effect in part by lowering intravascular volume. However, the primary diuretic effect of the class wears off in less than 24 hours and becomes less dramatic with continued use. The BP-lowering effects tend to last longer than the pharmacologic effect would suggest. Side effects include changes in serum potassium levels and at least temporary increases in urine output. Patients whose work limits their access to bathroom facilities may struggle to adhere to diuretic therapy.
- *Beta-blockers* work to lower BP by blunting the effect of epinephrine also called adrenaline. The baroreceptors in the great vessels work to increase BP via increased output from the sympathetic nervous system. The adrenal glands also respond to mental or physiologic stressors by increasing the output of epinephrine.
  - Negative considerations to the class include side effects such as fatigue, decreased exercise tolerance, and erectile dysfunction. Patients who have asthma treat it with beta-agonists like albuterol. Using a beta-blocker in such patients will prevent them from treating their bronchospasm effectively.

There are other classes of antihypertensives, but these are less likely to constitute a significant portion of a standardized test. The overwhelming majority of primary care patients can be brought to controlled levels with a combination of these four drug types.

Professional Considerations

- Treatment of secondary hypertension focuses on treating the secondary cause.
- Hypertensive emergencies should be treated with careful attention to the rate of BP reduction.
- Aortic dissection requires emergent surgical repair.

Table 2.1 Diseases to Consider When Choosing a HTN Treatment

Diseases to Consider when Treating HTM	Diuretic	Ca⁺ Channel Blocker	ACE Inhibitor	Angiotensin Rec Blocker	Beta-Blockers (need a compelling indication; not for all people with HTN)
Heart Failure—Edema	×		×	×	×
Post MI or High Coronary Dz. Risk			×		×
Diabetes			×	×	
Chronic Renal Disease: ACE and ARB Reduce Proteinuria			×	×	
Recurrent Stroke Prevention			×		

Hypertensive Emergencies and Urgencies

Pathophysiology

The control of HTN is rightly focused on the prevention of end-organ disease. The term *hypertensive emergency* refers to a patient with elevated BP readings in the presence of end-organ damage. Affected organs can be in cardiac, neurological, pulmonary, or renal systems. The presence of severe HTN (equal to or greater than 180 mmHg systolic or 110 mmHg diastolic) in the absence of end-organ damage is called a hypertensive urgency.

Clinical Presentation

Symptoms

Depending upon the affected organ system, symptoms can vary:

- Acute coronary syndrome presenting as chest pain
- Pulmonary edema presenting as shortness of breath
- Acute renal failure and diffuse or dependent edema
- Cerebral infarction presenting with stroke symptoms

Signs

- The physical exam may reveal abnormal lung sounds, focal neurological changes, or diffuse mental status changes.
- If the opportunity exists, a retinal exam may also show vascular changes consistent with acute or chronic hypertension.

NOTE

Do not delay diagnosis or treatment decisions trying to optimize a retinal exam.

Diagnostic and Lab Studies

- EKG, CXR, complete metabolic panel, UA, and cardiac enzymes, identifying any values that are abnormal. Some authors include a CBC, but that is less relevant in the acute phase of diagnosis.
- In theory, anemia supports the diagnosis of chronic kidney disease. Other authors report findings of red cell damage on the peripheral smear, likely due to erythrocytes being affected by damage to the endothelium.

Lab findings of interest would be the renal function, as well as abnormalities in sodium or potassium levels. Urinalysis may show proteinuria and red cell casts. The EKG may show changes consistent with myocardial ischemia; one may also see signs of left ventricular hypertrophy suggesting chronically poor control of BP.

Radiography of the chest can estimate heart size but is much better at looking for pulmonary edema. If history and exam suggest neurological changes, CT of the head may reveal chemical changes, but it is especially good at showing acute bleeding.

Differential Diagnosis/Formulating the Most Likely Diagnosis

In most care settings, BP will be measured before the patient even meets the clinician. As previously discussed, hypertensive urgency would be severe HTN in the absence of symptoms.

- Hypertensive encephalopathy refers to the presentation of severe HTN in the context of headache, with the possible addition of nausea, vomiting, mental status changes, or coma.

This is distinguishable from other end-organ damage in that the symptoms resolve soon after the BP normalizes. In the out-of-hospital setting, any patient with symptoms of end-organ damage should be moving toward the emergency department.

Do not belabor the differential diagnosis once symptoms such as chest pain and shortness of breath appear. As the diagnostic studies become available, refinement of the diagnosis is possible. In the case of hypertensive emergency, the diagnosis is typically clear.

Health Maintenance and Patient Education

Whenever a clinician is managing patients with HTN, the frequently asked questions is: "When should I call you?" "When should I call 911?" The literature generally describes 180/110 or higher (either number) as the action point. But if the patient calms themselves and then takes an inventory of any possible symptoms and finds none, that is a hypertensive urgency. The BP can be lowered safely as an outpatient, even 2–3 days after such a phone call. Rapidly lowering BP in these patients can even be harmful. The cerebral circulation has an autoregulation function. Simply explained, the brain maintains appropriate blood flow in the presence of the pressure that is available. If these autoregulatory mechanisms have been "clamped down" for weeks or months, and then suddenly the incoming blood pressure drops, the brain may experience an ischemic infarct.

Treatment (Pharmaceutical and Clinical Intervention)

"Time is tissue" is a frequently heard refrain in emergency medicine. When a patient with HTN develops symptoms of acute end-organ damage, immediate transfer to the ER is indicated. As diagnostic tests are pending, urgent reduction of the BP is appropriate.

- American Heart Association guidelines recommend no more than a 25% reduction in the systolic BP in the first hour, then cautiously approach readings of 160/100 in the next few hours.
  - Aim for normalization of the BP only at 24–48 hours.

- In the emergency department, pharmacologic interventions tend to be intravenous and rapidly acting. This allows titration to the desired BP level and remains available even if the patient is unconscious or obtunded.
  - Drug classes typically used are beta-blockers, CCBs, and nitrates.

Professional Considerations

Clear communication between the inpatient team and the outpatient practice is vital for continuity of care. In complex social circumstances, social workers may be needed to ensure the patient has access to transportation, filling prescriptions, etc.

Secondary Hypertension

Pathophysiology

Estimates of incidence vary, but it is certainly a higher percentage in younger patients. Across all age groups, roughly 10–15% of hypertensive disease is due to secondary causes. This refers to the presence of another disease state, which raises the BP reading apart from "essential" or "primary" hypertension.

Common causes of secondary HTN:

- Chronic kidney disease
- Sleep apnea
- Pregnancy (ranging from pregnancy-induced HTN to preeclampsia)
- Adrenaline secreting tumors
- Cushing's syndrome (cortisol hypersecretion)
- Drug use: both prescriptions like hormonal birth control and stimulants for ADHD and illegal drugs (e.g., cocaine and methamphetamine)
- Hyperthyroidism

In each of these disorders, one or more of the autoregulatory mechanisms for maintaining blood pressure are disrupted. In examples such as hyperthyroidism or adrenaline secreting tumors, direct action of the relevant hormones will increase cardiac output, vascular tone, or both. In cases of sleep apnea, the frequent nocturnal awakenings increase the secretion of adrenaline and other "stress" hormones. The subsequent effect is predictable. Pregnancy creates numerous physiologic changes in hormone levels, blood volume, and circulation. The complete understanding of pathologic BP rise in pregnancy is not fully understood.

Clinical Presentation

Diagnosis begins by suspecting secondary hypertension exists. Providers should exercise more caution to exclude secondary HTN in the following circumstances:

- History and exam features, which suggest any of the previously referenced diagnoses
- Early onset of HTN: interpreted as before age 30 and especially prior to puberty
- Absence of family history of HTN
- Severe HTN at onset
- Failure to gain control of BP with simultaneous use of two to three agents
- Sudden loss of BP control in previously stable patients
- Fifty percent rise in serum creatinine within a week of starting ACE-I or ARB therapy

NOTE

Many of these patients will be normotensive only a few days after delivery. When the BP rise persists, some authors suspect that primary HTN was simply recognized during the pregnancy.

Diagnostic and Lab Studies

Diagnostic testing should be targeted to address the suspected cause. For example, if polysomnography confirms sleep apnea, it is not cost-effective or necessary to exclude hormone-secreting tumors. In cases of renal bruit, or rise in serum creatinine, target the workup to examine renal blood flow. Doppler ultrasound may be adequate, and recognize that using contrast in other imaging studies may further jeopardize a diseased kidney. Hormonal testing can be challenging to interpret and is beyond the scope of this section.

Differential Diagnosis

As mentioned previously, the differential diagnosis is reasonably well circumscribed. Refer again to the previous section on pathophysiology in this chapter. At the bedside, review the mechanisms for generating and regulating blood pressure. Cardiac output is stroke volume times heart rate. Is there some external influence changing these? Regulation of BP occurs in the baroreceptors of the great vessels. Is there is dissection or coarctation? Careful auscultation may reveal a bruit over the affected vessel. Further regulation of blood volume and BP are regulated at the kidneys. Is there a risk factor for kidney dysfunction? Sleep apnea can be assessed by history and exam: Look for a large neck circumference and narrow oral airway. Pregnancy can be excluded by last menstrual period, but if there is any uncertainty, point-of-care testing is available in most office settings. Screen for substance abuse including prescription and street drugs and excess alcohol. Finally, a comprehensive review of all medications, supplements, etc., is in order. Consult a pharmacist or other reference if there are drugs that are not well known to the provider.

Treatment

Like so much of clinical medicine, treatment begins with a clear diagnosis. While the workup is underway, control of BP is an important goal. Even if the BP is not normalized, lowering the peak readings is of some value. After the diagnosis is clear, target the underlying disorder. In cases of pregnancy, most providers will defer to an expert.

One possible case for the boards is the patient who presents hypertensive after using illegal stimulants like cocaine. They are in an adrenaline-mediated crisis. Using an "unopposed beta-blocker" leaves the patient exposed to the effects of the alpha adrenal receptors. Vasoconstriction increases in these cases. Further rises in BP have been observed with disastrous effects. The preferred mode of treating these patients is to use nitroglycerin and CCBs, then add the alpha-blocker phentolamine before using a beta-blocker.

Health Maintenance and Patient Education

There is little to add to the information in the section regarding HTN.

- If the secondary cause is treatable, the patient can expect an improvement in BP control after that.
- If the secondary cause requires ongoing treatment, it is important for the provider to reinforce the link between the secondary cause and BP control.

Professional Considerations

Most patients will cooperate with the diagnosis and treatment of secondary HTN. The promise of better BP control and a reduction in the intensity of medical therapy is an attractive incentive. One major pitfall is to overlook the possibility of drug use. Prevalence is likely underestimated,

NOTE

In the interim before the consult, note that methyldopa (an alpha-adrenergic blocker), labetalol, and nifedipine are commonly considered safe in pregnancy.

and most users will be unwilling to reveal this behavior at the first opportunity. Advise the patient that you (typically) are not obligated to report illegal drug use in adults. Rapport at the bedside can be lifesaving.

Acute Pericarditis

Pathophysiology

- Typically idiopathic or due to viral infection
- Can be the result of:
  - Bacterial infection
  - Myxedema
  - Neoplasm
  - Chemotherapy
  - Radiation therapy
  - Cardiac surgery
  - Autoimmune or connective tissue disease
  - Pericardial effusion produces restrictive pressure on the heart

Clinical Presentation

- More common in males and those > 50 years old
- Sharp pleuritic substernal radiating chest pain relieved with sitting up and leaning forward
- Cardiac friction rub may be present
- Slowly progressive dyspnea, fatigue and weakness, accompanied by hepatomegaly, edema and ascites

Diagnostic and Lab Studies

- Elevated WBC count indicates infection.
- Echocardiography or chest X-ray reveals extent of cardiac effusion.
- ECG: diffuse ST segment elevation; pericardial effusion characterized by nonspecific T-wave changes and low QRS voltage.

Differential Diagnosis/Formulating the Most Likely Diagnosis

A cardiac friction rub is characteristic.

Health Maintenance and Patient Education

May be painful or painless and accompanied by cough and dyspnea.

Treatment (Pharmaceutical and Clinical Intervention)

- Pericardiodiocentesis
- Steriods or NSAIDS for inflammation
- Antibiotic therapy for infectious conditions

Professional Considerations

Cardiac tamponade usually presents with:
- Tachycardia
- Tachypnea

- Narrow pulse pressure
- Jugular venous distension
- Pulsus paradoxus

Valvular Disorders

Aortic Stenosis

Pathophysiology

Aortic stenosis is due to LV outflow tract obstruction due to restricted aortic valve leaflet motion from rheumatic valvular disease, congenitally abnormal valve, and calcific disease.

Clinical Presentation

Signs and Symptoms

- Dyspnea
- Orthopnea, fatigue
- PND
- Decreased exercise capability
- Heart murmur

Diagnostic and Lab Studies

- ECG: not useful for specific diagnosis
- Chest X-ray: left-sided atrial enlargement, ventricular hypertrophy

Turbulent blood flow across a stenotic aortic valve, best heard at the right upper sternal border; crescendo, decrescendo systolic murmur, late peaking, harsh, and radiating to the neck.

Practice Questions for Cardiovascular Review

1. Your patient is a 52-year-old male who presents with new onset peripheral edema, chest pain, shortness of breath, and extreme fatigue. He has no ongoing chronic medical conditions. He has mild hypertension, which has been well controlled on lisinopril. The patient reports that, two weeks ago, he was sick for about a week with fever, coughing, chest pain, and fatigue. He did not seek medical care and symptoms resolved. However, he reports that his ankles started swelling a few days ago and he has trouble walking even short distances without becoming extremely short of breath. He has been unable to work for the past few weeks. He denies fever. No nausea, vomiting, or diarrhea. No significant cough, although he has noticed he has a "wet-sounding" cough occasionally. He reports he is unable to sleep lying down and has had to rest in his recliner since becoming ill. On examination, you note tachycardia with a gallop rhythm and a pericardial friction rub. ECG shows sinus tachycardia. Chest X-ray is normal. Based on this presentation, your differential diagnoses includes

    (A) acute myocardial infarction.
    (B) dilated cardiomyopathy.
    (C) infectious myocarditis.
    (D) rheumatic fever.
    (E) community acquired pneumonia.

2. Acute pericarditis may be due to autoimmune conditions, systemic disease, or infectious causes. Diagnosis of acute pericarditis must include at least two of the following four findings: 1) pericardial chest pain, 2) pericardial rub, 3) new, widespread ST-elevation or PR depression, and 4)

    (A) cough.
    (B) hypertrophic myocardium.
    (C) bilateral pulmonary congestion.
    (D) widespread peripheral edema.
    (E) pericardial effusion.

3. The American College of Cardiology guidelines for treatment of hypertension recommend the threshold for starting pharmacotherapy (in patients with no increased cardiovascular risk) with a blood pressure of

    (A) > 130/80 mmHg.
    (B) > 140/80 mmHg.
    (C) > 140/90 mmHg.
    (D) > 150/90 mmHg.
    (E) > 160/80 mmHg.

4. Heart failure presenting with low cardiac output, dyspnea, and congestion is likely due to

    (A) right ventricular dysfunction.
    (B) left ventricular dysfunction.
    (C) infectious pathology.
    (D) restrictive cardiomyopathy.
    (E) chest wall trauma.

5. You are evaluating a pregnant patient who presents with exertional dyspnea, fatigue, orthopnea. She reports a history of rheumatic fever several years ago. On examination, you auscultate an "opening snap" following A2 heart sound. A diastolic murmur is heard at the apex with the patient lying in the left lateral position. You order an echocardiogram because you suspect

(A) mitral stenosis.
(B) bundle branch block.
(C) acute aortic regurgitation.
(D) mitral valve regurgitation.
(E) aortic stenosis.

6. Your patient is a 22-year-old male who presents to the ED with a chief complaint of "racing heart" associated with dizziness, diaphoresis, and mild dyspnea. He states this has happened before and usually lasts a few minutes and resolves spontaneously. He is worried he may be having a heart attack. On ECG, you note a narrow QRS complex with a heart rate of 200 beats per minute, which is regular. The patient is alert and oriented. He has no past medical history of severe or chronic disease. You suspect the patient is experiencing

(A) mitral regurgitation.
(B) aortic regurgitation.
(C) sinus tachycardia.
(D) paroxysmal supraventricular tachycardia (PSVT).
(E) acute myocardial infarction.

7. Telmisartan is used as pharmacotherapy for essential hypertension. This medication is a(n)

(A) ACE inhibitor.
(B) ARB.
(C) CCB.
(D) thiazide diuretic.
(E) beta-blocker.

8. Cigarette smoking is associated with the development of essential hypertension by increasing

(A) angiotensinogen levels.
(B) cortisol levels.
(C) cholesterol levels.
(D) heart rate.
(E) plasma norepinepherine levels.

9. Which of the following conditions should be suspected in the presentation of elevated blood pressure in young patients?

(A) Metabolic syndrome
(B) Atrial septal defect
(C) Coarctation of the aorta
(D) Patent foramen ovale
(E) Diabetes mellitus

10. There are five charcacteristic defects associated with tetralogy of Fallot. These include: over-riding aorta, right-sided aortic arch, concentric right ventricular hypertrophy, right ventricular outflow obstruction, and

    (A) atrial septal defect (ASD).

    (B) ventricular septal defect (VSD).

    (C) patent foramen ovale (PFO).

    (D) coarctation of the aorta (COA).

    (E) hypertrophic left ventricle.

Answers Explained

1. **(C)** Infectious myocarditis often ensues following an upper respiratory infection, and symptoms may include pleuritic chest pain or signs of heart failure. An echocardiogram is used to document cardiomegaly and contractile dysfunction. The intial heart size is usually normal; however, walls may be thickened. This condition is thought to be caused by the acute viral infection or a post-viral immune response. Biopsy is required for classification, including fulminany, subclinical, or chronic. The onset of heart failure symptoms may be gradual or abrupt. ECG changes are usually present with AMI and may be associated with ST-segment elevation (STEMI) or classified as non-ST-segment elevation (NSTEMI) in nature. Symptoms usually involve a worsening angina progressing in nature. Most MIs occur at rest (unlike angina) and in the early morning. Pain is similar to angina but is more severe and escalates quickly within minutes. Nitroglycerin has little effect when a patient is expderiencing an AMI. Associated symptoms include sweating, nausea, weakness, and apprehension. Patients also report light-headedness, dizziness, coughing, wheezing, and inability to lie still. The presentation above does not meet criteria for acute MI. Dilated cardiomyopathy often presents with gradual progression of symptoms of heart failure. The physical exam may reveal rales, S3 gallop, elevated JVP, peripheral edema, and ascites. Rheumatic fever is not seen commonly in the United States; it is most often in developing countries. RF is a systemic immune process resulting from infection with beta-hemolytic streptococcal infection. Peak incidence is between ages of 5 and 15 years.

2. **(E)** Diagnostic criteria for acute pericarditis includes pericardial chest pain, pericardial rub, new widespread ST-elevation or PR depresssion on ECG, and pericardial effusion. At least two of these findings must be present for diagnosis. Additional supportive findings include elevated serum inflammatory markers (WBC, CRP, ESR) and evidence of pericardial inflammation on CT or MRI. (A, B, C, D) These findings are not associated with diagnosis of acute pericarditis.

3. **(C)** The American College of Cardiology recommends starting pharmacotherapy for hypertension with a blood pressure of > 140/90. Guidelines vary according to organization. Evaluation of total cardiovascular risk is more important in determining treatment thresholds than individual blood pressure readings. The ACC provides an online toolkit for primary prevention: *https://tools.acc.org/ascvd-risk-estimator-plus/#!/calculate/estimate*. There is also an ASCVD Risk Estimator Plus: *https://www.acc.org/ASCVDApp*.

4. **(B)** Left ventricular heart failure may be due to either systolic or diastolic dysfunction. Presenting symptoms are those associated with low cardiac output and congestion and include dyspnea. Right heart failure presents with symptoms of fluid overload and is usually a result of left ventricular failure. Infectious pathology presents as pericarditis or cardiomyopathy. Restrictive cardiomyopathy is most commonly caused by amyloidosis and presents with pulmonary hypertension with predominant right heart failure (as opposed to left heart failure).

5. **(A)** Mitral stenosis is often presumed to be associated with a history of rheumatic fever and the sequelae of rheumatic heart disease. However, a known history of rheumatic fever is only found in about 30% of patients with mitral stenosis. A reported history of rheumatic fever should raise suspicion for mitral stenosis. A characteristic finding on exam is an "opening snap" following the A2 heart sound. This finding results from a stiff mitral valve. As the disease worsens, a localized diastolic murmur may be heard. Symptoms of mitral stenosis are

often precipitated by pregnancy or onset of atrial fibrillation. Bundle branch block is most often associated with an atrial septal defect. Acute aortic regurgitation usually occurs with aortic dissection or infective endocarditis. Left ventricular failure presents as pulmonary edema and may develop rapidly. Mitral valve regurgitation may be asymptomatic; however, severe disease may lead to left-sided heart failure, which usually presents as a pansystolic murmur that is maximal at the apex and radiates to the axilla.

6. **(D)** PSVT presents as rapid, regular tachycardia that develops abruptly and resolves spontaneously in most cases. PSVT is seen most often in young adults. Acute treatment includes having the patient perform the Valsalva maneuver. Having the patient lie supine and passively raising their legs following the maneuver increases its effectiveness in aborting the episode. (A) Mitral valve regurgitation is often asymptomatic, but severe disease may lead to left-sided heart failure and progressive exertional dyspnea and fatigue. (B) Aortic regurgitation is usually asymptomatic until middle age. AR may then present as left-sided heart failure and, rarely, chest pain. (C) Sinus tachycardia is defined as a heart rate faster than 100 beats/minute. It is a normal phsyiologic response to exercise or other conditions in which catecholamines are released. (E) An acute myocardial infarction is a heart attack, which is where the blood flow to the heart is cut off.

7. **(B)** Telmisartan belongs to a class of antihypertensive medications called angiotensin II receptor blockers (ARBs). These medications have been shown to improve cardiovascular outcomes in patients with heart failure and type 2 diabetes mellitus with nephropathy. ARBs rarely cause cough and are less likely to produce a skin rash or angioedema than other classes. However, they can cause hyperkalemia. (A) ACE inibitor medications include lisinopril and captopril. (C) Calcium channel blockers act by causing peripheral vasodilation and include diltiazem (nondihydropyridine agent) and amolodipine (dihydropridine agent). (D) Thiazide diuretics include hydrochlorothiazide (HCTZ). (E) Beta-blockers cause the heart to beat more slowly and with less force, and that helps to lower blood pressure.

8. **(E)** Cigarette smoking raises blod pressure by increasing plasma norepinephrine levels. Excessive use of alcohol raises blood pressure by increasing plasma catecholamines. Other risk factors/exacerbating factors include obesity, sleep apnea, NSAID use, increased salt intake, and low potassium intake. (A, B, C, D) These factors are not specifically associated with cigarette smoking.

9. **(C)** Coarctation of the aorta is an area of localized narrowing of the aortic arch just distal to the left subclavian vein origin.

10. **(B)** Tetralogy of Fallot includes five characteristic features: VSD, concentric RVH, RV outflow obstruction, right-sided aortic arch, and overriding aorta. (A, C, D, E) These findings are not found with tetralogy of Fallot.

3

Dermatology Review

Learning Objectives

In this chapter, you will review:

→ Acneiform eruptions
→ Desquamation
→ Disorders of the hair and nails
→ Infectious disease
   → Bacterial
   → Fungal
   → Parasitic
   → Viral
→ Keratotic disorders
→ Neoplasms
→ Papulosquamous disorders

Acneiform Eruptions

Acne Vulgaris

Pathophysiology

The pathogenesis of acne is multifaceted, and at least four factors have been identified. These features include:

- Follicular epidermal hyperproliferation
- Sebum production
- *Propionibacterium acne*s
- Inflammation and immune response

Each of these processes are interrelated and under hormonal and immune influence.

Clinical Presentation

- Gradual onset of lesions around puberty
- Hyperandrogenism should be considered in a female patient whose:
  ○ Acne is severe in the jawline or lower face distribution
  ○ Sudden in onset or associated with hirsutism or irregular menstrual periods

- A complete medication history is important.
  - The primary site of acne is the face and, to a lesser degree, the back, chest, and shoulders.
  - On the trunk, lesions tend to be concentrated near the midline.
  - Acne vulgaris is characterized by several lesion types:
    - Noninflammatory comedones (open or closed)
    - Inflammatory lesions (red papules, pustules, or nodules/cysts)

Diagnostic and Lab Studies

Laboratory workup may be indicated in patients with acne if hyperandrogenism is suspected, particularly in children with acne.

Differential Diagnosis/Formulating the Most Likely Diagnosis

The diagnosis is usually straightforward, but inflammatory acne may be confused with folliculitis, rosacea, or perioral dermatitis.

Health Maintenance and Patient Education

- Family history, body mass index, and diet may predict risk for development of moderate to severe acne.
- Variation in relation to the menstrual cycle

Treatment (Pharmaceutical and Clinical Intervention)

Using cleansing topical and antibiotic therapy, the treatment goal is to reverse the pathophysiology.

- Treatment options include medicated cleansers, topical retinoid (isoretinoin), and antibiotics (doxycycline, tetracycline).
  - Correct the altered pattern of follicular keratinization.
  - Decrease sebaceous gland activity.
  - Decrease the follicular bacterial population, particularly *P. acnes.*
  - Exert an anti-inflammatory effect.

Professional Considerations

Treatment regimens should be initiated early and be sufficiently aggressive to prevent permanent sequelae.

Rosacea

Pathophysiology

Rosacea is an inflammatory disorder of pilosebaceous glands. It is most common in 40-year-old women.

Clinical Presentation

- Erythema and telangectasias are seen on the cheeks, nose, chin, and ears.
- Patients frequently have exacerbation of affected areas by heat, hot drinks, spicy food, sunlight, exercise, alcohol, emotions, or menopausal flushing.
- Papules are common, and pustules may be associated.

Diagnostic and Lab Studies

None indicated.

Differential Diagnosis/Formulating the Most Likely Diagnosis

- Acne vulgaris
- Seborrheic dermatitis
- Perioral dermatitis
- Systemic lupus erythematosus
- Carcinoid
- Dermatomyositis

Health Maintenance and Patient Education

None indicated.

Treatment (Pharmaceutical and Clinical Intervention)

- Avoid triggers that may affect rosacea
- Metronidazole, 0.75% gel applied twice daily or 1% cream once daily, is the topical treatment of choice.
  - If metronidazole is not tolerated, topical clindamycin (solution, gel, or lotion) 1% used twice daily is effective; response is noted in 4–8 weeks.
- Oral tetracyclines should be used when topical therapy does not yield effective treatment.
- Minocycline or doxycycline, 50–100 mg once or twice daily orally, may also be effective.

Professional Considerations

Educate patients to avoid exacerbating factors such as poor hygiene and chemicals, stress, oils, and some topical medications. Patients should wear sunscreen with broad coverage.

Desquamation

Erythema Multiforme

Pathophysiology

This is an acute inflammatory mucocutaneous syndrome categorized into minor and major types.

- EM minor only involves the skin and lips.
- EM major involves the mucous membranes.

Most cases are related with infections, with herpes simplex virus being the most common cause followed by *Mycoplasma pneumoniae*. EM can be idiopathic. Medications are not a common cause of EM.

Clinical Presentation

A classic target lesion is often seen distally and spread centrally. The center of the lesion may become purpuric, necrotic, or develop into a vesicle or bulla. EM usually affects less than 10% of the body surface area. Mucosal lesions can be seen in up to 70% of patients and are not confined to the oral cavity; ocular lesions may be present. Prodromal symptoms of fever, cough, and rhinitis may be present, but in most cases are absent.

Diagnostic and Lab Studies

- Skin biopsy is diagnostic.
- In severe cases, labs may show an elevated erythrocyte sedimentation rate, leukocytosis, and mildly elevated liver aminotransferase.

Differential Diagnosis

Urticaria and drug eruptions, Stevens-Johnson syndrome, and toxic epidermal necrolysis must be differentiated from EM.

Health Maintenance and Patient Education

- EM minor usually last 2–6 weeks and may recur with subsequent HSV outbreaks.
- There may be transient skin discoloration.

Treatment

- Discontinue offending agent.
- Antihistamines and analgesics
- Proper skin care
- Topical corticosteroids can be used in the oral variant of EM.
- Systemic corticosteroids may shorten the duration of symptoms.
- Oral acyclovir prophylaxis of herpes simplex infections may be effective in preventing recurrent EM if HSV is a trigger.

Professional Considerations

Admission should be considered if oral lesions prevent adequate oral intake or if there are severe constitutional symptoms.

Stevens-Johnson Syndrome (SJS)/Toxic Epidermal Necrolysis (TEN)

Pathophysiology

A mucocutaneous reaction resulting in necrosis and detachment of the epidermis and mucosal epithelium. Apoptosis of keratinocytes results from cell-mediated cytotoxic reactions. Most often caused by medications (e.g., sulfonamides, NSAIDs, allopurinol, and anticonvulsants). The exposure to medication can be systemic or topical.

Clinical Presentation

- SJS presents with atypical target lesions.
  - There are only two zones of color change and a central blister or nonspecific purpuric macules with < 10% body surface area (BSA) detachment.
- TEN presents with similar lesions with > 30% BSA detachment. SJS/TEN overlap have between 10–30% BSA detachment.
  - Nikolsky sign (lateral pressure will displace the epidermis) is positive.
- Lesions evolve to blisters.

There is involvement of two or more mucosal surfaces, with oral and conjunctival mucosa most often affected. Additional symptoms of pain with eating, swallowing, and urination can indicate relevant mucosae involvement.

Prodromal symptoms are nonspecific and can include fever, malaise, headache, and URI symptoms.

Diagnostic and Lab Studies

Skin biopsy is diagnostic. Labs monitor for severity and management of the disease and should include evaluating for electrolyte imbalances, renal failure, hypoproteinemia, and lymphopenia.

Differential Diagnosis

Mycoplasma pneumoniae may trigger a reaction resembling SJS in children/young adults but does not progress to TEN and has good prognosis. SJS/TEN must be differentiated from other autoimmune bullous diseases (e.g., pemphigus, pemphigoid, and linear IgA bullous dermatosis), acute systemic lupus erythematosus, and vasculitis.

Health Maintenance and Patient Education

- Epidermal detachment can continue for 5–7 days and re-epithelialization can take days to weeks.
- Life-threatening complications can occur.

Treatment (Pharmaceutical and Clinical Intervention)

The most important part of treatment is to stop the offending medication. Consider tetanus prophylaxis. Patients with greater than 25–30% BSA should be transferred to an acute care unit (ICU or burn unit). Patients need to be provided with nutritional and fluid replacement with careful monitoring for infection and pain control.

Most treatments remain controversial:

- If corticosteroids are administered, they should be given prior to blistering and in high doses (prednisone, 1–2 mg/kd/day).
- Intravenous immunoglobulin (IVIG) at 1 g/kg/day for 4 days (total dose of at least 2 g/kg) may decrease mortality.
- Other systemic treatment options include cyclosporine (3–5 mg/kg/day for 7 days) and etanercept.
- Open wounds should be treated like second-degree burns.

Professional Considerations

The ABCD-10 and SCORTEN severity of illness scales predict mortality in SJS/TEN. The genetic marker HLA-B*1502 in patients of Southeast Asian ancestry can be correlated with carbamazepine induced SJS/TEN. There may also be an association with phenytoin. Testing for this genetic marker is recommended prior to initiation of treatment.

Measles

Pathophysiology

Measles is a single-stranded RNA virus that is a member of the Paramyxoviridae family. Transmission occurs via person-to-person contact or airborne respiratory secretions.

Clinical Presentation

Measles infection is characterized by an incubation period, prodrome, and exanthem.
- Prodrome of fever, cough, coryza, and conjunctivitis
- Koplik spots on the buccal mucosa are pathognomonic and begin as small, bright red macules that have a small blue-white speck within them and are typically found on the buccal mucosa.
- Koplik spots typically occur 48 hours prior to the onset of the rash and only last 12 to 72 hours.
- Skin eruption lasts 3 to 5 days.

Diagnostic and Lab Studies

The measles virus can be isolated using real-time reverse transcription polymerase chain reaction (PCR) from nasopharyngeal aspirates, throat swabs, blood, or urine. A positive serum immunoglobulin (Ig) M antibody for measles is diagnostic.

Differential Diagnosis/Formulating the Most Likely Diagnosis

- Drug hypersensitivity
- Rubella
- Rocky Mountain spotted fever
- Parvovirus
- Epstein-Barr virus

Health Maintenance and Patient Education

Uncomplicated measles last 10 to 12 days.

Treatment (Pharmaceutical and Clinical Intervention)

- The management of measles is supportive.
- Treatment focuses on antipyretics, fluids, and managing complications, if any should develop.

Professional Considerations

Prevention is key with initial vaccination at 12–15 months, followed by next vaccine at age 4–6 years old. Vitamins as a supplementation for all children with measles is a treatment consideration.

Infectious Disease—Bacterial/Fungal

Candidiasis

Pathophysiology

Although *Candida albicans* is the most commonly implicated *Candida* species in localized mucocutaneous candidiasis, an increasing number of other species have been implicated in mucocutaneous disease.

Risk factors for *Candida* infections include:

- Extremes of age
- Diabetes
- Obesity
- Pregnancy
- Glucocorticoids
- Immunodeficiency

Clinical Presentation

- Typically present with patchy erythema or erythematous plaques with associated itching and burning sensation.
- White plaques that bleed or erythematous when scraped
- Beefy-red patches and plaques often accompanied by satellite papules and pustules at the periphery
- Fissuring and crusting at the oral commissures may be seen in angular cheilitis
- In patients with vulvovaginitis, a thick, white, curdlike discharge is typical.

Diagnostic and Lab Studies

- Rapid confirmation achieved with potassium hydroxide (KOH) preparation from a scraping from an intact pustule, or a sample from a punch biopsy specimen demonstrating pseudo-hyphae and budding yeast infection.

Differential Diagnosis/Formulating the Most Likely Diagnosis

- Seborrheic dermatitis
- Tinea corporis/dermatophytosis
- Impetigo
- Erythrasma
- Intertrigo
- Irritant contact dermatitis
- Allergic contact dermatitis
- Atopic dermatitis
- Bacterial folliculitis
- Herpes simplex or herpes zoster
- Oral hairy leukoplakia

Health Maintenance and Patient Education

Most localized mucocutaneous *Candida* infections cause minor symptoms and respond readily to treatment.

Treatment (Pharmaceutical and Clinical Intervention)

Effective treatment includes one of the following:

- Ketoconazole 200–400 mg orally × 7 days
- Clotrimazole troches 10 mg dissolved orally × 5 days
- Fluconazole 100 mg orally × 7 days
- Nystatin rinses 3 × daily

Professional Considerations

For patients with recurrent disease, chronic suppressive dosing of fluconazole 150 mg orally three times weekly may be indicated. Also consider HIV testing if indicated.

Dermatophyte Infections

Pathophysiology

The molds that cause skin infections in humans include:
- Trichophyton
- Microsporum
- Epidermophyton

The characteristic ring shape of cutaneous lesions is the result of the organisms' outward growth in a centrifugal pattern in the stratum corneum.

Clinical Presentation

Dermatophyte infections occur more commonly in males than in females, and progesterone has been shown to inhibit dermatophyte growth. Dermatophyte infection of the skin is often called *ringworm* (trichophyton, microsporum, epidermophyton).

Diagnostic and Lab Studies

- Often diagnosed by their clinical appearance.
- If the diagnosis is uncertain, scrapings should be taken from the edge of a lesion with a scalpel blade, transferred to a slide to which a drop of potassium hydroxide is added, and examined under a microscope for the presence of hyphae.

Differential Diagnosis/Formulating the Most Likely Diagnosis

Characterized by ring-shaped lesions.

Health Maintenance and Patient Education

Affected areas should be kept as dry as possible.

Treatment (Pharmaceutical and Clinical Intervention)

Dermatophyte infections usually respond to topical therapy. In patients with extensive skin lesions, oral itraconazoles are recommended.

Professional Considerations

Named for body part affected:
- Tinea barbae
- Tinea capitis (head)
- Tinea pedis (feet)
- Tinea corporis (body)
- Tinea cruris (crotch)
- Tinea unguium (nails, although infection at this site is more often termed *onychomycosis*)

Infectious Disease—Viral

Herpes Simplex

Pathophysiology

Herpes simplex virus (HSV) infections are caused by closely related types of HSV. Their main clinical manifestations are mucocutaneous infections, with HSV type 1 (HSV-1) being mostly associated with orofacial disease, and HSV type 2 (HSV-2) usually being associated with genital infection.

Clinical Presentation

- Symptoms of primary oral herpes can include:
  - Painful grouped vesicles on erythematous base, which is hallmark
  - Ulcerative lesions involving the hard and soft palate
  - Tongue and buccal mucosa
  - Adjacent facial areas

The clinical course of acute first-episode genital herpes among patients with HSV-1 and HSV-2 infections is similar, and both are associated with extensive genital lesions in different stages of evolution, including vesicles, pustules, and erythematous ulcers that may require 2 to 3 weeks to resolve.

There is accompanying pain, itching, dysuria, vaginal and urethral discharge, and tender inguinal lymphadenopathy.

- Systemic signs and symptoms are common and include:
  - Fever
  - Headache
  - Malaise
  - Myalgias

Diagnostic and Lab Studies

The history and clinical findings may be sufficient. A Tzanck smear is a cytologic technique most often used in the diagnosis of herpesvirus infections. Lesion sample is placed on a glass slide, air-dried, and stained with Giemsa or Wright's stain. Multinucleated epithelial giant cells suggest the presence of HSV or VZV; culture, immunofluorescence microscopy, or genetic testing must be performed to identify the specific virus.

Differential Diagnosis/Formulating the Most Likely Diagnosis

The mostly likely differential diagnosis is an aphthous stomatitis.

Health Maintenance and Patient Education

- Primary infections can be severe, but subsequent infections are less symptomatic.
- Frequency typically decreases over time.

Treatment (Pharmaceutical and Clinical Intervention)

- Keep lesions clean and dry.
- Acyclovir may be warranted alternative treatment, along with valcyclovir or famcyclovir.

Professional Considerations

Antiviral treatment decreases symptomatic and subclinical shedding of HSV-2.

Varicella Zoster

Pathophysiology

Varicella-zoster virus (VZV) causes varicella (chickenpox) and herpes zoster (shingles). Transmission occurs via respiratory route, and viral replication leads to viremia.

Clinical Presentation

- Chickenpox presents as a rash, low-grade fever, and malaise; although a few patients develop a prodrome 1–2 days before onset.
- Lesions, or clusters of vesicles on erythematous base, which evolve from maculopapules to vesicles, appear on the trunk and face and rapidly spread to involve other areas of the body.
  - Most have an erythematous base with a diameter of 5–10 mm. Successive crops appear over a 2- to 4-day period.
  - Lesions can also be found on the mucosa of the pharynx and/or the vagina.
- Herpes zoster stems from virus activation of the dorsal root and occurs at all ages, but its highest incidence is among individuals in the sixth decade of life and beyond.
- Thoracic region is the most common area affected.
- Dermatomal distribution is hallmark.

Diagnostic and Lab Studies

Diagnosis usually made by history and physical exam. Other testing is warranted when presentation is atypical or when the patient has underlying medical conditions or lesions do not heal.

Differential Diagnosis/Formulating the Most Likely Diagnosis

Other viral infections that can imitate chickenpox include disseminated HSV infection in patients with atopic dermatitis and the disseminated vesiculopapular lesions sometimes associated with coxsackievirus infection.

Health Maintenance and Patient Education

Hygiene and daily cleansing of skin and lesions is greatly advised.

Treatment (Pharmaceutical and Clinical Intervention)

- Acyclovir (800 mg by mouth five times daily)
- Valacyclovir (1 g three times daily)
- Famciclovir (250 mg three times daily) for 5–7 days is recommended for adolescents and adults with chickenpox of ≤ 24-hour duration. This is for zoster only, not chickenpox.

Professional Considerations

A live-attenuated varicella vaccine is recommended for all children > 1 year of age (up to 12 years of age) who have not had chickenpox and for adults known to be seronegative for VZV. Two doses are recommended at 12–15 months of age and at ~4–6 years of age.

Practice Questions for Dermatology Review

1. A 34-year-old Caucasian female presents to your office with concerns about a facial rash that does not seem to be getting better. The rash has been progressively becoming more severe over several months. She reports flushing of the face when she gets out in the sunlight, exercises, eats spicy foods, or drinks alcohol. The rash primarily affects her cheeks, nose, chin, and ears. On exam, the rash covers the cheeks, nose, and chin and appears erythematous with pustular areas with telangiectasias. There are no systemic symptoms. No comedomes are seen. The patient denies any new medication use or exposure to new facial cleansers. She does not take oral contraceptives. She does state that the rash sometimes "stings" and burns. This presentation is consistent with which of the following diagnoses?

   (A) Acne vulgaris
   (B) Folliculitis
   (C) Miliaria
   (D) Molluscum contagiosum
   (E) Rosacea

2. A patient presents with complaints of severe itching and rash in body folds and the vulvar region. The patient is a 48-year-old female with a diagnosis of diabetes mellitus, type 2. She states her blood sugar has been high recently and she has not been strictly following her diet. This patient is morbidly obese and also carries diagnoses of hypertension and hypothyroidism. On examination of affected areas, superficial, beefy-red areas of redness are noted. Areas of satellite vesicopustules are seen around the periphery of affected areas. There are whitish, cheesy, curdlike secretions noted in these body folds as well as in the oral mucosa. Based on patient history and findings on physical exam, your differential diagnosis includes

   (A) erythema multiforme.
   (B) mucocutaneous candidiasis.
   (C) erysipelas.
   (D) cellulitis.
   (E) HSV 1.

3. Your patient is a 36-year-old male who is homeless and often stays in homeless shelters in the area. He reports a very itchy rash around his waist area, in the webs between the fingers, and in his wrist creases. On examination, small pruritic vesicles, pustules, and burrows are noted in the spaces between fingers and toes and the heels of the palms. Your differential diagnoses include scabies. First-line treatment for scabies includes

   (A) benzoyl peroxide topically.
   (B) systemic antibiotics for 7 days.
   (C) oral NSAIDs.
   (D) permethrin topically.
   (E) corticosteroids.

4. You are working in the ED and a patient presents with an abscess on his gluteal area. He states the area started with a "pimple" that has progressively become larger and more painful. On examination, a rounded abscess is seen with surrounding erythema and warmth. The lesion is fluctuant but no drainage is noted. First-line treatment is incision and drainage along with systemic antibiotics started at the time of the I&D. The patient denies medication allergies. You prescribe

   (A) TMP-SMZ 160/800 po BID for 10 days.
   (B) cephalexin 250 mg po TID for 7 days.
   (C) oral vancomycin 1 g po BID for 5 days.
   (D) amoxicillin 500 mg po TID for 10 days.
   (E) augmentin 500 mg BID for 5 days.

5. You are working in a clinic and a patient presents with fever blisters on her upper lip. She states the blisters are painful and making it difficult for her to drink liquids. She denies lesions elsewhere on her body but states she has had fever blisters before. Since this is not her first outbreak, and her disease is not severe, she declines systemic suppressive treatment at this time. You prescribe

   (A) valacyclovir 2 g po BID for 1 day.
   (B) famciclovir 500 mg po daily for 5 days.
   (C) pritelivir 100 mg po daily for 10 days.
   (D) valacyclovir 500 mg po TID for 5 days.
   (E) topical corticosteroid until lesions resolve.

6. Your patient is a 4-year-old male accompanied by his mom. Mom is requesting "an antibiotic" for an area of superficial blisters and weeping drainage on the patient's upper lip area. Mom reports the patient has been playing outside every evening and has multiple mosquito bites on his face, arms, and legs. On exam, you note an area of macules, pustules, blisters, and vesicles with a honey-colored crusting drainage. These findings are characteristic of

   (A) contact dermatitis.
   (B) porphyria.
   (C) impetigo.
   (D) acne vulgaris.
   (E) tinea.

7. You are seeing a 12-year-old girl for her annual wellness exam. Her exam findings are unremarkable, and she has no new complaints. You note several circular lesions with scaly borders present on her upper arms. She denies itching or pain and has no history of trauma or injury to the skin. A scraping of the lesions with application of KOH reveals a fungal dermatosis. Based on these findings, you suspect the cause might be

   (A) contact with an offending plant.
   (B) presence of a pet in the home.
   (C) her history of atopic dermatitis.
   (D) candida overgrowth of the skin.
   (E) exposure to poison oak plant.

8. The most common form of cancer is

   (A) breast cancer.
   (B) squamous cell carcinoma.
   (C) malignant melanoma.
   (D) lung cancer.
   (E) basal cell carcinoma.

9. Medications most often implicated in development of urticarial drug eruptions (dermatitis medicamentosa) include penicillins, cephalosporins, and

   (A) sulfonamides.
   (B) NSAIDs.
   (C) antihypertensives.
   (D) fluoroquinolones.
   (E) corticosteroids.

10. Your patient is a 45-year-old female who presents with painful nodules on the anterior aspect of both lower extremities. The patient states the lesions appeared several weeks ago and have become less red and somewhat less tender. Some of the areas now resemble contusions. Patient denies any trauma or prior history of rash. She does admit to feeling fatigued and tired more than usual and has experienced a few days of low-grade fever. Examination reveals the presence of multiple subcutaneous areas of nodules on the anterior lower legs that are tender. Lesions appear to be in various stages of resolution; however, no ulcerations are seen. This presentation is consistent with a diagnosis of

    (A) photodermatitis.
    (B) venous stasis ulcers.
    (C) cellulitis.
    (D) erythema nodosum.
    (E) basal cell carcinoma.

Answers Explained

1. **(E)** Rosacea is a common dermatologic condition that presents in adulthood. Patients with rosacea commonly present as noted above. In mild disease, redness and telangiectasis are seen on the cheeks only. No comedomes are present. With more severe rosacea, inflammatory papules are present and these may develop into pustules. Associated disorders include blepharitis, keratitis, and chalazion. (A) Acne vulgaris is a very common condition starting in puberty that may persist into adulthood. Characteristic findings are comedomes. The face, neck, and upper trunk area may be involved, and scarring may result from severe acne. (B) Folliculitis is frequently caused by staph infection and is seen more commonly in diabetic patients. Hot tub folliculitis is caused by *Pseudomonas aeruginosa*, and nonbacterial folliculitis may develop because of friction and oils. The lesions are typically tender, follicular, and pustular in nature, and treatment is directed by causation. (C) Miliaria is also known as "heat rash" and presents as a burning, itching rash on covered areas of skin typically. There may be aggregates of small vesicles, papules, or pustules present. (D) Molluscum contagiosum is an infection caused by a poxvirus resulting in a mild skin disease that is contagious but can be self-healing or treated with freezing off and medicated creams.

2. **(B)** Mucocutaneous candidiasis presents as a superficial fungal infection seen most often in patients with diabetes, who are pregnant, who are obese, or who are immunocompromised. Systemic antibiotics, oral corticosteroids, and hormone replacement therapy may contribute to development of mucocutaneous candidiasis in susceptible patients. (A) Erythema multiforme is caused by herpes simplex and presents as cutaneous lesions on the extensor surfaces, palms, soles, or mucous membranes. This eruption remains localized, and classic target lesions are seen on areas of involvement. (C) Erysipelas is a superficial type of cellulitis caused by beta-hemolytic streptococci. Presentation includes a circumscribed, edematous area on the face or lower extremity. The rash is very painful and patients appear systemically ill. (D) Cellulitis is a diffuse, spreading infection of the dermis and subcutaneous tissue. Cellulitis typically occurs on the lower leg and begins as a small, tender patch. The area expands within hours and systemic symptoms of fever, chills, and malaise develop. If untreated, septicemia may develop. (E) HSV 1 presents as painful single or grouped vesicles often around the mouth area.

3. **(D)** Scabies occurs as a result of *Sarcoptes scabiei* infestation. Close physical contact with affected individuals for 15–20 minutes is the typical mode of transmission. Patients report severe iching. The lesions occur on finger webs, wrist creases, umbilicus, waist crease, and elbows. First-line treatment is permethrin 5% cream topically. Treatment is a single application from the neck down for 8–12 hours then washed off. Treatment is often repeated in 1 week. Close contacts should be treated as well. (A, B, C, E) Benzoyl peroxide is used to treat acne vulgaris. Systemic antibiotics may be indicated for cellulitis. Oral NSAIDs are not indicated in treatment of scabies.

4. **(A)** First-line antibiotic treatment of furunculosis includes TMP-SMZ 160/800 po BID for 10 days. Alternatively, clindamycin 300 mg po TID for 10 days may be given. (B) Cephalexin, if used, should be dosed at 1 gram daily in divided doses for 10 days. (C) Oral vancomycin may be indicated to treat gastrointestinal carriage of *S. aureus*. (D, E) Because of pathogen resistance, amoxicillin and augmentin are not recommended in the treatment of furunculosis.

5. **(A)** Recommended treatment for mild episodic HSV 1 infection is valacyclovir 2 g po BID for 1 day. (B, C, D) These options represent maintenance or suppressive treatment options or episodic treatment for moderate disease. (E) Topical corticosteroids are not indicated in this scenario.

6. **(C)** Impetigo is a contagious, autoinoculable epidermal infection usually caused by staphylococci or streptococci. The lesions are typically vesicular, macular, pustular, and associated with classic "honey-colored" crusting. Treatment includes soaking and scrubbing the area and the use of topical agents such as mupiricin, retapamulin, and ozenoxacin. (A) Contact dermatitis presents with erythema and edema with itching, vesicles, bullae, and weeping and crusting lesions in a pattern consistent with contact with the irritating agent. (B) Porphyria cutanea tarda is characterized by development of noninflammatory blisters on sun-exposed areas, usually the dorsal surfaces of the hands. This condition is often associated with liver disease. (D) Acne vulgaris is a polymorphic condition usually starting in adolescence. Characteristic lesions are comedomes. (E) Tinea is a derm infection caused by a fungal infection of the skin.

7. **(B)** Tinea corporis or tinea circinata present as ring-shaped lesions with advancing scaly borders and central clearing. These lesions typically occur on exposed areas of the body such as the arms or face. Often a history of exposure to an infected pet may be elicited. The pet may have a scaly rash or patches of alopecia. (A) Contact with plant agents causing dermatitis is characteristic of contact dermatitis infections. (C) A history of atopic dermatitis is not specifically associated with increased risk for tinea corporis but may also be present. (D) Candidal rashes are bright red with macules and papules and, often, satellite lesions. These rashes frequently occur on mucus membranes or in skin folds or creases. (E) Exposure or contact with poison oak causes a contact dermatitis.

8. **(E)** Basal cell carcinoma is the most common form of cancer and presents as a pearly papule with an erythematous patch as an unhealing ulcer. BCC occurs most often on sun-exposed areas of the face, trunk, lower legs, or pinna of the ear. (B) Squamous cell carcinoma usually occurs on chronically sun-exposed areas and appears as a nonhealing ulcer or warty nodule. Individuals with fair skin, who sunburn easily, are at increased risk. (A) After skin cancer, breast cancer is the most common cancer diagnosed in women in the United States. Breast cancer can occur in both men and women, but it's far more common in women. (C) Malignant melanoma is the fifth most common form of cancer in the United States. It is the leading cause of death due to skin disease. Lesions may be flat or raised but have irregular borders. There may be varying colors, including red, white, blue, and black. These lesions often appear de novo, and appearance changes over time. Less than 30% of malignant melanomas arise from existing moles. (D) Lung cancer is the leading cause of cancer deaths and often presents with development of a new cough or a change in chronic cough. As the disease progresses, patients often develop dyspnea, hemoptytis, anorexia, and weight loss.

9. **(B)** The most common adverse reactions to medications are rashes, and penicillins, cephalosporins, and NSAIDs are the most common causes of urticarial drug eruptions. Maculopapular or morbilliform skin reactions are most often caused by antibiotics, anticonvulsants, allopurinol, and NSAIDs. Drug-induced hypersensitivity reaction (DIHS) is most often caused by anticonvulsants, sulfonamides, and allopurinol. (A, C, D, E) These classes of medications may cause drug eruptions but are less commonly implicated than those noted above.

10. **(D)** Erythema nodosum is actually a symptom complex associated with panniculitis. The condition is characterized by tender, erythematous nodules appearing most often on the anterior aspects of the lower legs. Lesions usually last for about 6 weeks and may recur. When EN is present, a systemic illness is usually the underlying factor, and a search for cause should be initiated. (A) Photodermatitis is characterized by painful or pruritic redness, edema, and/or blisters on sun-exposed areas of skin. (B) Venous stasis ulcers occur in the setting of venous insufficiency. There is a history of varicosities, thrombophlebitis, or postphlebitic syndrome. Ulcerations are irregular in shape and occur on the medial lower legs. There is accompanying edema of the leg, hyperpigmentation, and red, scaly areas (stasis dermatitis). (C) Cellulitis is an expanding, erythematous, edematous plaque of the lower leg frequently associated with systemic symptoms, such as pain, fever, and chills. (E) BCC presents as a crusting nonhealing ulcer on sun-exposed areas.

4

Endocrine Review

Learning Objectives

In this chapter, you will review:

→ Adrenal disorders
→ Diabetes mellitus
→ Hypogonadism
→ Neoplasms
→ Thyroid disorders
→ Parathyroid disorders
→ Hyperthyroidism

Adrenal Disorders

The adrenal disorders are typically divided into categories:

- Hyperfunction
- Hypofunction
- Neoplasm

Table 4.1 Categories of Adrenal Disorders

Adrenal Hyperfunction	Adrenal Hypofunction	Adrenal Neoplasm
Cushing's syndrome—Excess glucocorticoids	Primary adrenal insufficiency	Benign
Benign		
Hyperaldosteronism—Excess mineralocorticoids	Central adrenal insufficiency	Malignant
Malignant		
Congenital Adrenal Hyperplasia—Excess Androgens		
Pheochromocytoma—Excess catecholamines		

Adrenal Insufficiency

Pathophysiology

Adrenal insufficiency is a lack of hormones produced by the adrenal cortex. It can be due to a central hormonal deficiency in the pituitary or hypothalamus or a primary deficiency due to dysfunction of the adrenal gland itself. The adrenal gland is responsible for synthesis of a number of hormones, including cortisol, aldosterone, adrenal androgens that are made in the adrenal cortex, as well as catecholamines synthesized in the adrenal medulla.

Clinical Presentation

Patients with adrenal insufficiency can present with a variety of symptoms. Symptoms can range from mild symptoms to adrenal crisis. Patients with central adrenal insufficiency often present with less acute and more insidious symptoms due to the fact that the aldosterone system is still functional. Symptoms can range from fatigue, lethargy, gastrointestinal distress, and weight loss to severe illness manifesting as adrenal crisis. Presentation depends somewhat on the clinical situation and whether the individual has primary or secondary (central) adrenal insufficiency.

Symptoms
- Weakness
- Fatigue
- Anorexia
- Nausea
- Vomiting
- Nonspecific abdominal pain
- Salt craving
- Weight loss

Signs
- Physical exam findings may include hypotension or orthostatic hypotension, and in cases of primary adrenal insufficiency, may be associated with vitiligo and hyperpigmentation.
  - The hyperpigmentation seen in primary adrenal insufficiency is due to the elevated levels of melanocyte-stimulating hormone (aMSH).
  - The high level of aMSH is produced when proopiomelanocortin (POMC) is cleaved to produce ACTH, with aMSH as a biproduct.
- Patients with central adrenal insufficiency may demonstrate signs of other pituitary hormonal deficiencies, or if it is due to a pituitary tumor, they may show signs and symptoms related to mass effect such as headaches, visual field deficits, or cranial nerve abnormalities (CN 2, 4, 6 most likely).

Laboratory findings can include:

- Hyponatremia
- Hyperkalemia
- Hypoglycemia

> **NOTE**
>
> Adrenal crisis is associated with typically more severe symptoms and can include hypotension and vascular collapse, fever, and mental status changes.

Diagnosis and Lab Studies

Diagnosis is based on a combination of clinical findings and laboratory results.

- Adrenal insufficiency may be associated with hyponatremia, hypokalemia, hypoglycemia, and dehydration indicators, such as elevated creatinine or blood urea nitrogen (BUN). The gold standard for confirming the diagnosis of adrenal insufficiency is the ACTH stimulation test.
- This is performed by drawing a baseline blood sample for ACTH and cortisol, then injecting 250 mcg of ACTH either intraveneously or intramuscularly, and followed by a blood sample for cortisol at 30 and 60 minutes after the injection.
  - A normal response is a serum cortisol level > 18–20 at either of the time points. The baseline measurement of the ACTH will determine whether the adrenal insufficiency is primary or secondary.

- A high ACTH level indicates primary adrenal insufficiency, whereas a low or "inappropriately normal" ACTH indicates a central (hypothalamic/pituitary) cause.
- Additional laboratory tests may be obtained depending on whether the person has primary or secondary adrenal insufficiency.
  - For example, in primary adrenal insufficiency, checking adrenal autoantibodies or screening for other autoimmune disorders, such as primary hypothyroidism due to Hashimoto's thyroiditis, may be warranted.
- Adrenal imaging may be necessary in primary adrenal insufficiency to rule out a structural lesion of the adrenal gland. If a pituitary cause is identified, all the pituitary function should be assessed and brain imaging with a pituitary MRI would be indicated.

Table 4.2 Causes of Adrenal Insufficiency

Primary Adrenal insufficiency	Central Adrenal Insufficiency	
	Hypothalamic (Tertiary)	Pituitary (Secondary)
Autoimmune adrenalitis (80%) Infiltrative/destructive disorders		
Infiltrative: sarcoid, amyloid, hemochromatosis, adrenal hemorrhage, infarction, metastatic disease, surgery, radiation		
Infections: TB, HIV, CMV, fungus		
Drug-induced: enzyme inhibitors, cytotoxic agents, CTLA4 inhibitors, congenital adrenal hyperplasia, adrenal atrophy	Glucocorticoid therapy Opiates Tumors Radiation	Tumors: pituitary or other sellar lesions Radiation Infiltrative diseases Infarction/Apoplexy Trauma Hypophysitis

Treatment (Pharmaceutical and Clinical Intervention)

Treatment is replacement therapy with glucocorticoids. Patients with primary adrenal insufficiency (destruction of the adrenal gland) require both glucocorticoid and mineralocorticoid therapy whereas patients with central adrenal insufficiency typically only require glucocorticoid replacement since the aldosterone axis remains functional.

- Glucocorticoid replacement options include:
  - Hydrocortisone
  - Cortisone acetate
  - Prednisone with hydrocortisone the preferred drug option
- Fludrocortisone is used for mineralocorticoid replacement.
- The goal is to use the lowest dose replacement therapy that controls symptoms of adrenal insufficiency and avoids side effects or complications of over-replacement.
- Signs of over-replacement include:
  - Weight gain and related complications of hypertension
  - Hyperglycemia
  - Insomnia or sleep disturbances
  - Mood disturbances
  - Edema
  - Accelerated bone loss or osteoporosis
- Adrenal crisis can occur with severe illness without adequate replacement therapy.
- Treatment of adrenal crisis requires hospitalization, often with intensive care unit care.

NOTE

All patients should be advised to increase their baseline replacement doses for acute illness and wear medical alert jewelry in case of emergencies so that health care personnel are aware of their condition in case they are unable to speak. Family members should receive education as well so they may assist in an emergency.

- Patients should receive intravenous glucocorticoids (hydrocortisone), intravenous fluids, and treatment for the underlying crisis trigger such as infection, trauma, or dehydration.
- Hydrocortisone therapy should be tapered back to baseline physiologic doses as dictated by the patient's clinical status.

Adrenal Insufficiency Key Points

- Clinical presentation may vary in severity and include nonspecific symptoms.
- Diagnosis confirmed by ACTH stimulation test.
- It is important to differentiate primary vs. central adrenal insufficiency as different imaging may be necessary.
- Treatment is with glucocorticoid replacement using the lowest dose to control symptoms.
- Mineralocorticoid replacement typically only required in primary adrenal insufficiency.
- Use stress dose steroids when necessary, avoid over-replacement, and minimize side effects.

Additional Reading: Adrenal Insufficiency

Bornstein SR et al. Diagnosis and Treatment of Primary Adrenal Insufficiency: An Endocrine Society Clinical Practice Guideline. *J Clin Endocrinol Metab* 2016. 101: 364–389.

Adrenal Tumors

Pathophysiology

These tumors can be benign or malignant. They can also cause issues by secreting excessive amounts of one or more hormones. Most are benign, non-secreting/nonfunctional adenomas. They are often found incidentally on imaging done for evaluation of other symptoms (e.g., abdominal pain). The prevalence is approximately 2–3% of the population and increases with age. These tumors are very rare in children. The main evaluation of incidental adrenal tumors consists of determining malignant potential and assessing for excess hormonal secretion. Incidental adrenal tumors require evaluation for hormonal hypersecretion. Pheochromocytomas arise from the adrenal medulla and usually secrete both epinephrine and norepinephrine. MEN is associated with medullary thyroid carcinoma, pheochromocytomas, hyperparathyroidism, and cutaneous lichen amyloidosis.

Clinical Presentation

- Often present with secondary HTN
- Most patients with incidental tumors are completely asymptomatic and do not show specifical physical exam findings.
- Symptoms depend on size or hormonal hypersecretion.
- Clinical presentation of hormonally active adrenal tumors depends on which hormone(s) the tumor secretes.

Cushing's Syndrome: Syndrome of Excess Cortisol Production

Clinical presentation can vary dramatically, ranging from mild to very severe.

> **NOTE**
>
> In general, in cases where the adrenal lesion is not already known to exist, the biochemical diagnosis confirming states of hormonal hypersecretion should be performed BEFORE imaging.

Symptoms

- Central obesity
- Skin changes (thin skin, easy bruising, striae)
- Hirsutism
- Menstrual irregularities
- Weakness
- Mood changes
- Depression
- Insomnia
- Bone loss

Comorbidities

- Diabetes mellitus
- Obesity
- Hypertension
- Osteopenia/osteoporosis
- Obstructive sleep apnea

Signs

Physical exam findings include:

- Round face
- Central adiposity
- Supraclavicular dorsocervical fat accumulation ("buffalo hump")
- Plethora
- Striae (can be excessive and/or hyperpigmented)
- Hypertension
- Hirsutism
- Findings related to diabetes mellitus

If they have osteoporosis, then the patient may have evidence of fractures or kyphosis. They can have proximal muscle weakness. Laboratory findings include hyperglycemia, hypokalemia, and hypercortisolism.

Diagnostics and Lab Studies

- Confirm hypercortisolism using accepted screening tests (see section on Cushing's syndrome for more extended discussion of laboratory evaluation).
- It is critical to distinguish whether the etiology of the hypercortisolism is ACTH dependent (pituitary or ectopic tumor source) or ACTH independent (adrenal tumor source).
- The ACTH level differentiates the cause of hypercortisolism.
  - The ACTH will be suppressed if the adrenal gland is the source of excess cortisol production.
  - Once adrenal Cushing's is confirmed biochemically, adrenal imaging is performed for tumor localization.

Pheochromocytoma: Catecholamine-Producing Adrenal Tumor

- These tumors arise from chromaffin cells of neuroectoderm origin and are typically located in the adrenal medulla (80–85%).
- Less commonly they can be found in sympathetic ganglia (paraganglioma). The tumors secrete catecholamines.

> **NOTE**
>
> Patients have an increased risk of cardiovascular disease, cerebrovascular disease, and thromboembolic events.

- They are relatively rare and only account for a small fraction of cases of hypertension cases (0.2–0.6%) and are found in a minority of adrenal incidentalomas (~5%). Approximately 30–40% are hereditary and 40–50% show somatic mutations.
- Associated syndromes include multiple endocrine neoplasia (MEN) 2A and 2B.

Symptoms

Can be variable and often include spells of unusual symptoms. The classic symptoms include:

- Episodes of headache
- Diaphoresis
- Palpitations associated with hypertension
- Tremor
- Anxiety
- Weight loss
- Cardiac arrhythmias or other cardiac symptoms can also be noted.

Signs

- Hypertension

Diagnosis A

- Plasma free or urinary metanephrines are recommended as the initial screening test. Fractionated urinary catecholamines can also used in diagnosis. Unless evaluating an incidental adrenal tumor, it is recommended that the biochemical diagnosis be made before imaging.
- After the laboratory tests confirm the biochemical diagnosis, the adrenal CT scan is typically the first imaging study performed to localize the tumor.
- Additional imaging modalities are available including MRI and nuclear medicine scans such as meta-[123I]iodobenzylguanidine ([123I]MIBG) single-photon emission computed tomography (SPECT) or 68Gallium-labeled somatostatin receptor analogs positron emission tomography/computed tomography.

Primary Hyperaldosteronism: Excessive Production of Aldosterone Independent of the Renin-Angiotensin System

- Typically seen in an aldosterone-producing adrenal adenoma.

Differential Diagnosis

- Solitary aldosterone producing adenoma
- Bilateral adrenal hyperplasia/idiopathic hyperaldosteronism
- Primary unilateral adrenal hyperplasia
- Adrenal carcinoma
- Glucocorticoid remediable aldosteronism

Symptoms

- Hypertension
- Muscle weakness
- Muscle cramping
- Parasthesias
- Headaches

Signs

- Hypokalemia
- Metabolic alkalosis
- Hypomagnesemia

Diagnosis B

- There are screening and confirmatory tests.
- Typically screen for hyperaldosteronism using the aldosterone/renin ratio (cutoff depends on assay and if the lab uses conventional vs. SI units).
  - A ratio > 20–30 is suggestive of hyperaldosteronism.
- Confirmatory tests typically rely on salt loading, which should suppress aldosterone levels in the normal physiologic system (salt loading test, saline suppression test).
  - Tumors secreting too much aldosterone do not show the normal physiologic feedback and do not suppress aldosterone in response to a salt load.
- Adrenal imaging will usually confirm tumor location.

General Evaluation of an Incidental Adrenal Neoplasm

Need to assess malignant potential and determine if the lesion is secreting excess hormones.

1. Assess risk of malignancy: noncontrast CT scan of abdomen/adrenals. The lesion is usually benign if there are hounsfield units (HU) $\leq$ 10 indicating a lipid-rich tumor.
2. Screening tests for hormone excess

Cushing's Syndrome

Perform the 1 mg overnight dexamethasone suppression test to screen for hypercortisolism. A normal response is a morning cortisol < 1.8 ng/dL after taking 1 mg of dexamethasone the night before. Lack of suppression of morning cortisol following dexamethasone suggests autonomous cortisol production.

- Pheochromocytoma: plasma free or urinary metanephrines
- Aldosterone-secreting adrenal tumor: aldosterone/plasma renin activity ratio, particularly if the patient has hypertension or hypokalemia
- Androgen-secreting adrenal tumor: Androgens, sex steroids if clinical, or imaging features of adrenal cortical carcinoma

---

Treatment (Pharmaceutical and Clinical Intervention)

Adrenalectomy is recommended if the tumor is hormonally active, shows evidence of high risk for malignancy based on imaging, or is larger than 6 cm. Often tumors are monitored over time if they are smaller, nonfunctional, benign lesions.

Cushing's Syndrome

Pathophysiology

Cushing's syndrome is a syndrome of excess cortisol due to any etiology. The most common cause of the syndrome is exogenous steroid exposure. Cushing's disease refers specifically to an ACTH-secreting pituitary tumor and was named after the famous neurosurgeon Dr. Harvey Cushing who described the original disease.

Clinical Presentation

Can vary dramatically, ranging from mild to very severe.

Symptoms

- Central obesity/weight gain
- Skin changes (thin skin, easy bruising, striae)
- Hirsutism
- Menstrual irregularities
- Weakness
- Mood changes
- Depression
- Insomnia
- Bone loss

Comorbidities

- Diabetes
- Mellitus
- Obesity
- Hypertension
- Osteopenia/osteoporosis
- Obstructive sleep apnea

Patients have an increased risk of cardiovascular disease, cerebrovascular disease, and thrombo-embolic events.

Signs

Physical exam findings include:

- Round face
- Central adiposity
- Supraclavicular and dorsocervical fat accumulation ("buffalo hump")
- Plethora, striae (can be excessive and/or hyperpigmented)
- Hypertension
- Hirsutism
- Findings related to diabetes mellitus

If they have osteoporosis, then the patient may have evidence of fractures or kyphosis. They can have proximal muscle weakness. Laboratory findings include hyperglycemia, hypokalemia, and hypercortisolism.

Diagnostics and Lab Studies

The diagnosis of Cushing's syndrome can be very challenging. Cortisol is a stress hormone and can be variably elevated or elevated by non-tumor causes.

- Confirm hypercortisolism by using accepted screening tests.
  - Do not proceed to the next step without confirming cortisol excess (usually two or more screening tests).
- It is then critical to distinguish whether the etiology of the hypercortisolism is ACTH dependent (pituitary or ectopic tumor source) or ACTH independent (adrenal tumor source).
- The ACTH level differentiates the cause of hypercortisolism.
  - The ACTH will be suppressed if the adrenal gland is the source of excess cortisol production or normal/elevated in cases of ectopic or pituitary Cushing's disease.
- Biochemical diagnosis is critical before diagnostic imaging, as the laboratory tests will direct the body location to be imaged.

STEP 1 Document syndrome of hypercortisolism.

Screening tests for hypercortisolism include:

- 24-hour urine free cortisol
  - Will be elevated in Cushing's syndrome
- Late night salivary cortisol levels
  - Cortisol has a diurnal rhythm with lowest levels at night. Patients with Cushing's syndrome lose the diurnal variation and will have high levels at night.
- 1 mg overnight dexamethasone test
  - The synthetic steroid dexamethasone is given at 11 P.M. at night and should suppress the normal ACTH production leading to suppressed cortisol levels the next morning.
  - A normal response is a suppressed cortisol level of < 1.8 mcg/dL. Lack of suppression suggests autonomous cortisol production and dysfunction of the normal feedback mechanism.

STEP 2 Determine whether Cushing's syndrome is ACTH dependent or independent by measuring ACTH.

- If ACTH is suppressed, this suggests adrenal source. If ACTH is normal or elevated, this is consistent with ACTH-dependent causes (pituitary Cushing's disease or ectopic ACTH-producing tumor).
  - Bronchial carcinoid tumors are one of the more common causes of ectopic ACTH secretion.

STEP 3 Distinguish pituitary Cushing's disease from ectopic ACTH secretion with a pituitary MRI and/or inferior petrosal sinus sampling (IPSS).

- Start with a pituitary MRI first; if a tumor is identified, the diagnosis of Cushing's disease is confirmed and patient should be referred to a neurosurgeon for transsphenoidal pituitary tumor resection. Unfortunately, ACTH-producing pituitary tumors can be extremely small and difficult to see on MRI.
  - If a tumor is not visualized or is very small, the patient should undergo inferior petrosal sinus sampling (IPSS).
- IPSS is a procedure whereby blood samples are taken from the bilateral inferior petrosal sinuses to measure blood from the pituitary (central location) and compare to a peripheral location such as the inferior vena cava.
  - ACTH levels are higher from the pituitary sample compared to the peripheral site in Cushing's disease. This is not true if the tumor is ectopic and located outside the pituitary.
- CRH stimulation enhances the sensitivity of the test.
- A central to peripheral ACTH gradient greater than 2 in the basal state, or greater than 3 after CRH is consistent with pituitary Cushing's disease.
  - High levels of ACTH from both the sites, central and peripheral, suggests ectopic ACTH secretion.

STEP 4 Localize tumor and surgically remove.

- Surgery is the treatment of choice for all tumor causes of hypercortisolism.

Treatment (Pharmaceutical and Clinical Intervention)

The goal of treatment is tumor removal and resolution of the hypercortisolism with restoration of normal physiology. Normalization of cortisol levels should cause resolution or improvement of many of the symptoms and comorbidities associated with Cushing's syndrome. It is also important to manage the associated comorbidities, such as: hypertension, diabetes mellitus, mood disorders, and osteoporosis.

Surgery is the treatment of choice for all tumor causes of hypercortisolism. It's important to control the blood pressure preoperatively.

- ACTH-producing pituitary tumors—transsphenoidal pituitary tumor removal
  - Radiation is considered if the patient does not have a biochemical remission with surgery or has a tumor recurrence.
- Adrenal tumors—adrenalectomy
- Ectopic ACTH tumor—surgical removal once located

Medical Options

There are several medications available for treatment of Cushing's syndrome. Not all of them are FDA approved for use in Cushing's syndrome, but some are used "off label." Pituitary-directed therapies are reserved for pituitary patients who are unable to undergo or have failed transsphenoidal tumor resection. In these cases, radiation or even bilateral adrenalectomy may be considered to control the hypercortisolism. Medical therapy in Cushing's disease is often used while waiting for radiation to take effect.

- Pituitary-directed treatment
  - Cabergoline—dopamine agonist
  - Pasireotide—somatostatin analog
- Steroidogenesis inhibitors
  - Ketoconazole—inhibits side-chain cleavage, 17,20-lyase, and 11 β hydroxylase
  - Levoketoconazole—ketoconazole stereoisomer, experimental
  - Osilodrostat—inhibits 11 β hydroxylase
  - Metyrapone—inhibits 11 β hydroxylase
  - Mitotane (an adrenolytic agent, primarily used in adrenal cortical carcinoma)
  - Etomidate
- Glucocorticoid receptor antagonist
  - Mifepristone

Cushing's Syndrome Key Points

- The diagnosis and long-term management of Cushing's syndrome is often very challenging. Patient presentation can be quite variable.
- Repeated patient evaluations are not uncommon.
- Approach diagnosis in a stepwise fashion. Biochemistry before imaging.

STEP 1 Confirm hypercortisolism.
STEP 2 Determine ACTH dependent or independent.
STEP 3 Distinguish Cushing's disease from ectopic ACTH production.
STEP 4 Localize tumor and remove.

- Although surgery is the treatment of choice with the goal to normalize biochemistry, other modalities for treatment are available, including medical therapy.
- Cushing's disease is associated with increased risk for multiple comorbidities, and treatment should also attempt to reduce the risk for long-term complications.
- Lifelong follow-up is required.

Diabetes

Type 1 Diabetes Mellitus

Pathophysiology

Type 1 diabetes represents 5–10% of total diabetes cases:

- Majority of type 1 diabetes (95%) is due to autoimmune destruction of pancreatic beta-cells in the islet of Langerhans; less than 5% is idiopathic. Leads to an absolute deficiency of insulin, and if untreated, this leads to a catabolic state with ketosis. Most common in underweight or normal weight children with peak incidence at 10–14 years.
- Autoimmune (type 1A) incidence is highest in individuals with Scandinavian ancestry while idiopathic (type 1B) occurs primarily in individuals of African or Asian origin. Disease susceptibility is related to genetic predisposition (HLA-DR3, HLA-DR4, HLA-DQ genes). Environmental stimuli are thought to trigger the autoimmune process.

Patients with type 1 diabetes mellitus are at increased risk of other autoimmune diseases, including hypothyroidism and celiac disease.

Clinical Presentation

Symptoms
- Polyuria, polydipsia, polyphagia
- Nocturia
- Weight loss with normal or increased appetite
- Blurred vision
- Chronic skin infections are common. Generalized pruritus and symptoms of vaginitis are frequently the initial complaints of women. Inflammation of the foreskin and in uncircumcised males may occur.

Diabetic ketoacidosis in undiagnosed or untreated type 1 diabetes is associated with nausea, vomiting, dehydration, lethargy, mental status changes, and fruity-odor breath.

Diagnosis and Laboratory Studies

Diagnosis of diabetes mellitus can be met if any of the four following criteria are met. In absence of unequivocal hyperglycemia, result should be confirmed with repeat testing.

1. Fasting plasma glucose $\geq$126 mg/dL
   - Fasting for at least 8 hours on two separate occasions
2. Hemoglobin A1C $\geq$ 6.5%
3. 2-hour plasma glucose $\geq$ 200 mg/dL during oral glucose tolerance test (OGTT)
4. Random plasma glucose $\geq$ 200 mg/dL in a patient with classic diabetes symptoms

Patients are likely to have glucosuria. Some patients have ketonemia or ketouria. At diagnosis, all patients should have a complete physical examination, including fundoscopic examination, lipid profile, and tests for kidney and liver function. Patients should be screened for thyroid (TSH) and celiac disease (tTG, IgA).

Differential Diagnosis/Formulating the Most Likely Diagnosis

Differentiation of type 1 versus type 2 diabetes is typically made based on clinical presentation. In cases with uncertainty, insulin levels, c-peptide levels, and/or autoantibodies can be used.

- C-peptide levels of less than 0.2 nmol/L in combination with hyperglycemia is suggestive of type 1 diabetes but not diagnostic.
- Islet cell, glutamic acid decarboxylase (GAD-65), insulin, or tyrosine phosphatase 2 autoantibodies are associated with autoimmune type 1 diabetes.

Health Maintenance/Patient Education

Diabetes education and self-management by a multidisciplinary team, including diabetes educators and registered dieticians, is essential to care. Patients should be educated on the disease process and complications.

- Self-monitoring of blood glucose should be emphasized for all patients on insulin therapy to allow patients to manage fluctuations in carbohydrate intakes, as well as exercise and illness, which can both cause hypoglycemia.
- Self-monitoring of blood glucose is done through finger stick testing multiple times per day or continuous blood glucose monitoring devices (CGMs), which involve a subcutaneous catheter. CGMs communicate with insulin pumps and/or smartphone devices and have the advantages of avoiding finger sticks, as well as trending glucose levels.
- Patients and their families need to be taught to recognize signs/symptoms of and administer treatment for hypoglycemia. Hypoglycemia, defined as blood glucose < 70 mg/dL, is the most common complication of type 1 diabetes in children.

Signs/Symptoms of Hypoglycemia
- Tachycardia
- Diaphoresis
- Lethargy
- Headaches
- Behavior changes
- Severe cases can lead to unconsciousness.

Treatment in conscious patients should include 10–15 grams of simple carbohydrate (e.g., fruit juice, candy, glucose tabs). In unconscious patients or those unable to take oral therapy, treatment of choice is glucagon injection. After treatment for hypoglycemia, blood glucose should be rechecked every 15–20 minutes with repeat treatment if not normalized.

- Patients with diabetes should receive annual influenza vaccination.
- Children ≥ 2 years old should receive a single dose of pneumococcal polysaccharide vaccine (PPSV23).
- All other childhood vaccinations should be administered according to the recommended schedule.

Treatment (Pharmaceutical and Clinical Intervention)

Patients with type 1 diabetes require lifelong treatment with exogenous insulin. Goals of management include strict glycemic control in order to reduce the risk of long-term complications of hyperglycemia while avoiding severe hypoglycemia. The target A1C goal for most patients is < 7%. Less stringent goals of < 7.5% or < 8% can be considered in patients at high risk or history of hypoglycemic episodes. Initial and ongoing management requires a comprehensive approach to include pharmacotherapy, glucose monitoring, nutrition, psychosocial support, and monitoring for complications. Dietary guidance should be individualized to patients with a focus on consistent carbohydrate intake, carbohydrate counting, glycemic index of foods, impact of foods and activity on insulin needs, and healthy weight maintenance. There is not a specific diabetic diet that applies to all patients.

The aim of insulin therapy is to mimic physiology insulin, which requires combination of rapid-acting and long-acting insulin analogs in multiple injections per day or use of an insulin pump.

Insulin is administered via subcutaneous injection using syringes or injector pens. Typical regimens include once or twice daily injection of long-acting insulin plus rapid-acting insulin prior to each meal or snack. Total daily dose of insulin is typically 0.3–1 unit/kg/day.

- **Rapid-acting insulins** (lispro, aspart, glulisine) are given as premeal boluses 15 minutes prior to eating. Doses are calculated based on anticipated carbohydrate intake (carbohydrate ratio) plus correction for blood glucose above goal (correction factor). Peak effect occurs 60–90 minutes after dosing, and duration of action is 4 hours.
- **Long-acting insulins** (glargine, detemir, degludec) provide background or "basal" insulin coverage. Dosing is weight-based and makes up approximately 50% of the total daily dose of insulin. Duration of action is ~24 hours and typically peakless, which confers low risk of hypoglycemia.

Insulin pumps deliver a continuous infusion of rapid-acting insulin, which is supplemented with boluses for meals and snacks. Some insulin pumps (closed loop systems) can integrate with continuous glucose monitors.

- **Intermediate-acting insulin** (NPH) with onset of action in 2–4 hours and duration of action for 10–20 hours can be used in place of long-acting insulin to provide basal coverage. It has the disadvantage of twice daily dosing and a peak effect at 6–7 hours with associated hypoglycemia risk. The advantage is lower cost, particularly in underinsured patients.
- **Regular insulin** is short acting with an onset of action in 30–60 minutes and an effective duration of 3–6 hours. It can be used for mealtime coverage, though has the inconvenience of needing to be administered at least 30 minutes prior to eating. It is less costly than rapid-acting insulins.

The primary role of regular insulin is in the treatment of acute, severe hyperglycemia such as diabetic ketoacidosis (DKA) or hyperosmolar hyperglycemic state (HHS). It is also used in hospitalized patients via sliding scale dosing, particularly in patients who cannot have oral intake. It can be given subcutaneously or by intravenous bolus or continuous infusion.

Patients with diabetes should have follow-up visits at least four times per year. At each visit, A1C should be checked. A1C value and self-monitoring blood glucose logs should be used to adjust insulin doses. Close monitoring of blood pressure, psychosocial concerns, and growth parameters should occur at each visit.

Starting 5 years after diagnosis, patients need to be screened annually for micro- and macrovascular complications.

- Dilated eye examination for retinopathy
- Foot examination with vibratory sensation and monofilament testing for neuropathy
- Lipid profile for cardiovascular risk assessment
- Urine albumin:creatinine ratio (spot assessment) for nephropathy

Most common side effects of insulin therapy include weight gain and hypoglycemia.

Somogyi effect is nocturnal hypoglycemia followed by secretion of counter-regulatory hormones, which leads to gluconeogenesis by the liver and causes a reactive hyperglycemia so patient awakes in the morning with hyperglycemia. This effect can be detected by having patient check blood glucose in the middle of the night. Management can include decreasing bedtime insulin dose, adding a bedtime snack, or lowering nocturnal basal insulin rate for patients with insulin pumps.

Type 2 Diabetes Mellitus

Pathophysiology

Type 2 diabetes mellitus accounts for more than 90% of all diabetes. It is predominantly found in adults, but incidence is increasing in children and adolescents. Characterized by insulin resistance and abnormal insulin secretion due to progressive loss of beta cell function. In early stages, glucose tolerance is maintained through increased secretion of insulin from the pancreas. Disease progression results in pancreatic islet cell failure with resulting decline in insulin secretion and overt hyperglycemia. The highest risk factor is obesity. Other risk factors for development include age > 45 years old, race/ethnicity (African-American, Latino, Native American, Asian American, Pacific Islander), family history of diabetes, personal history of gestational diabetes, physical inactivity, hyperlipidemia, and hypertension.

Clinical Presentation

Due to insidious onset of hyperglycemia, many patients with type 2 diabetes are asymptomatic and diagnosed during routine laboratory studies. Some patients may present with increased thirst or urination. Ketonuria and weight loss are rare. Skin manifestations including generalized pruritus, recurrent candidal vulvovaginitis, and chronic skin infections are common. Acanthosis nigricans, hyperpigmentation, and hyperkeratosis of the groin, axilla, and back of neck is associated with insulin resistance. In patients with long-standing hyperglycemia, signs of neuropathic or cardiovascular complications may be present.

Diagnosis and Laboratory Studies

The diagnostic criteria for type 2 diabetes are the same as for type 1 diabetes:

- Fasting plasma glucose $\geq$ 126 mg/dL **OR**
- A1C $\geq$ 6.5% **OR**
- 2-hour plasma glucose $\geq$ 200 mg/dL during oral glucose tolerance test (OGTT) **OR**
- Random plasma glucose $\geq$ 200 mg/dL in a patient with classic diabetes symptoms

The preferred method for screening for, diagnosing, and monitoring diabetes is hemoglobin A1C as it does not require fasting and provides an estimate of glucose control for the preceding 2–3 months.

- The ADA recommends screening patients for diabetes every 3 years starting at age 45 years old. Screening should start at an earlier age in patients who are overweight (BMI > 25 kg/m^2) and have one or more additional risk factors.
- Patients with prediabetes that is diagnosed with A1C values 5.7%-6.4% are at high risk of developing diabetes.
- At diagnosis, all patients should have a complete physical examination including fundoscopic examination, lipid profile, and tests for kidney and liver function.
- Routine self-monitoring of blood glucose is not indicated in patients with type 2 diabetes but may be considered in patient.

Differential Diagnosis/Formulating the Most Likely Diagnosis

Persistent hyperglycemia is uncommon in adults. Transient hyperglycemia can occur in patients with severe illness, which is caused by hormone-mediated increased gluconeogenesis and glycogenolysis.

Health Maintenance/Patient Education

- Patients with newly diagnosed type 2 diabetes should receive comprehensive education on disease state process, medical nutrition therapy, exercise, weight reduction, and prevention of complications.
- Self-management of diabetes is essential to successful glycemic control.
  - Major emphasis should be on reduced caloric intake, increased physical activity, and behavior modification with the goal of weight reduction in patients who are overweight (BMI $\geq$ 25–29 kg/m^2) or obese (BMI $\geq$ 30 kg/m^2).
  - Patients with diabetes should receive annual influenza vaccination. Adults ages 19–64 years should receive a single dose of pneumococcal polysaccharide vaccine (PPSV23).

Treatment (Pharmaceutical and Clinical Intervention)

Approach to therapy in type 2 diabetes should be centered on controlling hyperglycemia, reducing occurrence of microvascular complications while limiting episodes of hypoglycemia and adverse effects of medications.

Glycated hemoglobin (A1C) levels are used to monitor diabetes control. Target A1C should be individualized to patient needs.

For most adults, A1C < 7% is a reasonable goal. A more stringent goal (A1C < 6.5%) may be considered in younger patients, those without comorbid conditions, or those who are newly diagnosed. A less stringent goal (A1C > 8%) may be considered in patients with history of hypoglycemia, limited life expectancy, extensive comorbidity, or long-standing uncontrolled diabetes.

As with type 1 diabetes, lifestyle modifications are a key component in treatment of type 2 diabetes. There is no specific diet recommended by the American Diabetes Association. Focus should be placed on nutrient-dense foods in appropriate portions.

- Carbohydrate intake should emphasize nutrient-dense carbohydrates that are high in fiber. Sugar-sweetened beverages should be avoided, and consumption of foods with added sugars should be limited.
- Other metabolic needs should be considered particularly in patients with hypertension, hyperlipidemia, or nephropathy. Fat intake should consist of polyunsaturated fats and omega-3 fatty acids with avoidance of saturated fats.

Numerous medications are available to treat type 2 diabetes. Each class is discussed in detail below. In most cases, pharmacotherapy is initiated utilizing oral agents. Metformin is the initial pharmacotherapeutic agent for most patients with type 2 diabetes.

- Initial injectable therapy (GLP-1 agonist or insulin) therapy is indicated in patients with symptomatic hyperglycemia, ketonuria, or A1C $\geq$ 9–10%.
- Patients with A1C $\geq$ 1.5% above target should be considered initial dual agent therapy.

Patients should be reassessed every 3–6 months for A1C level, adherence, and adverse effects. For patients in whom metformin is contraindicated or not tolerated, as well as patients who do not meet A1C target with metformin monotherapy, selection of next pharmacotherapy agent is based on patient factors. Pharmacotherapy is generally additive; some medications are available as combination products with metformin to assist with adherence.

- In patients with established or high risk for atherosclerotic cardiovascular disease (ASCVD), GLP-1 agents should be prioritized.
- In patients with heart failure or chronic kidney disease, SGLT-2 inhibitors are preferred.
- For other patients, consideration for individualizing therapy should be given to risk of hypoglycemia, need to minimize weight gain, or promotion of weight loss and cost.

Biguainides

Metformin, a biguanide, acts to reduce hepatic glucose production.

Benefits of this medication include:

- No risk of hypoglycemia
- Possible promotion of weight loss
- Decreased triglycerides
- Low cost

Metformin should be started at a low dose and titrated slowly to maximum dose. Patients should be counseled on high incidence of GI side effects, which are limited with dose titration and abate over time. Metformin is not recommended for use in females with SCr > 1.4 mg/dL or males with SCr > 1.5 mg/dL due to risk of lactic acidosis. Metformin can interfere with vitamin B12 absorption so baseline and periodic vitamin B12 levels should be obtained.

GLP-1 receptor agonists (exenatide, dulaglutide, liraglutide, lixisenatide, semaglutide) act as incretin mimetics to increase glucose-dependent insulin secretion, decrease glucagon secretion, and slow gastric emptying. GLP-1 agonists have proven benefit in reducing cardiovascular disease, as well as promoting modest weight loss. Most GLP-1 agonists are injected; some agents are available in extended release requiring only once weekly dosing. Semaglutide has been approved in an oral formulation. Side effects are primarily gastrointestinal including nausea and early satiety as well as less commonly pancreatitis. There is an association with thyroid tumors and it should not be used in patients with a history of thyroid cancer. Risk of hypoglycemia is small.

- **Sodium-glucose cotransporter-2 (SGLT2) inhibitors** (canagliflozin, dapagliflozin, empagliflozin) prevent reabsorption of glucose in kidneys resulting in increased urinary excretion of glucose. These oral agents have proven benefit in atherosclerotic cardiovascular disease (ASCVD), heart failure, and chronic kidney disease. There is no hypoglycemia risk and they are associated with weight loss. Adverse events include genitourinary infections, volume depletion/hypotension, amputation, bone fractures, and increased LDL cholesterol. Efficacy is decreased in patients with reduced kidney function.
- **Dipeptidyl peptidase IV (DPP-4) inhibitors** (sitagliptin, saxagliptin, linagliptin, alogliptin) prolong endogenous action of GLP-1, increase insulin secretion, and suppress glucagon release. These oral medications are well tolerated, weight neutral, and not associated with hypoglycemia. Side effects include respiratory and dermatologic symptoms.
- **Thiazolidinediones** (rosiglitazone, pioglitazone) increase tissue sensitivity to insulin, decrease hepatic glucose production, and increase hepatic glucose uptake. Benefits include relative low cost and no hypoglycemia when used as monotherapy. Risks include weight gain, edema, potential for new or exacerbation of heart failure, fractures, and bladder cancer.
- **Sulfonylureas** (glipizide and glimepiride) increase insulin secretion from the pancreas. These agents are administered orally, highly efficacious, and very low cost. They are associated with weight gain and high rate of hypoglycemia.

Meglitinides

Alpha-Glucosidase Inhibitors

Insulin therapy in type 2 diabetes can be additive to oral agents, in place of oral agents or initial therapy. Most insulin therapy in type 2 diabetes begins with basal insulin regimen dosed at bedtime (glargine, detemir, degludec) or twice daily (NPH). Dosing is weight-based 0.2 units/kg/day and titrated to fasting plasma glucose 80–130 mg/dL. Risks of insulin therapy include weight gain and hypoglycemia. Patients who require prandial insulin with short or rapid-acting insulin are at higher risk for hypoglycemia and should be counseled accordingly.

At diagnosis and annually, patients with type 2 diabetes should be assessed for microvascular complications:

- Spot assessment of urinary albumin:creatinine ratio for nephropathy; patients with urinary albumin > 30 mg/g creatinine or eGFR < 60 should have monitoring increased to every 6 months.
- Foot exam with vibratory testing and monofilament exam for peripheral neuropathy
- Dilated retinal exam for retinopathy

Patients with type 2 diabetes are at high risk for ASCVD. All patients should be counseled on tobacco cessation. Hyperlipidemia management should be based on risk assessment and utilize statin therapy. Blood pressure should be controlled with a target of < 130/80 (American College of Cardiology/American Heart Association) or < 140/90 (ADA). Preferred agents in treatment of hypertension in patients with diabetes are ACE inhibitors.

Hypogonadism

Klinefelter Syndrome

Klinefelter syndrome (KS)is the most common human sex chromosome disorder and occurs in approximately 1 in 500–1,000 males. It is characterized by supernumerary X chromosomes in an XY male.

Pathophysiology

It is not inherited and occurs due to a random nondisjunction error during division of the sex chromosomes in the egg or sperm. The majority (90%) of cases present with a 47, XXY karyotype. Mosaicism (46, XY/47, XXY), meaning that some cells have an extra X chromosome and other cells do not, higher-grade aneuploidy (48, XXXY; 49, XXXXY), and structurally abnormal X chromosomes account for the rest. It is the most common cause of primary hypogonadism in males, and clinical presentation is highly variable.

Clinical Presentation

Symptoms

- There are no distinct dysmorphic features, and presentation may vary according to the degree of gonadal dysfunction.
- Diagnosis is often made prenatally, through prenatal screening for chromosomal abnormalities, at puberty due to abnormalities in development or at adulthood as a result of infertility.
- In infancy and preschool age, deficits in motor, speech, and behavioral development may be present, and in later years, difficulties with language, learning, social, and executive function may be exhibited. Individuals may also be asymptomatic until puberty.
- In adulthood, presentation is often for evaluation of infertility.

Signs

- Long bone abnormality causing increased length; taller than peers
- Small firm testes. This is a consistent finding and regarded as a hallmark of diagnosis. Cryptorchidism, small phallus (micropenis), and hypospadias may also be present.
- Evidence of hypogonadism in postpubertal males: sparse body hair, gynecomastia, female body habitus, and gynoid aspect of hips (broad hips)

There is increased thromboembolic risk and also increased risk of testicular cancer, which may be multifactorial and linked to X-linked gene susceptibility, abdominal adiposity, diabetes mellitus, abdominal adiposity, and autoimmune diseases, such as systemic lupus erythematosus.

Diagnostic and Lab Studies

- Karyotype is confirmatory.
- Evaluation for androgen deficiency.
- Labs typically are consistent with primary hypogonadism, with elevated gonadotrophins FSH and LH, and with low testosterone levels.

Evaluation for infertility with seminal analysis may reveal azoospermia and oligospermia with hyalinization and fibrosis of the seminiferous tubules.

Differential Diagnosis/Formulating the Most Likely Diagnosis

Kallmann syndrome, characterized by a complete or partial loss of smell and secondary hypogonadism. Laboratory evaluation shows a low or inappropriately normal FSH and low testosterone levels. Both men and women share the failure to experience puberty and the complete or partial loss of the sense of smell.

Health Maintenance and Patient Education

Lifelong follow-up is important due to the multisystemic involvement and the risk for complications.

Treatment (Pharmaceutical and Clinical Intervention)

- Testosterone treatment is the main treatment. There have been suggestions that early testosterone therapy may improve the neurodevelopmental outcome for boys with Klinefelter syndrome.
- Orchipexy in infancy for individuals with cryptorchism.
- In individuals with gynecomastia, surgical reduction or treatment with aromatase inhibitors to block the increased aromatization of testosterone to estradiol may be utilized.
- Fertility potential declines with age, hence sperm retrieval and cryostorage should be considered during adolescence.
- Multidisciplinary care inclusive of pediatricians, speech therapists, psychologists, endocrinologists, reproductive specialists, and urologists may be required.

Professional Considerations

Individuals with Klinefelter syndrome have an increased predilection for autoimmune diseases, insulin resistance, dyslipidemia, obesity, osteoporosis, and bone fractures.

Specific cancers (breast cancer, extragonadal germ cell tumors) are also more frequently seen, hence surveillance strategies (imaging, serum tumor markers, self-examination) are utilized for screening and monitoring.

Syndrome of Inappropriate Anti Diuretic Hormone (SIADH)

Pathophysiology

Antidiuretic hormone (ADH) is also known as vasopressin hormone. It is produced in the hypothalamus and transported to the posterior pituitary, where it is stored and released in response to physiologic signals. Osmoreceptors in the hypothalamus regulate the amount of ADH released in response to low plasma osmolality, which is the typical stimulus. ADH secretion can also occur in states of hypovolemia. Baroreceptors in the left atrium, carotid artery, and aortic arch detect sudden reduction in blood pressure, thus directly stimulating the release of ADH from the posterior pituitary. Release of antidiuretic hormone has effects systematically by increasing vascular tone via V1a and V1b receptors, which are involved in vasoconstriction and adrenocorticotropic hormone release.

In the kidney, the antidiuretic response is mediated by V2 receptors. ADH increases the transcription and the insertion of aquaporin-2 channels in the distal convoluted tubules and collecting ducts, thus allowing movement of water across the previously impermeable membrane, increasing water reabsorption, and restoring plasma osmolality and blood volume.

Inappropriate secretion of ADH occurs in a situation of ADH release in the absence of its appropriate stimuli, resulting in a state of water excess and increased sodium loss.

Clinical Presentation

- SIADH, the syndrome of inappropriate antidiuretic hormone, is characterized by clinical findings of normal volume status and biochemical findings of low serum sodium with a non-dilute urine.
- Clinical exam should reveal a normal volume status and a normal blood pressure. Biochemically, labs should show hyponatremia.
  - Clinical conditions that increase the risk of SIADH fall into the following main categories: medications; pulmonary diseases; CNS diseases such as infection, trauma, and stroke; malignancy; and other causes such as HIV infection, surgery, pain, nausea, and intense exercise.
  - Also, hereditary cases have been described and attributed to function mutation in the vasopressin 2(V2) receptors in the kidneys.

The most common drugs include carbamazepine, oxcarbazepine, cyclophosphamide, chlorpropamide, and selective serotonin reuptake inhibitors (SSRI).

Carbamazepine and oxcarbazepine act in part by increasing the sensitivity to ADH. Less commonly, chemotherapeutic agents, such as methotrexate, vincristine, vinblastine, and imatinib, as well as interferons, opiates, nonsteroidal anti-inflammatory drugs (NSAIDs), ciprofloxacin, and haloperidol have all been associated with SIADH.

Symptoms

- Clinical symptoms could range from an asymptomatic state in mild-to-moderate hyponatremia to severe neurologic deficits such as coma with severe hyponatremia.

Other Symptoms

- Nausea
- Vomiting
- Personality changes such as confusion, hallucinations, combativeness, seizures

Signs

- Normal blood pressure. The absence of findings is suggestive of dehydration or hypovolemia.
- Hyponatremia, which could be mild 130–134 mEq/L, moderate 125–129 mEq/L, or severe < 125 mEq/L

Diagnostic and Lab Studies

- Hyponatremia should be confirmed, and sodium level should be corrected for hyperglycemia, paraproteinemia, and hypertriglyceridemia, if present.
- In severe cholestatic disease, elevated levels of an abnormal lipoprotein, lipoprotein X, may be present.
    - The presence of these substances creates an osmotic gradient, leading to displacement of water from the intracellular into the extracellular space, and lower measured serum sodium level than what is present.

A good clinical rule is to remember that when there is an abnormality in the serum sodium (salt) level, a review of the serum glucose (sugar) serum albumin and globulin fractions (proteins) and triglyceride (fat) levels are also important to ensure that the hyponatremia is present prior to further extensive tests.

Commonly used formulae for estimation

- Change of 1.6 mEq/L in sodium for every 100 mg/dL increase in glucose concentration. For example, a measured serum sodium is 130 meq/L with a corresponding glucose value of 200 mg/dL. The corrected sodium level is approximately 132 meq/L.
- Change in sodium level by a conversion of 0.002 of the value of triglycerides. For example, a triglyceride level of 500.
- $(500 \times 0.002) = 1$ meq/L should be added to the measured sodium level.
- Change in sodium level for hyperproteinemia is calculated by (serum protein − 8) $\times$ 0.25; hence, a serum total protein of 10g/dL, will result in a 0.50 meq/L addition to the measured sodium level.

The Schwartz and Bartter criteria for SIADH is helpful for diagnosis, and the criteria includes:
- Hyponatremia and euvolemic status
- Decreased serum osmolality: < 275 mOsm/kg
- Inappropriately concentrated urine: > 100 mOsm/kg
- Elevated urine sodium: urine NA > 20 meq/L

Exclusion of other causes of hyponatremia:
- Laboratory evaluation should include a comprehensive metabolic panel, liver function, and renal function.
- A random urine sodium, as well as serum and urine osmolality, should be obtained concomitantly at the same time for ease of interpretation of the results.

Other endocrine causes of hyponatremia should be excluded by thyroid function tests and screening for adrenal insufficiency with early morning cortisol.

In specific situations, imaging of the head, chest, abdomen, and pelvis may be appropriate.

Differential Diagnosis/Formulating the Most Likely Diagnosis

Differential diagnosis of SIADH includes all causes of hyponatremia.
- Hypervolemic states such as congestive heart failure, renal failure or impairment, and chronic liver disease
- Hypovolemic states such as dehydration, nausea, and vomiting. A careful review of medications is imperative. Medications such as diuretics often cause renal salt wasting and may cause hyponatremia.

Central salt wasting is another differential of SIADH. It is characterized by hypovolemia and elevated urine sodium in the context of central nervous system assault, such as head injury, intracranial surgery, hemorrhage, tumors, or infection. Etiology is not well understood. Treatment typically involves hydration and, in severe cases, salt repletion.

Health Maintenance and Patient Education

Potential contributory factors such as tobacco use, inadequate pain control, and age-appropriate cancer screening should be addressed.

Treatment (Pharmaceutical and Clinical Intervention)

Once a diagnosis of SIADH is made, the identification and treatment of the underlying cause is paramount.

Treatment options include:
- Fluid restriction
- Hypertonic saline
- Salt tablets with or without diuretics
- Urea and vasopressin receptor antagonists

Oral urea increases urinary free water excretion; however, bitter taste may limit use. Treatment of the hyponatremia often involves water restriction, to less than 1 L/day in mild to moderate or asymptomatic cases.

In severe cases of hyponatremia, or with neurologic symptoms, urgent treatment with 3% hypertonic saline 100 mL given over 3 to 4 hr is indicated, and this can be repeated if needed to improve clinical status or raise sodium levels to a safe level.

Sodium should be monitored closely, as there is the risk of central pontine myelinolysis if hyponatremia is corrected too rapidly. Correction of 10 meq/L/24 hr or less than 1 meq/L every 2 hr is recommended.

Vasopressin receptor (V2 receptor) antagonists: Conivaptan (IV) and tolvaptan (oral) are indicated for severe persistent SIADH.

Professional Considerations

Fluid restriction may be difficult for patients, and a multidisciplinary approach and specialist expertise is often required, especially in severe cases.

The cost of the vasopressin receptor antagonist can be prohibitive to the patients.

Thyroid Disorders

Hypothyroidism

Pathophysiology

- Primary hypothyroidism accounts for over 95% of hypothyroidism. In iodine-sufficient locations, most common causes are autoimmune (Hashimoto's) and iatrogenic (iodine therapy and surgical thyroidectomy).
- Worldwide, iodine deficiency is still a leading cause; other causes include amyloidosis and medications (amiodarone, lithium, interferon).
- Overt hypothyroidism increases with age and is more common in females than males (4:1).
- Subclinical hypothyroidism is associated with an increased risk of developing overt hypothyroidism (4% annually).

- Causes of secondary hypothyroidism in which the disorder occurs outside the thyroid gland include neoplasms of the hypothalamus or pituitary, pituitary necrosis (Sheehan syndrome), and hypopituitarism.

Clinical Presentation

Onset is typically insidious, and a wide range of nonspecific symptoms are associated with hypothyroidism.

Most common symptoms include:
- Weakness
- Lethargy
- Weight gain
- Feeling cold
- Dry skin
- Constipation
- Cognitive dysfunction
- Depression

Most common signs include:
- Coarse skin
- Facial or periorbital edema
- Delayed relaxation of deep tendon reflexes
- Bradycardia

Hypothyroidism is often associated with other autoimmune disorders.
- Myxedema crisis—a severe and life-threatening presentation of hypothyroidism; hallmark is mental status changes, which are accompanied by significant hypothermia, hyponatremia, hypoglycemia, hypotension, and hypercapnia.
- Myxedema crisis is most common in elderly female patients and can be triggered by acute illness, prolonged cold exposure, and medications.

Diagnosis and Lab Studies

- Best screening test is thyroid-stimulating hormone (TSH).
- Elevated TSH with low free T4 levels is diagnostic for overt primary hypothyroidism.

Table 4.3

Diagnosis	TSH	Free T4
Euthyroid state (normal)	Normal	Normal
Primary hypothyroidism	Elevated	Low
Secondary hypothyroidism	Low/normal	Low
Subclinical hypothyroidism	Elevated	Normal

- Additional associated laboratory findings include hypercholesterolemia, hyponatremia due to SIADH, anemia, and hypoglycemia.
- Imaging is not indicated in patients with hypothyroidism.

Differential Diagnosis/Formulating the Most Likely Diagnosis

- Due to the nonspecific symptoms, the differential diagnosis of hypothyroidism is broad.
- Narrowing the concerns to the thyroid is best accomplished by ordering a TSH.

Health Maintenance and Patient Education

- Hypothyroidism requires lifelong treatment and regular monitoring of TSH.
- Absorption of synthetic levothyroxine can vary between manufacturers so patients should ideally continue with the same product.

Treatment

- Preferred treatment is synthetic levothyroxine. Dosing is weight-based with full replacement on average at 1.6 mcg/kg/day.
  - Doses are titrated based on clinical response and serum TSH (checked every 4–6 weeks during dose titration).
- Lower initial doses (25–50 mcg/day) should be used in the elderly and patients with coronary artery disease.
- Subclinical hypothyroidism does not require treatment unless patient is symptomatic, less than 30 years old, actively trying to conceive, or has markedly elevated TSH (typically greater than 20 µIU/mL).
- Pregnant women with hypothyroidism typically require an increased in their levothyroxine dosage; adequate levothyroxine is essential to fetal development.
- Goal of treatment is to maintain TSH in low-normal range.
- Myxedema crisis is typically treated with higher dose intravenous levothyroxine, warming, and correction of electrolyte abnormalities.

Hyperthyroidism

Pathophysiology

Thyrotoxicosis refers to the clinical manifestations of excess thyroid hormone.

- The most common causes are Graves' disease, toxic multinodular goiter, and toxic adenomas.
  - Graves' disease is an autoimmune condition that affects TSH receptors and causes 60–80% of hyperthyroidism cases.
  - More common in females than males (8:1) with a typical onset between 20 and 40 years old.

Clinical Presentation

Symptoms
- Anxiety
- Weakness
- Unexplained weight loss
- Sweating
- Heat intolerance
- Fine tremor
- Loose stools
- Muscle cramps
- Menstrual irregularity is common in females.

Cardiovascular effects can include:

Tachycardia

Palpitations

PVCs

Atrial fibrillation

- Ophthalmopathy is specifically associated with Graves' disease and can present as upper eyelid retraction, periorbital swelling, protrusion of the eyes, and lid lag.
- Enlargement of the thyroid gland with or without palpable nodules consistent with hyperthyroidism.
  - Thyroid bruit is associated with Graves' disease.

Thyroid storm (thyrotoxic crisis): severe and life-threatening clinical presentation of hyperthyroidism; patients have high fever, arrhythmias including severe tachycardia and ventricular fibrillation, heart failure, vomiting, diarrhea, and dehydration. Thyroid storm can be associated with amiodarone or stopping hyperthyroidism treatment.

Diagnostics and Lab Studies

- Free and unbound T4 (thyroxine) and T3 (triiodothyronine) are elevated in Graves' disease.
  - In a small percentage of patients, T4 may be normal with T3 elevated (T3 toxicosis).
- TSH is very low or undetectable in primary hyperthyroidism.
- Thyroid-stimulating immunoglobulin (TSI) and thyroid peroxidase antibodies (TPO) are the most specific test for Graves' disease and are not typically detected in toxic multinodular goiter.
- Radioactive iodine uptake imaging is used where increased diffuse uptake is seen and when the etiology of hyperthyroidism is uncertain but is contraindicated in pregnancy or breastfeeding.

Health Maintenance and Patient Education

Treatment of hyperthyroidism requires regular monitoring for both symptom control and thyroid function. Particular consideration should be given to females of childbearing age as the preferred treatment for hyperthyroidism differs in pregnant women.

Treatment

- Beta-blockers, particularly propranolol, are used for symptomatic control in hyperthyroidism and are the initial treatment of choice in thyroid storm.
- Thiourea drugs including methimazole and prophythiouracil (PTU) are first-line to achieve remission in younger patients, patients with mild thyrotoxicosis, small goiters and in whom radioactive isotopes are contradindicated.

Patients should be cautioned about and monitored for agranulocytosis and hepatitis.

- Methimazole is typically preferred due to higher efficacy, less dosing frequency, and lower risk of hepatic necrosis.
- PTU is the medication of choice in pregnancy and breastfeeding.
- TSH and free T4 levels should be checked 4–6 weeks after therapy initiation for treatment response and dose adjustment.

- Radioactive iodine is used patients unable to tolerate or adhere to methimazole/PTU, relapse, and treatment failure.
  - It is contraindicated in pregnancy and breastfeeding. Dosing is based on radioactive uptake imaging.
  - There is a high incidence of posttreatment hypothyroidism, and patients should have life-long monitoring of thyroid function tests.
- Partial or total thyroidectomy can be used in patients with very large goiters, treatment failures, or contraindications to radioactive iodine therapy.
  - Patients should be euthyroid prior to surgery.

Risks of surgery include damage to recurrent laryngeal nerve and hypoparathyroidism.

- Patients should have calcium levels followed closely in the postoperative period.

Thyroiditis

Acute (Suppurative) Thyroiditis

Pathophysiology

- Rare condition due to bacterial infection of the thyroid gland
- Most common *S. aureus*
- Most common in children with piriform sinus

Clinical Presentation

- Includes painful, tender thyroid gland, febrile, fever, dysphagia, and small fluctuant goiter.
- Thyroid function tests are normal; fine needle aspiration with Gram stain and culture are diagnostic.
- Increased WBCs

Treatment

Antibiotics and possible surgical drainage of abscess, if present.

Subacute Thyroiditis (de Quervain Thyroiditis, Granulomatous Thyroiditis)

Pathophysiology

Affects females more than males with most common age group being 30 to 50 years old. Etiology is likely viral and presentation is often preceded by upper respiratory infection; peak incidence is in summer months.

Clinical Presentation

- Symptoms are painful dysphagia, jaw pain, tender thyroid, and low-grade fever
- Thyroid function tests follow a pattern of
  - Mildly elevated free T4 and T3, and low TSH during early stages
  - Hypothyroid symptoms
  - Recovery over a period of 6–12 months
- ESR is markedly elevated. Thyroid antibody titers are low.

Treatment

- Treatment of choice is aspirin for 6–8 weeks.
- Propranolol may be used to control thyrotoxic symptoms.
- Thyroid function tests and ESR should be monitored during treatment.

Painless (Silent) Thyroiditis

Pathophysiology

Occurs in patients with underlying autoimmune thyroid disease. Can be classified as postpartum thyroiditis if this occurs within 1–6 months after delivery; up to 5% incidence.

Clinical Presentation

The thyroid is typically enlarged and firm, and symptoms are related to thyroid hormone levels as clinical course is similar to subacute thyroiditis with initial thyrotoxicosis followed by hypothyroidism.

- TPO antibodies are present and ESR is normal.

Treatment

- Treatment can include propranolol for severe symptoms.
- Thyroid replacement with levothyroxine may be used but should be limited in duration to 6–9 months.

Patients should have thyroid function tests monitored annually if they are at risk of developing permanent hypothyroidism.

Drug-Induced Thyroiditis

Pathophysiology

- Most commonly caused by amiodarone or interferon
- Mostly causes painless thyroiditis or hypothyroidism.

Hashimoto (Autoimmune) Thyroiditis

Pathophysiology

Most common type of thyroiditis; frequently progresses to overt hypothyroidism.

Clinical Presentation

- Thyroid gland is firm with variable size goiter and typically painless.
- Autoimmune etiology with TPO antibodies and/or thyroglobulin antibodies is typically high.

Treatment

Thyroid ultrasound and fine needle aspiration can be used to distinguish Hashimoto thyroiditis from multinodular goiter or malignancy. Fine needle aspiration reveals lymphocytes and cellular changes. Levothyroxine replacement is used if hypothyroidism is present. Decrease any radioactive uptake.

Riedel Thyroiditis

Pathophysiology

- Rare, most often in middle-aged females
- Likely due to a systemic fibrotic syndrome

Clinical Presentation

- Presents with painless, hard goiter, which then enlarges and can cause compression of neck structures including trachea and esophagus
- Thyroid function is normal and diagnosis often requires open biopsy.

Treatment

Give tamoxifen and surgical decompression as part of treatment.

Practice Questions for Endocrine Review

1. A patient presents to the ED with nausea, vomiting, diarrhea, weakness, and abdominal pain. The patient is a 36-year-old female who reports symptoms started a few months ago and continue to get worse. She also reports that she hasn't had a period for 3 months, which is unusual for her. On physical examination, you note increased skin pigmentation in skin folds and creases and low blood pressure. Included in your differential diagnoses list is adrenal insufficiency. You order a serum ACTH stimulation test. The results indicate a serum cortisol level of 160. Based on this finding, you suspect the patient may be diagnosed with

   (A) Wilson's disease.
   (B) type 2 diabetes.
   (C) hypothyroidism.
   (D) diabetes mellitus.
   (E) primary adrenal insufficiency.

2. Characteristic findings in patients with adrenal tumors include hypokalmeia, hypomagnesemia, and

   (A) metabolic acidosis.
   (B) metabolic alkalosis.
   (C) refractory hypertension.
   (D) Cushing's syndrome.
   (E) metabolic failure.

3. Initial screening tests for Cushing's syndrome should include

   (A) random cortisol levels.
   (B) BUN/creatinine ratio level.
   (C) dexamethasone suppression testing.
   (D) MRI of the adrenal gland.
   (E) X-ray.

4. Physical exam findings of central adiposity, round face, striae, hirsutism, and supraclavicular and dorsocervical fat accumulation are consistent with

   (A) adrenal carcinoma.
   (B) diabetes mellitus.
   (C) hypothyroidism.
   (D) androgen secretion.
   (E) Cushing's syndrome.

5. A 10-year-old patient presents to the clinic with complaints of nocturnal enuresis, weight loss, and increased thirst. The patient was previously at 50th percentile on the BMI-for-age growth chart. Random blood glucose is 260 mg/dL. What is the most likely etiology for this patient's condition?

   (A) Random blood glucose levels
   (B) Insufficient insulin secretion with peripheral insulin resistance
   (C) Hyperglycemia due to elevated levels of cortisol and epinephrine
   (D) Deficiency of antidiuretic hormone
   (E) Insulin deficiency due to autoimmune destruction of beta cells

6. Diagnostic criteria for diabetes mellitus type 1 includes

   (A) fasting plasma glucose of > 126 mg/dL.
   (B) random glucose of > 150 mg/dL.
   (C) positive glucose found in urine.
   (D) positive ketones found in urine.
   (E) hypoglycemia.

7. Your patient is a young adult male who is very tall and has long arms. On physical exam, you note testicular size is smaller than average and the testes are very firm in density. Hypospadius and small penis size are also present. Body hair is sparse and gynecomastia is present. These findings are characteristic of Klinefelter syndrome. You discuss with the patient that, in order to confirm this diagnosis, which of the following testing should be done?

   (A) Complete blood count
   (B) DEXA scan
   (C) Karyotype
   (D) Androgen levels
   (E) Urinalysis

8. Patients with diabetes mellitus, who are administering insulin to control blood glucose, may experience the Somogyi effect. This phenomenon is characterized by

   (A) early morning hypoglycemia followed by a rebound hyperglycemia immediately after the first meal.
   (B) episodes of hypoglycemia followed by hyperglycemia occurring randomly throughout the day.
   (C) nocturnal hypoglycemia and early morning hyperglycemia.
   (D) early morning hypoglycemia unrelieved by eating.
   (E) late afternoon hypoglycemia.

9. The syndrome of inappropriate anti-diuretic hormone (SIADH) may be caused by medications. The most common drugs associated with inducing SIADH include carbamazepine, oxcarbazepine, cyclophosphamide, chlorpropamide, and

   (A) angiotensin-receptor blockers (ARBs).
   (B) beta-blockers (BBs).
   (C) sulfonamide antibiotics.
   (D) selective serotonin reuptake inhibitors (SSRIs).
   (E) antidepressants.

10. Hypothyroidism is a common disease, most often associated with autoimmune destruction or inflammation of the thyroid gland. Iodine deficiency is a leading cause in developing nations. Three medications are specifically associated with development of hypothyroidism. These include amiodarone, interferon, and

    (A) lithium.
    (B) carbamazepine.
    (C) allopurinol.
    (D) potassium chloride (HcL).
    (E) iodine.

Answers Explained

1. **(E)** Primary adrenal insufficiency is also called Addison's disease and is caused by dysfunction of the adrenal gland. These patients, with chronic disease, often have mineralocorticoid deficiency, especially hyponatremia, hyperkalemia, and volume depletion. ACTH stimulation test is the gold standard for ruling out adrenal insuffieciency. Normal cortisol level is > 18–20. A high ACTH level indicates primary adrenal insufficiency. (A) Wilson's disease is an autosomal recessive disorder characterized by deposits of copper in the liver and brain. This accumulation of copper within the liver causes mitochondrial damage of hepatic cells. Wilson's disease often presents as liver disease in adolescents or neuropsychiatric disease in young adults. (C) Hypothyroidism is a common disorder, most often caused by autoimmune disease of the gland. Symptoms include fatigue, cold intolerance, depression, dry skin, menstrual irregularities, and hoarseness. The FT4 level is usually low. (D) Diabetes mellitus is characterized by elevated serum glucose levels. Symptoms of polyuria and polydipsia are usually present.

2. **(B)** Characteristic findings associated with adrenal tumors include hypokalemia, hypomagnesemia, and metabolic alkalosis. (A) Because of lowered levels of potassium, the metabolic abberration will be alkalotic instead of acidotic in nature. (C) Refractory hypertension in young adults and middle-aged adults is often caused by primary aldosteronism. (D) Cushing's syndrome often presents as central obesity, muscle wasting, purple striae on the torso, and hirsutism. These findings are not necessarily associated with adrenal tumors. (E) Complete metabollic failure is an inability of cells to perform normal processes and that just does not apply here.

3. **(C)** The overnight dexamethasone suppression test is used to screen for hypercortisolism. (A) Random serum corticol levels are not helpful in ruling out or screening for Cushing's syndrome. (B) BUN/creatinine ratio is helpful in evaluation of kidney function in patients with chronic disease such as diabetes mellitus. (D) MRI of the adrenal gland is not indicated for screening for Cushing's syndrome. (E) An X-ray is only used for detection of certain infections.

4. **(E)** Classic findings associated with Cushing's syndrome include a round face, central adiposity, striae, hypertension, hirsutism, and supraclavicular and dorsocervical fat accumulation ("buffalo hump"). (A) Adrenal carcinoma is most often found through abnormal metabolic levels and mineralocorticoid abberations. (B) Diabetes mellitus may present with evidence of metabolic syndrome and symptoms of polyuria and polydipsia. (C) Hypothyroidism presents with fatigue, cold intolerance, dry skin, bradycardia, constipation, weight gain, hoarseness, menorrhagia, and depression. (D) Androgen secretion is a symptom of Cushing's syndrome.

5. **(E)** This patient is displaying classic symptoms of diabetes mellitus—polyuria, polydipsia, weight loss. Given age and previously healthy weight, the most likely diagnosis is type 1 diabetes. Majority of type 1 diabetes is autoimmune mediated. Type 2 diabetes is associated with insulin resistance. Stress hyperglycemia is seen in critically ill patients due to elevated stress hormones. Diabetes insipidus is caused by deficiency of antidiuretic hormone, which is not associated with hyperglycemia.

6. **(A)** A fasting plasma glucose of 126 mg/dL or greater on more than one occasion serves as a diagnostic criteria for diabetes mellitus. (B) A random glucose of 200 mg/dL or greater is also considered diagnostic; 150 mg/dL is not. (C) Glucose in the urine is a common finding and is not useful in diagnosing diabetes mellitus. (D) Ketonuria may be been in patients with diabetes if their disease is not under good control; however, this finding is seen in other conditions and is not diagnostic for diabetes mellitus. (E) Hypoglycemia is when blood sugar levels fall too low.

7. **(C)** Klinefelter syndrome is characterized by hypergonadotropic hypogonadism with small testes. The disorder reveals a 47,XXY karyotype, which is confirmatory. (A, E) Complete blood count and urinalysis may be included in an overall metabolic workup, however this test does not add to the diagnosis of Klinefelter syndrome. (B) DEXA scan is used to screen for and serially monitor bone loss disorders such as osteopenia and osteoporosis. (D) Androgen levels may be ordered in patients who present with findings of Klinefelter syndrome, and they are often low. However, androgen level is not a confirmatory diagnostic test.

8. **(C)** The Somogyi effect presents as nocturnal hypoglycemia, which prompts the liver to produce more glucose during the night. Early morning hyperglycemia is then seen. (A, B, D, E) These presentations are not consistent with the Somogyi effect.

9. **(D)** SSRIs may cause SIADH along with the other medications listed above. (A, B, C, E) These classes of medications have not been implicated in causing SIADH.

10. **(A)** Lithium has been associated with inducing hypothyroidism in certain individuals; therefore, patients taking lithium need regular thyroid studies performed. (B, C, D, E) These specific medications have not been implicated in causing hypothyroidism.

5

Eyes, Ears, Nose, and Throat Review

Learning Objectives

In this chapter, you will review:

→ Conjunctival
→ Retinal
→ Traumatic disorders
→ Vision abnormalities
→ External ear disorders
→ Inner and middle ear disorders
→ Hearing impairment
→ Abnormalities for the ears
→ Foreign bodies
→ Sinus disorders
→ Oropharyngeal disorders
→ Diseases
→ Traumas for the nose and throat

Eye Disorders

Conjunctival Disorders

Conjunctivitis

Pathophysiology

Conjunctivitis is inflammation of the mucous membrane that lines the cornea and inner eyelids and can be acute or chronic. Most cases are due to viral or bacterial infections. Adenovirus is the most common cause of viral conjunctivitis. The organisms isolated most commonly in bacterial conjunctivitis are staphylococci, including methicillin-resistant *S. aureus* (MRSA); streptococci, Haemophilus species; Pseudomonas; and Moraxella.

Clinical Presentation

- **Viral:** There is usually sequential bilateral disease with copious watery discharge and a follicular conjunctivitis. The active viral conjunctivitis lasts up to 2 weeks, with the immune-mediated keratitis occurring later. Infection with adenovirus types 3, 4, 7, and 11 is typically associated with pharyngitis, fever, malaise, and pre-auricular adenopathy.
- **Bacterial:** All may produce purulent discharge and eyelid matting. Blurring of vision and discomfort are mild. In severe cases, examination of stained conjunctival scrapings and cultures is recommended, particularly to identify gonococcal infection that requires emergent treatment.

The disease is usually self-limited, lasting about 10–14 days if untreated. Most topical antibiotics hasten clinical remission. This infection is typically self-limited, and no topical antibiotic has proven superiority over another.

- **Allergic:** the patient complains of conjunctival hyperemia and edema. The patient complains of (dry eye) dryness, redness, foreign body sensation, and variable vision. There may also be discomfort, photophobia, difficulty in moving the lids, and excessive mucus secretion.

Diagnostic and Lab Studies

- Fluorescein stain
- Culture of discharge
- Schirmer test
- Differential Diagnosis/Formulating the Most Likely Diagnosis
- Viral conjunctivitis
- Bacterial conjunctivitis
  - Gonoccocal
  - Chlamydial
  - Inclusion
- Allergic
- Dry Eyes

Health Maintenance and Patient Education

Most cases are due to viral or bacterial (including gonococcal and chlamydial) infection.

Advise patients of modes of transmission to reduce incidence. The mode of transmission of infectious conjunctivitis is usually via direct contact of contaminated fingers or objects to the other eye or to other persons. It may also be spread through respiratory secretions or contaminated eye drops.

Treatment (Pharmaceutical and Clinical Intervention)

- Viral conjunctivitis:
  - Self-limited, if HSV-acyclovir
- Bacterial conjunctivitis:
  - Gonoccocal—1-g dose of intramuscular ceftriaxone plus azithromycin 1,000 mg orally
  - Chlamydial—1-g dose of oral azithromycin
  - Inclusion—1-g dose of oral azithromycin
  - Allergic—oral antihistamines
  - Dry eyes—Artificial tear preparations

Professional Considerations

Conjunctivitis must be distinguished from other red eye etiologies such as: acute uveitis, acute glaucoma, and corneal disorders and cataracts.

A cataract is a clouding of the lens, which reduces vision. Most cataracts develop slowly, as a result of aging, leading to gradual impairment of vision.

Clinical Presentation

- Progressive loss of vision
- Lens opacity

Cataracts can be detected by noting an impaired red reflex when viewing light reflected from the fundus with an ophthalmoscope or by examining the dilated eye with the slit lamp.

Diagnostic and Lab Studies

No other diagnostics than pupil dilation.

Differential Diagnosis/Formulating the Most Likely Diagnosis

Age-related cataracts are the most common. Consider other etiologies and systemic disease; traumatic, diabetes mellitus, atopic dermatitis, corticosteroid treatment; uveitis, radiation exposure.

Health Maintenance and Patient Education

Most persons over age 60 have some degree of lens opacity. Cigarette smoking increases the risk of cataract formation. Multivitamins and dietary antioxidants may prevent the development of age-related cataract.

Treatment (Pharmaceutical and Clinical Intervention)

The only treatment for cataract is surgical extraction of the opacified lens.

Professional Considerations

Cataract surgery improves quality of life and prevents falls.

Corneal Ulcer

Pathophysiology

Etiology of corneal ulcers are due to bacteria, viruses, fungi, or amoebas. A corneal ulcer is an inflammatory and ulcerative keratitis. Common infectious etiologies include bacteria (Staphylococcus, Streptococcus, Pseudomonas) and viruses (HSV, adenovirus). Bacterial corneal ulcers are commonly associated with extended-wear contact lenses. Rare causes of corneal ulcers include fungal infections. Fungal infections may also arise from trauma involving vegetable matter such as a tree branch. Other causes include inadequate lid closure, severe dry eye, severe allergic eye disease, and inflammatory disorders.

Clinical Presentation

Patients complain of pain, photophobia, tearing, and reduced vision. The conjunctiva is injected, and there may be purulent or watery discharge. The corneal appearance varies according to the underlying cause.

Diagnostic and Lab Studies

- Stains and cultures should be obtained as expeditiously as possible.
- Differential Diagnosis/Formulating the Most Likely Diagnosis.
- Consider history and other causes of red eye.

Health Maintenance and Patient Education

A contact lens wearer must discontinue contact lens wear. Contact lens use is a risk factor for corneal ulcer.

Treatment (Pharmaceutical and Clinical Intervention)

Topical treatment using antibiotics is the most effective treatment route, initially given every 30 to 60 minutes. For mild cases, a single fluoroquinolone is advised. For more severe cases, dual therapy using a cephalosporin or vancomycin plus an aminoglycoside is recommended; steroids and eye patching are contraindicated.

Professional Considerations

A corneal ulcer is an ophthalmologic emergency.

Infectious

Pathophysiology

Eye infections are named for their anatomical site, that is, conjunctivitis affects the conjunctiva, uveitis affects the uveal tract (iris, ciliary body, choroid, and retina), and endophthalmitis affects the vitreous or aqueous humor that occupies most of the space within the eye. Adjacent structures can be involved in which case the compound names are used, such as keratoconjunctivitis and chorioretinitis.

Conjunctivitis is typically caused by an infection of the conjunctiva, but consider allergic and chemical conjunctivitis also. It is useful to consider infectious conjunctivitis according to the age of the patient (neonatal vs. adult).

Clinical Presentation

The most common clinical manifestations are a red eye (hyperemia) and discharge. The discharge in bacterial conjunctivitis is typically copious and purulent. Itching, lid edema, and light sensitivity may also occur. In viral conjunctivitis, the discharge usually consists of a small amount of watery fluid that can cause matting of the eyelashes. Viral conjunctivitis is often called "pink eye."

Diagnostic and Lab Studies

Most diagnoses are made based on clinical assessment. If serious bacterial conjunctivitis is suspected, microbiologic diagnosis of conjunctivitis can be made by Gram stain and culture of a specimen of the discharge.

Polymerase-chain reaction (PCR) assay may be considered to support diagnosis (especially *C. trachomatis*, HSV1, and HSV2).

Differential Diagnosis/Formulating the Most Likely Diagnosis

Most eye infections are caused by bacteria and viruses, although some are also caused by fungal and parasitic infections. Some symptoms associated with "a red eye" can be caused by other diseases such as autoimmune uveitis, acute angle glaucoma, and traumatic corneal ulcer.

Health Maintenance and Patient Education

Mild cases of conjunctivitis often resolve without treatment.

Treatment (Pharmaceutical and Clinical Intervention)

- Bacterial neonatal conjunctivitis can be prevented by the application of erythromycin ointment to the eyes of the neonate.
- In mild cases of bacterial conjunctivitis, topical ophthalmic antibiotics can be used. Conjunctivitis, such as that caused by *N. gonorrhoeae*, should be treated with systemic ceftriaxone in both the neonate and adult.
- Conjunctivitis caused by HSV-1 can be treated with oral acyclovir.

Professional Considerations

Most diagnoses are made based on clinical assessment. A patient with an acute painful red eye and corneal abnormality should be referred emergently to an ophthalmologist.

Keratitis

Pathophysiology

Keratitis is an inflammatory lesion of the cornea, most often caused by infection. Keratitis related to contact lens use is primarily caused by Pseudomonas. Other contributing factors include trauma to the eye, surgical procedures, and contaminated eye solutions. Systemic diseases such as diabetes, Sjögren syndrome, and immunodeficiencies play a role. Viral keratitis is often related to reactivation of latent infection by HSV-1 and VZV.

Clinical Presentation

Common symptoms include pain, redness, photophobia, and discharge. Slit-lamp examination shows damage to the corneal epithelium and sometimes a cloudy anterior chamber. A corneal ulcer and a hypopyon may occur.

Diagnostic and Lab Studies

Gram stain visualization of the organisms in the Gram stain of corneal scraping is used to guide therapy. Giemsa stain can assist in the diagnosis of *C. trachomatis*. A microbiologic diagnosis of keratitis is made by culture of the specimen or by PCR assay, which is useful to identify viruses, fungi, and Acanthamoeba.

Differential Diagnosis/Formulating the Most Likely Diagnosis

Consider all etiologies of red eye diagnosis and ocular discharge.

Health Maintenance and Patient Education

- The shingles vaccine can reduce reactivation of VZV.
- Proper contact lens cleaning and wearing practices are important.
- Wearing safety glasses to prevent injury to the cornea is also important.

Treatment (Pharmaceutical and Clinical Intervention)

Bacterial keratitis should be treated with antibiotic therapy. Pseudomonas keratitis in a contact-lens user can be treated with a topical fluoroquinolone. Herpes simplex keratitis and keratitis caused by VZV should be treated with oral acyclovir.

Professional Considerations

Trachoma-related keratitis is one of the leading causes of blindness.

Pterygium

Pathophysiology

A pterygium is an extensive growth of fibrovascular tissue on the surface of the eye extending onto the cornea. The etiology of pterygium is not thoroughly understood; however, chronic UV exposure is accepted as a causative agent. Chronic inflammation may also play a role in the development of pterygium.

Clinical Presentation

- Fibrovascular tissue growing onto the cornea in a triangular or bird wing shape from the nasal aspect of the eye is a classic presentation.
- Redness, itching, and/or irritation of the involved eye may be present.
- Visual blurring if the pterygium grows over the visual axis.

Diagnostic and Lab Studies

Pinguecula is a yellowish patch or nodule on the conjunctiva and does not extend onto the cornea. Conjunctivitis is conjunctival infection with discomfort and eye discharge. Consider carcinoma when a unilateral growth is noted on the temporal side or there are irregular blood vessels on the surface of the eye.

Health Maintenance and Patient Education

Advise patients to wear sunglasses with 100% UV protection to protect eyes from UV damage.

Treatment (Pharmaceutical and Clinical Intervention)

Nonprescription artificial tears and/or topical lubricating drops to soothe the inflammation. Pterygia are usually treated when they interfere with vision or when they cause significant irritation or pain. Surgical removal may be advised when growth impairs vision.

Professional Considerations

Most pterygia do not require surgical treatment. Pterygia that interfere with vision and are removed have a high chance of recurrence. Consider monitoring vision during annual examinations because of the increased risk of age-related macular degeneration.

Lacrimal Disorders

Dacryocystitis

Pathophysiology

Dacryocystitis is an inflammation of the lacrimal sac, positioned immediately distal to the canaliculi and proximal to the nasolacrimal duct. Inflammation is usually secondary to obstruction of the nasolacrimal duct. It may be acute or chronic and occurs most often in infants and in patients over 40 years. It is usually unilateral. As a consequence of the obstruction, infection occurs. Infection is typically with *S. aureus* and streptococci in acute dacryocystitis and *Staphylococcus epidermidis*, streptococci, or gram-negative bacilli in chronic dacryocystitis.

Clinical Presentation

Clinical findings include swelling over the lacrimal sac, redness, tearing, eyelash matting and crusting, and conjunctival redness. Tears and mucopurulence may be expressed; pressure is applied over the lacrimal sac.

Diagnostic and Lab Studies

None advised. Clinical assessment is diagnostic. As a consequence of the obstruction, infection occurs:

- *S. aureus* is the most common etiology.
- Streptococcus species and *Escherichia coli* can also be involved.

Differential Diagnosis/Formulating the Most Likely Diagnosis

History and physical exam support the formulation of this diagnosis.

Health Maintenance and Patient Education

Eye hygiene advised for adult patients.

Treatment (Pharmaceutical and Clinical Intervention)

- Oral clindamycin for 7 to 10 days is recommended for management.
- Unresolved nasolacrimal duct obstruction requires lacrimal duct probing by the ophthalmologist.

Professional Considerations

Complications include conjunctivitis and orbital or preseptal cellulitis.

Lid Disorders

Blepharitis

Pathophysiology

Blepharitis is a common chronic bilateral inflammatory condition of the lid margins and may be infected by staphylococci, or occur in association with seborrhea of the scalp, brows, and ears. Anterior blepharitis involves the lid skin, eyelashes, and associated glands. Posterior blepharitis results from inflammation of the meibomian glands and may be associated with acne rosacea.

Clinical Presentation

Symptoms are irritation, burning, and itching. In anterior blepharitis, the eyelids are red and scales may be seen adhered to the lashes. In posterior blepharitis, the lid margins are hyperemic with telangiectasias, and the meibomian glands and their orifices are inflamed. The lid margin is frequently rolled inward to form a mild entropion, and the tear film may be frothy or greasy.

Diagnostic and Lab Studies

There are no diagnostics to run or lab studies to review.

Differential Diagnosis/Formulating the Most Likely Diagnosis

Carefully review history and other eyelid disorders. Lid erythema and inflammation guides the diagnosis.

Health Maintenance and Patient Education

Patients should be advised on appropriate eyelid hygiene.

Treatment (Pharmaceutical and Clinical Intervention)

Anterior blepharitis is usually controlled by eyelid hygiene. Warm compresses help soften the scales and warm the meibomian gland secretions. Eyelid cleansing can be achieved by gentle eyelid massage and lid scrubs with baby shampoo. In acute exacerbations, an antibiotic eye ointment (e.g., erythromycin) is applied daily to the lid margins. Mild posterior blepharitis may be controlled with regular meibomian gland expression and warm compresses. Inflammation of the conjunctiva and cornea is treated with long-term low-dose oral antibiotic therapy; short-term (5–7 days) topical corticosteroids may also be indicated. Topical therapy with antibiotics may be helpful but should be restricted to short treatment course.

Professional Considerations

Blepharitis is a common cause of recurrent conjunctivitis.

Chalazion

Pathophysiology

A chalazion is a granulomatous inflammation of a meibomian gland that may follow an internal hordeolum.

Clinical Presentation

Appears as a hard, nontender swelling on the upper or lower lid with redness and swelling of the adjacent conjunctiva.

Diagnostic and Lab Studies

None; diagnosis is made by history and physical exam.

Differential Diagnosis/Formulating the Most Likely Diagnosis

Review other lid lesions to identify discriminating features.

Health Maintenance and Patient Education

An antibiotic ointment applied to the lid every 3 hours may be beneficial during the acute stage.

Treatment (Pharmaceutical and Clinical Intervention)

Initial treatment is with warm compresses. If resolution has not occurred by 3 weeks, incision and curettage is the appropriate next step. Corticosteroid injection may be effective.

Professional Considerations

A chalazion resembles a sty in appearance but is not infectious.

Ectropion

Ectropion is an outward turning of the lid margin common in elderly patients and following facial nerve palsy.

Clinical Presentation

Symptoms of tearing and irritation resulting in exposure keratitis may occur.

Diagnostic and Lab Studies

None; diagnosis is made by history and physical exam.

Differential Diagnosis/Formulating the Most Likely Diagnosis

Lid tumor may be a cause of ectropion, which needs to be evaluated.

Health Maintenance and Patient Education

Patient should seek early evaluation of this condition.

Treatment (Pharmaceutical and Clinical Intervention)

Surgical correction is indicated.

Professional Considerations

Trauma and inflammation may also be etiologies.

Entropion

Pathophysiology

Entropion is an inward turning of the lid margin usually due to laxity related to aging.

Clinical Presentation

Inward turning of the lid margin is evident on physical exam.

Diagnostic and Lab Studies

None; diagnosis is made by history and physical exam.

Differential Diagnosis/Formulating the Most Likely Diagnosis

Distinguish entropion from epiblepharon, where the pre-tarsal skin and orbicularis muscle cause the lashes to rotate around the tarsal border.

Health Maintenance and Patient Education

- Patient should seek early evaluation of this condition.
- Eyelashes may need to be removed or shortened.

Treatment (Pharmaceutical and Clinical Intervention)

Correction of entropion may be achieved by surgical lid tightening, repair of the lower lid retractors, or rotation of the lid margin. Botulinum toxin may be effective for lid tightening.

Professional Considerations

Chronic inflammatory lid diseases, such as blepharitis may also cause scarring of the lash follicles and subsequent misdirected growth. It causes corneal irritation and may result in corneal ulceration.

Hordeolum

Pathophysiology

A hordeolum is a painful infection of the Zeiss or Moll glands of the eyelid, usually caused by bacteria. *Staphylococcus aureus* is the causative agent in most cases.

Clinical Presentation

- Tenderness and erythema localized to a point on the eyelid.
- Conjunctival injection may be present.
- Chalazion is a nontender nodule on the eyelid.

Diagnostic and Lab Studies

Laboratory tests are generally not indicated.

Differential Diagnosis/Formulating the Most Likely Diagnosis

Differential for eyelid masses:

- *Basal cell carcinoma*—pearly nodule, often with telangiectasias or central ulceration; more common on lower medial eyelid
- *Herpes zoster ophthalmicus*—vesicular lesions on an erythematous base
- *Hidrocystoma*—benign cystic lesion that grows on the edge of the eyelids
- *Molluscum contagiosum*—waxy nodules with central umbilication and clear fluid
- *Sebaceous cell carcinoma*—rare cancer difficult to distinguish from recurrent chalazion or unilateral chronic blepharitis without biopsy
- *Xanthelasma*—yellowish plaques, generally near medial canthus

Health Maintenance and Patient Education

Hordeolum commonly responds to warm soaks and topical antibiotics. It can recur and can develop into a chronic chalazion, which needs treatment with surgical removal or a steroid injection.

Treatment (Pharmaceutical and Clinical Intervention)

- Warm soaks, three to four times a day
- Topical antibiotics

If above are ineffective, then incision and drainage is warranted.

Professional Considerations

Treatment is often effective; however, when it recurs, it can develop into a chronic chalazion, which may need to be treated with surgical removal or a steroid injection.

Neuro-Ophthalmologic Disorders

Nystagmus

Pathophysiology

Nystagmus occurs in both peripheral lesions and central lesions. In testing the horizontal tracking function, anything other than a smooth horizontal eye movement is assumed to be indicative of vestibulocerebellar pathology. During the vertical tracking test, a superimposed horizontal eye movement (i.e., a saccadic intrusion) may occur in patients with a central oculomotor lesion.

Clinical Presentation

Oculomotor function is tested by asking patients to gaze at the tip of the clinician's index finger. Clinicians should first hold their finger 25 cm away from the patient's eyes and then move the finger laterally and vertically, assessing whether the patient's eye movements are conjugate or disconjugate. If the patient does not have spontaneous nystagmus, the examiner should perform a provocative maneuver to test for positional nystagmus.

Diagnostic and Lab Studies

Vertical nystagmus is a central vestibular sign that usually warrants MRI. A unidirectional horizontal nystagmus that includes a slight torsional component is more likely caused by a peripheral abnormality. Upbeating nystagmus seen only on upward gaze is usually a benign finding.

Differential Diagnosis/Formulating the Most Likely Diagnosis

Vestibular disorders may present once a patient has been admitted for an unrelated ailment involving peripheral disorders, including vestibular neuritis, benign paroxysmal positional vertigo, and Ménière's disease, as well as central disorders, including vestibular migraine, medication-induced dizziness and vertigo, and stroke.

Health Maintenance and Patient Education

The history is the most critical first step in distinguishing vertigo from other causes of dizziness, paying attention to underlying systemic diseases and risk factors, as well as possible medication-related dizziness and vertigo.

Treatment (Pharmaceutical and Clinical Intervention)

Dependent on underlying cause.

Professional Considerations

The examiner should check for orthostatic vital signs, perform a cardiovascular and neurologic examination, and make an assessment of the patient's overall health.

Optic Neuritis

Pathophysiology

Optic neuritis is an inflammation of the optic nerve.

Clinical Presentation

- Usually unilateral visual loss
- Pain exacerbated by eye movements.
- Optic disk normal appearing in acute stage but subsequently develops pallor.
- Field loss is usually central.
- Loss of color vision and an afferent pupillary defect

Diagnostic and Lab Studies

Patients with continuing deterioration of vision or persisting pain after 2 weeks should undergo MRI of the head and orbits.

Differential Diagnosis/Formulating the Most Likely Diagnosis

Associated with lupus and sarcoid.

Health Maintenance and Patient Education

Visual acuity usually improves within 2–3 weeks and returns to near original visual acuity.

Treatment (Pharmaceutical and Clinical Intervention)

IV prednisone followed by oral prednisone.

Professional Considerations

All patients with optic neuritis should be referred urgently for ophthalmologic or neurologic assessment with evaluation for multiple sclerosis.

Papilledema
Pathophysiology

Papilledema refers to optic disc swelling related to increased intracranial pressure.

Clinical Presentation

Patients present a blurring of the optic disc and spontaneous venous pulsations.

Diagnostic and Lab Studies

Patients with papilledema should have an MRI and possible cerebral spinal fluid culture.

Differential Diagnosis/Formulating the Most Likely Diagnosis

Pseudopapilledema or optic disc drusen is an optic nerve anomaly that elevates the optic disc surface and blurs the disc margins, which can be caused by calcifications in the optic nerve head. Optic neuropathies are swelling of all or parts of one or both discs, which can be caused by ischemia or demyelination (as in multiple sclerosis) and may be seen in patients with diabetes mellitus type 1 or 2. Elevated intracranial pressure can also be caused by obstructing lesions, medical conditions, or medications.

Health Maintenance and Patient Education

Maintenance of ideal body weight may prevent papilledema. Patients should report any visual changes immediately.

Treatment (Pharmaceutical and Clinical Intervention)

Refer to an ophthalmologist to guide therapy. Treatment may be required to lower the intracranial pressure to prevent optic nerve damage and irreversible loss of vision.

Professional Considerations

Advise patients with new papilledema of the need for an evaluation for dangerous causes of increased intracranial pressure.

Orbital Disorders
Orbital Cellulitis
Pathophysiology

Infection of the orbit is commonly caused by *S. pneumoniae*, the incidence of which has been reduced by the administration of pneumococcal vaccine; other streptococci, *H. influenzae*; and, less commonly, *S. aureus* including MRSA.

Clinical Presentation

Physical exam findings include fever, proptosis, restriction of extraocular movements, and swelling with redness of the lids.

Diagnostic and Lab Studies

Diagnosis is usually made based on clinical evaluation.

- Leukocytosis and an increased sedimentation rate are often present but are not specific.
- Blood cultures may be positive.
- Non-contrast coronal CT scans provide a rapid and effective means to assess all the paranasal sinuses and to identify areas of greater concern.

Differential Diagnosis/Formulating the Most Likely Diagnosis

Infection of the paranasal sinuses is the usual underlying cause. Clinicians should rule out other etiologies.

Health Maintenance and Patient Education

Immediate treatment with intravenous antibiotics is necessary to prevent optic nerve damage and spread of infection to the cavernous sinuses, meninges, and brain.

Treatment (Pharmaceutical and Clinical Intervention)

Penicillinase-resistant penicillin is recommended, together with metronidazole or clindamycin, to treat anaerobic infections. The response to antibiotics is typically effective, but surgery may be required to drain the paranasal sinuses or orbital abscess.

Professional Considerations

All patients with suspected orbital cellulitis should be referred emergently to an ophthalmologist.

Retinal Disorders

Macular Degeneration

Pathophysiology

Age-related macular changes.

Clinical Presentation

- Appears in patients > 70 years old
- Acute or chronic deterioration of central vision in one or both eyes
- Distortion or abnormal size of images in one or both eyes
- No pain or redness
- Macular abnormalities noted on exam
- Other associated factors
- Race (usually caucasian)
- Sex (female predominance)
- Family history
- Hypertension
- Hypercholesterolemia

- Cardiovascular disease
- Farsighted
- Light iris color
- Smoking

On ophthalmoscopic examination, various abnormalities are visualized in the macula.

Diagnostic and Lab Studies

Fundal photography is often required; may need fluorescein.

Differential Diagnosis/Formulating the Most Likely Diagnosis

Age-related macular degeneration is categorized as dry or wet.

Health Maintenance and Patient Education

Age-related macular degeneration results in loss of central vision in the majority of patients.

Treatment (Pharmaceutical and Clinical Intervention)

- Dry age-related macular degeneration: no specific treatment
- Wet age-related macular degeneration
- Low-vision aids are important.
- Inhibitors of vascular endothelial growth factors
- Long-term repeated intraocular injections may be warranted.

Professional Considerations

Patients should be advised to stop smoking. Older patients with sudden visual loss, central distortion, or scotoma with preservation of central acuity should be referred urgently to an ophthalmologist.

Retinal Detachment

Pathophysiology

Retinal detachments caused by retinal tears or holes can be associated with trauma, previous ocular surgery, nearsightedness, family history of retinal detachment, and Marfan disease.

Clinical Presentation

Patients present with loss of vision in one eye that is usually rapid, "curtain" visualized across field of vision. There is no pain or redness. Detachment seen by ophthalmoscopy. On an ophthalmoscopic examination, the retina may be seen elevated in the vitreous cavity with an irregular surface.

Diagnostic and Lab Studies

On ophthalmoscopic examination, the retina may be seen elevated in the vitreous cavity with an irregular surface.

Differential Diagnosis/Formulating the Most Likely Diagnosis

Nearsightedness and cataract extraction are the two most common predisposing causes. Retinal detachment may also be caused by penetrating or blunt ocular trauma.

Health Maintenance and Patient Education

The presence of gas within the eye is a contraindication to air travel, mountaineering at high altitude, and nitrous oxide anesthesia. These gases persist in the globe for weeks after surgery.

Treatment (Pharmaceutical and Clinical Intervention)

Treatment of retinal detachments requires closing all of the retinal tears and holes by forming a permanent adhesion between the retina, the retinal pigment epithelium, and the choroid with laser photocoagulation to the retina or cryotherapy to the sclera.

Professional Considerations

All cases of retinal detachment should be referred urgently to an ophthalmologist. During transportation, the patient's head should be positioned so that the retinal tear is placed at the lowest point of the eye.

Retinopathy

Pathophysiology

Non-proliferative diabetic retinopathy:

- Microvascular changes are limited to the retina.
- Proliferative diabetic retinopathy: New blood vessels grow on the surface of the retina, optic nerve, or iris.

Clinical Presentation

Non-proliferative retinopathy exam findings:

- Microaneurysms
- Retinal hemorrhages
- Retinal edema
- Hard exudates

In mild non-proliferative retinopathy, there are retinal abnormalities without visual loss. Reduction of vision is most commonly due to diabetic macular edema, which may be due to macular ischemia.

Proliferative retinopathy:

- Characterized by neovascularization, usually arising from the optic disc
- Vitreous hemorrhage is a common sequela.

Diagnostic and Lab Studies

- Fundus photography, preferably after pupillary dilation
- Slit-lamp examination after pupillary dilation

Fluorescein angiography in patients with severe non-proliferative retinopathy can help determine whether laser photocoagulation should be undertaken prophylactically by determining the extent of retinal ischemia.

Differential Diagnosis/Formulating the Most Likely Diagnosis

Retinopathy increases in prevalence and severity with increasing duration and poorer control of diabetes.

Health Maintenance and Patient Education

Optimize blood glucose, blood pressure, kidney function, and serum lipids. Vitrectomy is necessary for removing persistent vitreous hemorrhage.

Treatment (Pharmaceutical and Clinical Intervention)

Optimize blood glucose, blood pressure, kidney function, and lipid levels.

Professional Considerations

Untreated, the visual prognosis in proliferative retinopathy is generally much worse than in non-proliferative retinopathy.

Traumatic Disorders

Blowout Fracture

Pathophysiology

Orbital blowout fractures most commonly involve the orbital floor in caucasians and the medial wall in Afro-Caribbean and Asian patients.

Clinical Presentation

Clinical findings may include: enophthalmos, diplopia in upward gaze, limitation of ocular movement in the upward gaze, and decreased or absent sensation over the maxilla.

Diagnostic and Lab Studies

CT scan of the orbit reveals orbital floor disruption. If a metallic foreign body is suspected, the initial study can be an orbital radiograph. MRI is contraindicated if the history suggests a possible metal foreign body.

Differential Diagnosis/Formulating the Most Likely Diagnosis

All patients with an orbital blowout fracture will present with pain, and the vast majority will present with periorbital ecchymosis. Fractures of other orbital bones should be ruled out.

Health Maintenance and Patient Education

The patient should not blow his/her nose. If there is no enophthalmos or entrapment, then discharge with close outpatient follow-up is acceptable.

Treatment (Pharmaceutical and Clinical Intervention)

Apply a topical antibiotic. Apply cold compresses and a sterile eye patch.

Professional Considerations

Early consultation with an ophthalmologist is advised, especially for entrapment of muscles. Initial treatment includes appropriate tetanus prophylaxis and pain control, as well as avoiding any Valsalva maneuvers.

Corneal Abrasion

Pathophysiology

Corneal abrasions are corneal epithelial defects and can be traumatic, spontaneous, acquired, or genetic.

Clinical Presentation

- History of ocular trauma
- History of contact lens wear
- History of ocular or perioral herpesvirus infection
- Symptoms of pain, eye redness, photophobia, and a foreign-body sensation
- Foreign body evident with direct visualization or a slit lamp

Diagnostic and Lab Studies

During examination with fluorescein stain and UV light, the corneal abrasion appears as a bright green area indicating disruption in the corneal epithelium.

Differential Diagnosis/Formulating the Most Likely Diagnosis

Acute-Angle Closure Glaucoma
- Cloudy cornea and scleral injection
- Eye pain with ipsilateral headache
- Severe vision loss
- Acutely elevated intraocular pressure

Bacterial and Fungal Keratitis or Corneal Ulcerations
- Diffuse erythema
- Discharge
- Pain
- Photophobia
- Vision loss

Conjunctivitis
- Conjunctival erythema and eye discharge
- Foreign body

Uveitis or Iritis
- Usually unilateral injection, eye pain, photophobia, and vision loss

Health Maintenance and Patient Education

Advise patients with corneal abrasions that healing usually occurs simultaneously, and they should report symptoms such as persistent pain, redness, and photophobia. Eye protection should be worn for high-risk occupations. Contact lens wearers should follow recommendations for use.

Treatment (Pharmaceutical and Clinical Intervention)

- Remove any foreign bodies
- Consider topic NSAIDs
- Consider topical antibiotics

Professional Considerations

Immediate referral with complicated abrasions is advised.

Globe Rupture

Pathophysiology

Emergent situation, usually a result of trauma causing disruption of the eye and contents.

Clinical Presentation

- Penetrating wound of cornea
- Subconjunctival hemorrhage

Periorbital ecchymosis and maxillofacial fractures, along with limitation of extraocular muscle movement, should raise one's suspicion for globe rupture. Examination of the eye may reveal decreased visual acuity, an irregular or teardrop-shaped pupil, an afferent pupillary defect, shallow anterior chamber, hyphema, positive Seidel test, and lens dislocation.

Diagnostic and Lab Studies

Slit-lamp exam, and if using ultrasound to evaluate for trauma, do not apply significant pressure on the globe.

Differential Diagnosis/Formulating the Most Likely Diagnosis

Diagnosis is supported by history and physical examination.

Health Maintenance and Patient Education

Administer antiemetics to prevent increased intraocular pressure and extrusion of intraocular contents from vomiting. Avoid any topical eye solutions, and give the patient nothing by mouth in anticipation of surgery.

Treatment (Pharmaceutical and Clinical Intervention)

Metal eye shield (or paper cup) placed in suspected globe rupture prior to surgical repair.

Professional Considerations

Eye examination must be careful and gentle. Do not measure intraocular pressure.

Hyphema

Pathophysiology

A hyphema is a collection of blood in the anterior chamber, usually resulting from trauma.

Clinical Presentation

- Layered blood in the anterior chamber
- History of eye trauma
- Possible increased intraocular pressure
- Decreased vision

Diagnostic and Lab Studies

Consider laboratory tests to evaluate for bleeding disorders: bleeding time, electrophoresis for sickle cell trait, platelet count, prothrombin and partial thromboplastin time, and liver function studies. Consider CT imaging if a mechanism of injury suggests an orbital fracture or need to evaluate for orbital or intraocular foreign body.

Differential Diagnosis/Formulating the Most Likely Diagnosis

- Blood clotting disturbances
- Bleeding
- Medication
- Melanoma
- Neovascularization
- Trauma

Health Maintenance and Patient Education

Usually resolves spontaneously within 7 days.

Treatment (Pharmaceutical and Clinical Intervention)

Oral antifibrinolytic agents can be used. Avoid aspirin and nonsteroidal anti-inflammatory drugs (NSAIDs), which have been associated with higher rates of rebleeding. Surgical intervention is recommended for patients with persistent hyphema or prolonged elevated intraocular pressure.

Professional Considerations

Evaluate or refer for evaluation for elevated intraocular pressure and other associated injuries. Urgent referral if concern for globe rupture.

Vascular Disorders

Retinal Vascular Occlusion

Pathophysiology

Retinal vascular occlusions are typically ischemic or embolic.

Clinical Presentation

Central retinal artery occlusion causes sudden, severe loss of vision without pain. Transient visual loss (amaurosis fugax) may be reported and is suggestive of giant cell arteritis or retinal emboli. Branch retinal artery occlusion also causes sudden painless visual loss and impairment of visual field that usually is permanent.

Diagnostic and Lab Studies

Retinal imaging.

Differential Diagnosis/Formulating the Most Likely Diagnosis

The patient usually presents with sudden, painless loss of vision at the time of the occlusion, when the clinical appearance varies from a few small, scattered retinal hemorrhages and cotton-wool spots to a hemorrhagic appearance with both deep and superficial retinal hemorrhage.

Health Maintenance and Patient Education

Patients are usually over 50 years of age, and many have associated cardiovascular disease. Maintenance of stable cardiovascular conditions are important patient education components.

Treatment (Pharmaceutical and Clinical Intervention)

Irreversible retinal damage occurs within a few hours of retinal artery occlusion. Treatment options include ocular massage, anterior chamber paracentesis, medications to reduce intraocular pressure, and vasodilators.

Professional Considerations

A foveal cherry-red spot develops, surrounded by the pale swollen retina of the rest of the macula. The fundal abnormalities resolve within 4–6 weeks, leaving a pale optic disk as the major ophthalmoscopic finding.

Vision Abnormalities

Amaurosis Fugax

Pathophysiology

Transient retinal ischemia due to emboli; carotid artery disease is the most common source.

Clinical Presentation

Monocular visual loss with full recovery after 5–10 minutes, with the beginning and end often described as a curtain passing vertically across the visual field.

Diagnostic and Lab Studies

None indicated.

Differential Diagnosis/Formulating the Most Likely Diagnosis

Cardiac causes such as atrial fibrillation, mitral or aortic valve disease, or infective endocarditis particularly need to be considered in patients with a history of cardiac disease or age under 40 years. Examine the fundus for emboli and auscultate for carotid bruits and cardiac murmurs. Evaluate pulse for atrial fibrillation.

Health Maintenance and Patient Education

Arrange for evaluation of the carotids, including for underlying risk factors and cardiac disease as indicated.

Treatment (Pharmaceutical and Clinical Intervention)

Management of cardiovascular risk factors and diagnoses.

Professional Considerations

Monitor patient overall cardiovascular status.

Amblyopia

Pathophysiology

Reduced visual acuity beyond that explained by structural, ocular, or visual pathway disease. Strabismus, impairing binocular function, is a common cause.

Clinical Presentation

Cover/uncover test reveals strabismus. As the cover is removed from the eye following the cover test, the eye emerging from under the cover is observed by the examiner. If the position of the eye changes, strabismus can be noted. Corneal light reflection may be altered.

Diagnostic and Lab Studies

No diganostics are indicated.

Differential Diagnosis/Formulating the Most Likely Diagnosis

Several types of strabismus exist. Diagnosis is made by evaluation of visual limitations.

Health Maintenance and Patient Education

Parental involvement needed to support treatment.

Treatment (Pharmaceutical and Clinical Intervention)

The goals of treatment in children are to prevent and/or reverse the effects of strabismus (e.g., amblyopia, suppression, loss of stereopsis) and to correct any cosmetic conditions. Nonsurgical treatment of strabismus includes treatment of amblyopia, the use of optical devices (prisms, glasses), pharmacologic agents, and orthoptics.

Professional Considerations

Consultation with an ophthalmologist will guide treatment decisions.

Glaucoma

Pathophysiology

Types
Chronic glaucoma is characterized by gradually progressive excavation "cupping" of the optic disk with loss of vision progressing from slight visual field loss to complete blindness. In chronic open-angle glaucoma, intraocular pressure is elevated due to reduced drainage of aqueous fluid through the trabecular meshwork.

- *In angle-closure glaucoma,* flow of aqueous fluid into the anterior chamber angle is obstructed.
- *In normal-tension glaucoma,* intraocular pressure is not elevated but the same pattern of optic nerve damage occurs.

Clinical Presentation

No symptoms in early stages.

- Insidious progressive bilateral loss of peripheral vision, resulting in tunnel vision; visual acuities preserved until advanced disease; pathologic cupping of the optic discs.
- Intraocular pressure is usually elevated.

Diagnostic and Lab Studies

None indicated.

Differential Diagnosis/Formulating the Most Likely Diagnosis

Increased intraocular pressure is a usual finding for glaucoma.

Health Maintenance and Patient Education

All persons over age 50 years may benefit from intraocular pressure measurement and optic disc examination every 3–5 years.

Treatment (Pharmaceutical and Clinical Intervention)

Medical treatment is directed toward lowering intraocular pressure. Prostaglandin analog eye drops are commonly used as first-line therapy because of their efficacy, lack of systemic side effects, and convenient once-daily dose. Laser therapy and surgery may be warranted.

Professional Considerations

Early diagnosis and treatment can preserve vision throughout life. Screening for chronic open-angle glaucoma should be targeted at individuals with an affected first-degree relative, at persons who have diabetes mellitus, and at older individuals with African or Hispanic heritage. Screening may also be warranted in patients taking long-term oral or combined intranasal and inhaled corticosteroid therapy.

Scleritis

Pathophysiology

Scleritis and episcleritis are inflammatory conditions causing congestion of the conjunctival, episcleral, and scleral plexuses overlying the avascular sclera.

Causes of Scleritis

Systemic autoimmune diseases such as:

- Rheumatoid arthritis
- Polyarteritis nodosa
- Systemic lupus erythematosus (SLE)

Infections

- Pseudomonas
- Tuberculosis
- Syphilis
- Herpes zoster

Less Common Causes

- Behçet syndrome
- Gout
- Sarcoidosis
- Idiopathic

Clinical Presentation

Scleritis is painful, destructive, and potentially blinding. The pain is constant and may radiate to the face and periorbital region. Associated features include tearing, photophobia, globe tenderness to palpation, and painful eye movement.

Diagnostic and Lab Studies

Slit-lamp microscopy.

Differential Diagnosis/Formulating the Most Likely Diagnosis

Causes of red eye, other than scleritis and episcleritis:

- Acute-angle closure glaucoma
- Conjunctivitis
- Keratitis or corneal ulcerations
- Uveitis or iritis

Health Maintenance and Patient Education

Scleritis is frequently associated with systemic disease cases, most commonly rheumatoid arthritis. Pain is exacerbated with ocular movements because the extraocular muscles insert into the sclera itself.

Treatment (Pharmaceutical and Clinical Intervention)

Treatment varies according to underlying disease (if present) and can involve NSAID therapy, glucocorticoids, and immunosuppressive medications.

Professional Considerations

Ophthalmology consultation is required.

Strabismus

Pathophysiology

Strabismus is associated with various abnormal sensory phenomena, including diplopia (double vision), visual confusion, retinal correspondence, amblyopia, and fixation.

Clinical Presentation

In the presence of strabismus, each fovea receives a different image.

Important questions for patient history:

- Direction
- Laterality
- Duration
- Frequency
- Modifying factors
- Associated symptoms
- Past ocular history
- Past medical history
- Family history

On physical exam, inspection can show whether strabismus is constant or intermittent, alternating or non-alternating, and variable. Associated ptosis and abnormal position of the head should be noted. Nystagmus indicates unstable fixation and usually reduced visual acuity.

Diagnostic and Lab Studies

None indicated.

Differential Diagnosis/Formulating the Most Likely Diagnosis

There are multiple forms of strabismus, and an ophthalmology support is suggested.

Health Maintenance and Patient Education

Multiple forms of strabismus exist. PAs should start with cover/uncover tests during pediatric evaluations.

Treatment (Pharmaceutical and Clinical Intervention)

Orthoptic exercises may relieve symptoms in individuals with difficulty maintaining normal convergence with near viewing tasks such as reading. Treatment for amblyopia or strabismus should be instituted as soon as the diagnosis is made. Results are favorably influenced by early realignment of the eyes, preferably by age 2.

Professional Considerations

Treatment for strabismus should be instituted as soon as the diagnosis is made. Results are favorably influenced by early realignment of the eyes, preferably by age 2.

Ear Disorders

External Ear

Pathophysiology

The clinical presentation of atopic dermatitis of the ear is thought to be secondary to skin barrier breakdown and allergic inflammation.

Clinical Presentation

Lesions present on the ear are often pruritic and erythematous. Lesions typically persist for more than 1 month.

Diagnostic and Lab Studies

No specific laboratory or histologic markers.

Differential Diagnosis/Formulating the Most Likely Diagnosis

The differential diagnosis is broad and includes seborrheic dermatitis, psoriatic dermatitis, candidiasis, contact dermatitis, dermatitis herpetiformis, lichen simplex chronicus, and urticaria.

Health Maintenance and Patient Education

Patients may have a personal or family history of allergy.

Treatment (Pharmaceutical and Clinical Intervention)

Topical corticosteroids are first-line prescription therapy.

Professional Considerations

Atopic dermatitis is defined by pruritic erythematous patches or weeping plaques. Psoriasis may affect the ear with oval salmon-pink plaques. Contact dermatitis presents with pruritic, indurated, and erythematous lesions after exposure to irritant.

Cerumen Impaction

Pathophysiology

In most cases, cerumen impaction is self-induced through efforts at cleaning the ear.

Clinical Presentation

- Fullness in ear
- Conductive hearing loss when canal is blocked

Diagnostic and Lab Studies

None indicated.

Differential Diagnosis/Formulating the Most Likely Diagnosis

Diagnosis made by otoscopic inspection.

Health Maintenance and Patient Education

Use of jet irrigators (i.e., WaterPik oral cleaner) should not be used to prevent tympanic membrane rupture.

Treatment (Pharmaceutical and Clinical Intervention)

- Ear drops
- Mechanical removal
- Suction or irrigation

Otitis Externa

Pathophysiology

Otitis externa usually results from a combination of heat and retained moisture, with desquamation and maceration of the epithelium of the outer ear canal. The disease exists in several forms: localized, diffuse, chronic, and invasive. It's primarily bacterial in origin, with *P. aeruginosa* and *S. aureus* the most common pathogens.

Clinical Presentation

Acute diffuse otitis externa is also known as swimmer's ear. Heat, humidity, and the loss of protective cerumen lead to excessive moisture and elevation of the pH in the ear canal, which in turn lead to skin maceration and irritation. Infection may then follow. Repeated irritation, such as insertion of cotton swabs or other foreign objects into the ear canal, can lead to this condition. Chronic otitis externa typically presents as erythematous, scaling dermatitis in which the predominant symptom is pruritus.

Diagnostic and Lab Studies

None indicated.

Differential Diagnosis/Formulating the Most Likely Diagnosis

Other conditions that produce a similar clinical picture include atopic dermatitis, seborrheic dermatitis, psoriasis, and dermatomycosis.

Health Maintenance and Patient Education

Antibiotics are most effective when given topically.

Treatment (Pharmaceutical and Clinical Intervention)

- Cleaning ear canal
- Penicillin
- Incision and drainage in cases of abscess formation

Professional Considerations

Therapy consists of identifying and treating or removing the offending process, although successful resolution is frequently difficult.

Trauma

Pathophysiology

Etiology of penetrating trauma or barotrauma.

Clinical Presentation

- History of trauma to ear or foreign body insertion into the ear
- Symptoms of pain and hearing loss
- Bloody otorrhea

Diagnostic and Lab Studies

None indicated.

Differential Diagnosis/Formulating the Most Likely Diagnosis

The Weber tuning-fork test should be performed to verify that sound radiates to the affected ear, and eyes should be checked for nystagmus.

Health Maintenance and Patient Education

If no evidence of sensorineural hearing loss is found, no specific treatment is required because traumatic TM perforations, especially central perforations, typically heal spontaneously.
Strict dry ear precautions should be followed to prevent water from getting into the ear.
    Instructions to the patient include no swimming and use of a cotton ball thoroughly.

Treatment (Pharmaceutical and Clinical Intervention)

If no evidence of sensorineural hearing loss is found, no specific treatment is required because traumatic TM perforations, especially central perforations, typically heal spontaneously.

Professional Considerations

An audiogram should be performed after about 3 months to verify that hearing has returned to normal.

Inner Ear

Pathophysiology

Diseases of the cochlea result in sensory hearing loss, a condition that is usually irreversible. Most cochlear diseases result in bilateral symmetric hearing loss.

Clinical Presentation

Presbyacusis, or age-related hearing loss, is the most frequent cause of sensory hearing loss and is progressive, predominantly high-frequency, and symmetrical.

Diagnostic and Lab Studies

Audiometry is useful.

Differential Diagnosis/Formulating the Most Likely Diagnosis

Noise trauma, physical trauma, and ototoxicity are other conditions in the differential diagnosis.

Health Maintenance and Patient Education and Treatment

The most important treatment of inner ear conditions is avoidance of exposure to excessive noise, ototoxic agents, and other factors that may cause cochlear damage.

Professional Considerations

When the tympanic membrane is perforated, use of potentially ototoxic ear drops should be avoided.

Acoustic Neuroma

Pathophysiology

Eighth nerve schwannomas are among the most common of intracranial tumors.

Clinical Presentation

Typical auditory symptoms are unilateral hearing loss with deterioration of speech discrimination exceeding that predicted by the degree of pure-tone loss. Vestibular dysfunction more often takes the form of continuous disequilibrium.

Diagnostic and Lab Studies

Diagnosis is made by MRI.

Differential Diagnosis/Formulating the Most Likely Diagnosis

Schwannoma, meningioma, and epidermoids.

Health Maintenance and Patient Education

Hearing loss is present in 95% of patients.

Treatment (Pharmaceutical and Clinical Intervention)

- Observation
- Microsurgical excision
- Stereotactic radiotherapy

Professional Considerations

Any individual with a unilateral or asymmetric sensorineural hearing loss should be evaluated for an intracranial mass lesion.

Barotrauma

Pathophysiology

Persons with poor eustachian tube function may be unable to equalize the barometric stress exerted on the middle ear by air travel, rapid altitudinal change, or underwater diving.

Clinical Presentation

- Hemorrhage
- Emesis
- Sensory hearing loss or vertigo

Diagnostic and Lab Studies

None indicated.

Differential Diagnosis/Formulating the Most Likely Diagnosis

Diagnosis is based on symptoms in a patient who has recently undergone recent increase or decrease in ambient pressure.

Health Maintenance and Patient Education

Patients should be warned to avoid diving when they have upper respiratory infections or episodes of nasal allergy.

Treatment (Pharmaceutical and Clinical Intervention)

- Oral decongestants
- Myringotomy

Professional Considerations

Repeated barotrauma in patients who must fly frequently may be alleviated by insertion of ventilating tubes.

Labyrinthitis

Pathophysiology

In the setting of middle ear infection, bacterial infection can invade through the round window causing acute labyrinthitis. From the labyrinth, bacteria move to the cochlear aqueduct, forming a conduit between the perilymph and the cerebrospinal fluid (CSF) resulting in meningeal infiltration.

Clinical Presentation

Patients present with sudden sensorineural hearing loss, severe vertigo, and nystagmus, nausea, and vomiting. Complications include conductive hearing loss and speech/language delay.

Diagnostic and Lab Studies

None indicated.

Differential Diagnosis/Formulating the Most Likely Diagnosis

Is a complication of acute otitis media.

Health Maintenance and Patient Education

Diagnosis and appropriate, timely management of AOM and OME are essential for reducing complications and improving overall patient quality of life.

Treatment (Pharmaceutical and Clinical Intervention)

Antibiotic therapy.

Professional Considerations

It is important to diagnose and treat labyrinthitis early in order to prevent the subsequent development of meningitis.

Vertigo

Pathophysiology

Causes can be determined based on the duration of symptoms (seconds, hours, days, months) and whether auditory symptoms are present.

Causes include:
- Anticonvulsants
- Antibiotics
- Hypnotics
- Analgesics
- Tranquilizing drugs and ETOH

Clinical Presentation
Patient has a sensation of motion when there is no motion or an exaggerated sense of motion in response to movement.

- **Peripheral:** Onset is sudden; often associated with tinnitus and hearing loss; horizontal nystagmus may be present.
- **Central:** Onset is gradual; no associated auditory symptoms.

Diagnostic and Lab Studies

An audiogram and electronystagmography (ENG) or videonystagmography (VNG) and MRI.

Differential Diagnosis/Formulating the Most Likely Diagnosis

Must differentiate peripheral from central causes of vestibular dysfunction.

Health Maintenance and Patient Education

Various etiologies.

Treatment (Pharmaceutical and Clinical Intervention)

- Medications
- Diazepam
- For acute phases of vertigo only
- Discontinue as soon as feasible to avoid long-term dysequilibrium.
- Ménière's disease
- Low-salt diet
- Diuretic
- For acute attacks, valium
- Labyrinthitis
- Antibiotics if patient is febrile or has symptoms of bacterial infection
- Vestibular suppressants

Professional Considerations

For refractory cases: intratympanic corticosteroid injections.

Middle Ear

Cholesteatoma

Pathophysiology

Factors that appear to be associated with formation of cholesteatoma retractions of the TM include history of poor eustachian tube function and chronic inflammation of the middle ear, as in chronic otitis media or recurrent acute otitis media.

Clinical Presentation

Patients with acquired cholesteatomas typically present with recurrent or persistent purulent otorrhea and hearing loss. Tinnitus is also common. In primary acquired cholesteatoma, there will be a retraction of the pars flaccida in most cases, and less commonly in the pars tensa.

Diagnostic and Lab Studies

Physical findings are usually diagnostic in cases of acquired cholesteatoma. CT or MRI may be indicated.

Differential Diagnosis/Formulating the Most Likely Diagnosis

Chronic otitis media without cholesteatoma; otitis externa; malignant external otitis; neoplasms such as squamous cell carcinoma of the ear or other rare tumors, such as adenomas, adenocarcinoma, adenoid cystic carcinoma, and cerebrospinal fluid otorrhea.

Health Maintenance and Patient Education

There is a high rate of recurrent and/or residual cholesteatoma disease after primary surgical intervention.

Treatment (Pharmaceutical and Clinical Intervention)

The initial goal of treatment for cholesteatomas is to reduce the level of the inflammatory and infectious activity in the involved ear. Surgical excision follows medical treatment. Regular examinations over a course of 10 years or more after definitive treatment remain a critical part of the patient's care.

Professional Considerations

Although the pathogenesis of primary acquired cholesteatoma is not clearly understood, if it is assumed that eustachian tube dysfunction (ETD) is one of the factors that may foster its formation, restoring eustachian tube function may help prevent the formation of this type of cholesteatoma.

Otitis Media

Pathophysiology

Chronic infection of the middle ear and mastoid generally develops as a consequence of recurrent acute otitis media. Common organisms include *P. aeruginosa*, Proteus species, *Staphylococcus aureus*, and mixed infections.

Clinical Presentation

- Chronic otorrhea with or without ear pain
- Tympanic membrane perforation with conductive hearing loss
- Conductive hearing loss results from destruction of the tympanic membrane or ossicular chain, or both.

Diagnostic and Lab Studies

None indicated.

Differential Diagnosis/Formulating the Most Likely Diagnosis

Formulating the diagnosis is clear with an effective history and physical exam.

Health Maintenance and Patient Education

Pain is uncommon except during acute exacerbations.

Treatment (Pharmaceutical and Clinical Intervention)

Medical treatment includes regular removal of infected debris, use of earplugs to protect against water exposure, and topical antibiotic drops and consideration of oral antibiotics. Surgical management is definitive.

Professional Considerations

Ciprofloxin, effective against Pseudomonas, 500 mg twice a day for 1–6 weeks, may help dry a chronically discharging ear.

Tympanic Membrane Perforation

Pathophysiology

Acute tympanic membrane (TM) perforations may be caused by direct penetrating trauma, barotrauma, otitis media, chemicals, thermal injuries, or iatrogenic causes.

Clinical Presentation

Patients with a tympanic membrane perforation complain of a sudden onset of ear pain, vertigo, tinnitus, and altered hearing. Physical examination of the tympanic membrane reveals a tear or perforation with an irregular border, often with blood along the margins. Chronic perforations may have smooth margins and a round or ovoid shape.

Diagnostic and Lab Studies

None indicated in primary evaluation. Myringotomy may be considered.

Differential Diagnosis/Formulating the Most Likely Diagnosis

Careful evaluation for possible underlying causes. Diagnosis is made by history and physical exam.

Health Maintenance and Patient Education

Patients are instructed to avoid water in the ear while the perforation is healing and to return if symptoms of infection appear.

Treatment (Pharmaceutical and Clinical Intervention)

Treatment should be trailed to the mechanism of injury. Systemic antibiotics should be reserved for perforations associated with OM, penetrating injury, and possibly water-sport injuries.

Professional Considerations

While most TM perforations heal spontaneously, all perforations require referral to an otolaryngologist for follow-up. Topical steroids impede perforation healing and should not be used.

Other Abnormalities of the Ear

Mastoiditis

Pathophysiology

Mastoiditis is an infection of the mastoid air cells often resulting from extension of purulent OM.

Clinical Presentation

- Patients present with fever, chills, postauricular ear pain, and otorrhea.
- Patients may have tenderness, erythema, swelling, and fluctuance over the mastoid process; proptosis of the pinna and otorrhea.

Diagnostic and Lab Studies

Complete blood count and sedimentation rate. Contrast CT of the head or mastoid sinus may reveal bone erosion.

Differential Diagnosis/Formulating the Most Likely Diagnosis

Initial evaluation includes a thorough head, neck, and cranial nerve examination.

Health Maintenance and Patient Education

Otorrhea of at least 2 months in duration is a symptom of chronic mastoiditis, and patients should be advised to seek care if symptoms reoccur.

Treatment (Pharmaceutical and Clinical Intervention)

- Oral penicillinase-resistant penicillins
- Amoxicillin-clavulanic acid
- Third-generation cephalosporins
- Macrolides

Professional Considerations

Mastoiditis requires immediate consultation and close follow-up.

Ménière's Disease

Pathophysiology

The cause of Ménière's disease is attributed to anatomic, infectious, immunologic, and allergic etiologies.

Clinical Presentation

Occurs as episodic attacks lasting for several hours.

Signs and Symptoms

- A unilateral, fluctuating sensorineural hearing loss
- Vertigo that lasts minutes to hours
- A constant or intermittent tinnitus typically increasing in intensity before the vertiginous attack
- Aural fullness

Diagnostic and Lab Studies

Ménière's disease is a clinical diagnosis. The diagnostic evaluation includes audiometry and a fluorescent treponemal antibody absorption (FTA-ABS) test to rule out syphilis.

Differential Diagnosis/Formulating the Most Likely Diagnosis

Syphilis may imitate Ménière's disease and it's important to rule this out (FTA-ABS). MRI with gadolinium contrast allows the exclusion of retrocochlear conditions. Dizziness may be caused by poor vision, decreased proprioception (diabetes mellitus), cardiovascular insufficiency, strokes, neurological conditions (migraines, multiple sclerosis), metabolic disorders, and the side effects of medications.

Health Maintenance and Patient Education

The acute attack is also associated with nausea and vomiting, and following the acute attack, patients are exhausted for a few days.

Treatment (Pharmaceutical and Clinical Intervention)

The primary management of Ménière's disease involves a sodium-restricted diet and diuretics. Intratempanic gentamycin therapy may be appropriate in refractory cases.

Professional Considerations

Ménière's disease is characterized by remissions and exacerbations, making it difficult to predict the disease course and pattern. The initial manifestation is vertigo or hearing loss, but within 1 year of onset, attacks of vertigo, tinnitus, fluctuating hearing loss, and aural fullness are present.

Tinnitus

Pathophysiology

Bilateral tinnitus may occur with damage to the conductive hearing system from environmental (prolonged noise exposure) or systemic (medications that damage the cochlear hairs) causes. Unilateral tinnitus with conductive hearing loss results from tympanic membrane damage, recurrent unilateral ear infections, ossicle damage, or trauma.

Clinical Presentation

- Men > women
- Caucasian > non-Caucasian

Tinnitus is highly associated with depression, anxiety, and other personality disorders. Perception of tinnitus is altered by the patient's attention to the sounds, level of stress, and ambient noise level.

Diagnostic and Lab Studies

Weber test, Rinne test warranted during physical exam. Audiometry may be evaluated.

Differential Diagnosis/Formulating the Most Likely Diagnosis

Increasing prevalence with age. Most tinnitus coexists with conductive (recurrent infections or otosclerosis) or sensorineural (cochlear damage from medications, loud music) hearing loss. A lesion anywhere along the auditory pathway can cause tinnitus.

Health Maintenance and Patient Education

Ruling out a cause that results in deafness is essential.

Treatment (Pharmaceutical and Clinical Intervention)

Difficult to treat effectively.

Professional Considerations

If initial evaluation based on history, physical examination, and initial diagnostic testing is unrevealing, consider referring to an otolaryngologist.

Foreign Bodies

Neoplasms (Benign/Malignant)

Pathophysiology

Basal cell carcinoma is the most common malignant neoplasm of the ear. The five subtypes are: nodular-ulcerative, cystic, superficial multicentric, micronodular, and morpheaform. Chronic sun exposure is the predominant risk factor for BCC, and the incidence of cancer increases with age.

Clinical Presentation

Patients may initially present with a skin lesion that is nodular, ulcerated, and/or bleeding. BCCs of the auricle typically occur on the helix and in the preauricular area due to sun exposure.

Diagnostic and Lab Studies

The diagnosis of any suspicious lesion should be confirmed with biopsy. CT or MRI may be warranted.

Differential Diagnosis/Formulating the Most Likely Diagnosis

The differential diagnosis includes benign nevi, melanomas, squamous cell carcinomas, eczema, and scleroderma.

Health Maintenance and Patient Education and Treatment

- Topical 5-fluorouracil
- Immiquimod
- Surgical removal

Professional Considerations

In addition to the patient's age and overall immune status, the prognosis for SCC is dependent on the histologic subtype, size, and location of the tumor.

Nose/Sinus Disorders

Epistaxis

Pathophysiology

Epistaxis is an extremely common problem in the primary care setting. Bleeding is most common in the anterior septum where a confluence of veins creates a superficial venous plexus (Kiesselbach plexus).

Clinical Presentation

Predisposing factors include nasal trauma, rhinitis, nasal mucosal drying from low humidity or nasal oxygen, deviation of the nasal septum, atherosclerotic disease, hereditary hemorrhagic telangiectasia (Osler-Weber-Rendu syndrome), inhaled drug, and alcohol abuse.

Diagnostic and Lab Studies

None aside from thorough history and physical exam, unless other diagnosis is uncovered.

Differential Diagnosis/Formulating the Most Likely Diagnosis

Careful nasal examination should be performed to rule out neoplasia.

Health Maintenance and Patient Education

Poorly controlled hypertension is associated with epistaxis.

Treatment (Pharmaceutical and Clinical Intervention)

Most cases of anterior epistaxis may be successfully treated by direct pressure on the site for 15 minutes.

Professional Considerations

When direct pressure is ineffective, topical sympathomimetics and nasal tamponade methods are usually effective.

Nasal Polyps

Pathophysiology

The precise cause of nasal polyp formation is unknown, although allergies are perceived to play a role.

Clinical Presentation

- Variable size
- Smooth and translucent
- Color ranging from nearly none to deep erythema
- The middle meatus is the most common location.
- Frequently bilateral

Diagnostic and Lab Studies

In young patients with multiple polyps, sweat test to rule out cystic fibrosis. CT of the nose and paranasal sinuses may be indicated.

Differential Diagnosis/Formulating the Most Likely Diagnosis

- Papilloma
- Meningoencephalocele
- Nasopharyngeal carcinoma
- Pyogenic granuloma
- Chordoma
- Glioblastoma

Health Maintenance and Patient Education

Nasal polyps are benign and tend to recur.

Treatment (Pharmaceutical and Clinical Intervention)

Surgical excision is often required to relieve symptoms. Consider immunotherapy for patients with allergies.

Professional Considerations

Periodic reevaluation advised because of recurrence incidence.

Rhinitis

Pathophysiology

Allergen exposure in the presence of allergen-specific IgE.

Clinical Presentation

Clear rhinorrhea, sneezing, tearing, eye irritation, and pruritus.

Associated Symptoms
- Cough
- Bronchospasm
- Eczematous dermatitis

On physical examination, the mucosa of the turbinates is usually pale or purple.

Diagnostic and Lab Studies

None indicated.

Differential Diagnosis/Formulating the Most Likely Diagnosis

Mucosal turbinates are erythematous with viral conditions. Nasal polyps, which are yellowish boggy masses of hypertrophic mucosa, are associated with long-standing allergic rhinitis.

Health Maintenance and Patient Education

In some cases, allergic rhinitis symptoms are inadequately relieved by medication and avoidance measures. These patients have a strong family history of atopy and may also have lower respiratory manifestations, such as allergic asthma. Referral to an allergist for immunotherapy may be appropriate.

Treatment (Pharmaceutical and Clinical Intervention)

Intranasal corticosteroids are the primary treatment of allergic rhinitis. Antihistamines offer temporary, but immediate, control of symptoms.

Professional Considerations

Vasomotor rhinitis is a common cause of rhinorrhea in older patients.

Sinusitis

Pathophysiology

- **Infection:** most commonly viral
- **Noninfectious obstruction:** allergic, polyps, barotrauma, chemical irritants, tumors

Clinical Presentation

Facial pain and pressure over affected sinus along with viral URI symptoms. Most sinus infections involve the maxillary sinus.

Diagnostic and Lab Studies

Routine culture of nasopharyngeal mucosa is not recommended unless the patient is immuno-compromised.

Differential Diagnosis/Formulating the Most Likely Diagnosis

The diagnosis is based on the clinical picture with typical symptoms listed.

Health Maintenance and Patient Education

For chronic rhinosinusitis, inflammation is documented objectively using anterior rhinoscopy, nasal endoscopy, or CT.

Treatment (Pharmaceutical and Clinical Intervention)

Treat for these microorganisms if condition is not self-limited and etiology is considered bacterial: *Streptococcus pneumoniae*, *Haemophilus influenzae*, *Moraxella catarrhalis*, and *Staphylococcus aureus*.

Professional Considerations

Potentially life-threatening complications include subperiosteal orbital abscess, meningitis, epidural, or cerebral abscess.

Trauma

Pathophysiology

Fracture of the nasal bone.

Clinical Presentation

Fracture is suggested by crepitance or palpably mobile bony segments. Epistaxis, pain, and soft-tissue hematomas are common.

Diagnostic and Lab Studies

X-ray may be helpful but is not necessary in uncomplicated nasal fractures.

Differential Diagnosis/Formulating the Most Likely Diagnosis

Rule out septal hematoma.

Health Maintenance and Patient Education and Treatment

- Surgical reduction
- Packing for 2–5 days is often helpful.
- Antibiotics with ant-istaphylococcal coverage should be given for 3–5 days or the duration of the packing.

Professional Considerations

In case of motor vehicle accidents, evaluation for other fractures is important.

Oropharyngeal Disorders

Diseases of the Teeth/Gums

Pathophysiology

Gingival abscesses result from entrapment of food and plaque debris bacterial overgrowth.

Clinical Presentation

Swelling, erythema, tenderness, and fluctuance in the space between the tooth and gingiva. There may be spontaneous purulent drainage from the gingival margin.

Differential Diagnosis/Formulating the Most Likely Diagnosis

Evaluate for periapical infection.

Health Maintenance and Patient Education

Update tetanus if needed.

Treatment (Pharmaceutical and Clinical Intervention)

Oral antibiotic therapy, analgesics, and dental follow-up are indicated.

Professional Considerations

Oral antibiotic therapy, analgesics, and dental follow-up are indicated.

Infectious/Inflammatory Disorders

Aphthous Ulcers

Pathophysiology

Cause is uncertain, although an association with human herpesvirus 6 has been suggested. Stress is a predisposing factor.

Clinical Presentation

- Found on freely moving mucosa
- May be single or multiple, are usually recurrent, and appear as small, round, painful ulcerations with yellow-gray fibrinoid centers surrounded by red halo

Diagnostic and Lab Studies

Based on clinical appearance. When the diagnosis is not clear, incisional biopsy is indicated.

Differential Diagnosis/Formulating the Most Likely Diagnosis

Ulcers may be secondary to the following conditions:

- Erythema multiforme or drug allergies
- Acute herpes simplex
- Pemphigus
- Bullous lichen planus
- Behçet disease
- Inflammatory bowel disease

Health Maintenance and Patient Education

Minor ulcers usually heal in 10–14 days.

Treatment (Pharmaceutical and Clinical Intervention)

- Topical corticosteroids
- A 1-week course of topical steroids may be indicated.

Professional Considerations

Correlated to URI symptoms.

Candidiasis

Pathophysiology

Oral candidiasis is usually painful and looks like creamy-white curd-like patches overlying erythematous mucosa.

Clinical Presentation

Oral candidiasis is commonly associated with the following: (1) use of dentures, (2) poor oral hygiene, (3) diabetes mellitus, (4) anemia, (5) chemotherapy or local irradiation, (6) corticosteroid use, and (7) broad-spectrum antibiotics.

Diagnostic and Lab Studies

The diagnosis is made clinically. A wet preparation using potassium hydroxide will reveal spores.

Differential Diagnosis/Formulating the Most Likely Diagnosis

Leukoplakia or lichen planus (patches are fixed).

Health Maintenance and Patient Education

Rapid resolution of symptoms with appropriate treatment.

Treatment (Pharmaceutical and Clinical Intervention)

Antifungal therapy may be achieved with fluconazole 100 mg orally daily for 7 days or ketoconazole 200–400 mg orally.

Professional Considerations

Candidiasis is often the first manifestation of HIV infection, and HIV testing should be considered in patients with no known predisposing cause for symptoms.

Deep Neck Infection

Pathophysiology

Deep neck abscesses most commonly originate from dental infections. Bacteria include: streptococci, staphylococci, Bacteroides, and Fusobacterium. Patients with diabetes may have different flora, including Klebsiella, and a more aggressive clinical course. Ludwig angina is the most commonly encountered neck space infection.

Clinical Presentation

Patients with deep neck abscesses usually present with marked neck pain and swelling. Fever is common. Patients with Ludwig angina have edema and erythema of the upper neck under the chin and often of the floor of the mouth.

Diagnostic and Lab Studies

Contrast-enhanced CT usually supports the clinical examination and outlines the extent of the infection.

Differential Diagnosis/Formulating the Most Likely Diagnosis

Other possible causes include lymphadenitis, pharyngeal infection, trauma, pharyngeal or esophageal foreign bodies, cervical osteomyelitis, and intravenous injection of the internal jugular vein.

Health Maintenance and Patient Education and Treatment

Recurrent deep neck infection may suggest an underlying congenital lesion, such as a branchial cleft cyst.

Professional Considerations

Abscesses are emergencies because rapid airway compromise may occur.

Epiglottitis

Pathophysiology

May be viral or bacterial in origin.

Clinical Presentation

- Sudden onset of sore throat
- Odynophagia that is disproportional to apparently minimal oropharyngeal findings on examination

Diagnostic and Lab Studies

Lateral plain film radiographs may demonstrate an enlarged epiglottis (the epiglottis "thumb sign"). Swollen, erythematous epiglottis on laryngoscopy.

Differential Diagnosis/Formulating the Most Likely Diagnosis

Careful history and thorough physical will guide the diagnosis.

Health Maintenance and Patient Education

When epiglottitis is recognized early in the adult, it is usually possible to avoid intubation.

Treatment (Pharmaceutical and Clinical Intervention)

- Hospital admission
- Intravenous antibiotics, followed by oral antibiotics
- Dexamethasone
- Corticosteroid (tapered as signs and symptoms resolve)

Professional Considerations

Laryngoscopy is safe for adults.

Herpes Simplex

Pathophysiology

HSV-1 causes acute gingivostomatitis, recurrent herpes labialis (cold sores), keratoconjunctivitis (keratitis), and encephalitis, primarily in adults. Herpes simplex virus is a virus of the nerve roots, which has dermatologic manifestation.

Clinical Presentation

HSV infection presents as grouped vesicles on an erythematous base. Recurrent HSV is typically less severe than the primary infection. The vesicles progress to pustules and crusted erosions.

A prodrome is frequently noted with fever, malaise, anorexia, and regional lymphadenopathy.

Diagnostic and Lab Studies

PCR assay.

Differential Diagnosis/Formulating the Most Likely Diagnosis

Prodrome of viral symptoms is a distinguishing feature.

Health Maintenance and Patient Education

Recurrences of vesicles frequently reappear at the same site.

Treatment (Pharmaceutical and Clinical Intervention)

Acyclovir (Zovirax) is the drug of choice for orolabial herpes.

Professional Considerations

Laryngitis is characterized by hoarseness. Drugs do not eradicate the latent state, but prophylactic, long-term administration of acyclovir, valacyclovir, or famciclovir can suppress clinical recurrences.

Laryngitis

Pathophysiology

Many respiratory viruses have been implicated in acute viral laryngitis, including rhinovirus, influenza virus, adenovirus, coxsackievirus, coronavirus, and RSV. Acute laryngitis can also be associated with acute bacterial respiratory infections such as group A Streptococcus.

Clinical Presentation

Laryngitis is characterized by hoarseness; usually occurs in association with other symptoms and signs of URI, including rhinorrhea, nasal congestion, cough, and sore throat.

Diagnostic and Lab Studies

None indicated.

Differential Diagnosis/Formulating the Most Likely Diagnosis

Chronic disease often includes mucosal nodules and ulcerations visible on laryngoscopy; these lesions are sometimes mistaken for laryngeal cancer.

Health Maintenance and Patient Education

- Concurrent URI symptoms are often present.
- Most cases of acute laryngitis occur in the setting of a viral URI.

Treatment (Pharmaceutical and Clinical Intervention)

Acute laryngitis is usually treated with humidification and voice rest. The choice of therapy for chronic laryngitis depends on the pathogen, whose identification usually requires biopsy with culture.

Professional Considerations

Laryngitis due to *Mycobacterium tuberculosis* is often difficult to distinguish from laryngeal cancer, due to absence of signs, symptoms, and radiographic findings typical of pulmonary disease.

Peritonsillar Abscess

Pathophysiology

When infection extends to the tonsil and the surrounding tissues, peritonsillar cellulitis results.

Clinical Presentation

Peritonsillar abscess and cellulitis present with severe sore throat, odynophagia, trismus, medial deviation of the soft palate and peritonsillar area, and an abnormal muffled ("hot potato") voice.

Diagnostic and Lab Studies

Ultrasound may be a useful to support clinical suspicion, but imaging is not required for the diagnosis.

Differential Diagnosis/Formulating the Most Likely Diagnosis

The existence of an abscess may be confirmed by aspirating pus from the peritonsillar fold superior to the upper pole of the tonsil.

Health Maintenance and Patient Education

Tonsillectomy may be considered.

Treatment (Pharmaceutical and Clinical Intervention)

Patients with peritonsillar abscess present to the emergency department and receive a dose of parenteral amoxicillin (1 g). Less severe cases and patients who are able to tolerate oral intake may be treated for 7–10 days with oral antibiotics.

Professional Considerations

Be sure the abscess is adequately treated, since complications such as extension to the retropharyngeal, deep neck, and posterior mediastinal spaces are possible.

Salivary Disorders and Sialadenitis

Pathophysiology

Typically presents with acute swelling of the gland, increased pain and swelling with meals, and tenderness and erythema of the duct opening (parotid or submandibular gland).

Clinical Presentation

Sialadenitis often occurs in the setting of dehydration or in association with chronic illness.

Ductal obstruction, often by a mucous plug, is followed by salivary stasis and secondary infection.

Diagnostic and Lab Studies

None indicated.

Differential Diagnosis/Formulating the Most Likely Diagnosis

Underlying Sjögren syndrome and chronic periodontitis may be present.

Health Maintenance and Patient Education and Treatment

Treatment consists of intravenous antibiotics, such as nafcillin (1 g intravenously every 4–6 hours), and measures to increase salivary flow, including hydration, warm compresses.

Professional Considerations

If no response to rehydration and intravenous antibiotics; incision and drainage to resolve the infection may be indicated.

Parotitis

Pathophysiology

Salivary gland enlargement can indicate local or systemic disease. Bacterial parotitis presents as a unilateral swelling, where the gland is swollen and tender and usually produces pus at the Stensen's duct.

Clinical Presentation

- **Suppurative:** Acute bacterial parotid infection is seen in debilitated, immunosuppressed, and previously irradiated patients. The gland is swollen, tender, and painful; induration and pitting edema are often present, accompanied by high fever. The duct orifice discharges pus.
- **Non-suppurative:** There is induration of the parotid region, with swelling in front of the tragus and behind the mandible and earlobe. The skin is warm and painful, accentuated by mouth opening or chewing and exquisite tenderness. Fever is common. The duct orifice can be red, occasionally discharging pus.

Diagnostic and Lab Studies

Serum and urinary amylase rise during the first week of parotitis.

Health Maintenance and Patient Education and Treatment

The best way to treat parotitis is directly through intravenous (IV) hydration, analgesics, and 7 to 10 days of IV antibiotics.

Trauma

Pathophysiology

Patient's tooth/teeth are loose.

Clinical Presentation

Multiple methods exist for describing injuries to teeth. The simplest that has clinical applicability is that teeth may be:

- Subluxed (loose, but without change in position)
- Luxated (loose and in a different position than normal)
- Fractured (missing a part of the tooth)
- Avulsed (missing)

Diagnostic and Lab Studies

None indicated.

Differential Diagnosis/Formulating the Most Likely Diagnosis

Focused to history and physical findings of patient.

Health Maintenance and Patient Education and Treatment

If the tooth appears longer than the others, try to push it back firmly into the socket with steady, gentle pressure. If the tooth seems to be pushed ahead of or behind the other teeth (lateral displacement), try to firmly realign.

Professional Considerations

If tooth changes color or if signs of an abscess develop, refer for extraction.

Other Oropharyngeal Disorders

Leukoplakia

Pathophysiology

Histologically, they are keratoses occurring in response to chronic irritation.

Clinical Presentation

A white lesion that cannot be removed by rubbing the mucosal surface. Alcohol and tobacco use are the major epidemiologic risk factors.

Diagnostic and Lab Studies

None indicated.

Differential Diagnosis/Formulating the Most Likely Diagnosis

The differential diagnosis may include oral candidiasis, hyperplasia, median glossitis, and erosive lichen planus.

Health Maintenance and Patient Education

- **Oral lichen planus:** Most commonly presents as lacy leukoplakia but may be erosive; definitive diagnosis requires biopsy.
- **Oral cancer:** Early lesions appear as leukoplakia or erythroplakia; more advanced lesions will be larger, with invasion into the tongue and a mass lesion that is palpable. Ulceration may be present.
- **Oropharynx cancer:** Unilateral throat masses, typically presenting with painful swallowing.

Treatment (Pharmaceutical and Clinical Intervention)

Any area of erythroplakia, enlarging area of leukoplakia, or a lesion that has submucosal depth on palpation should have an incisional biopsy. Fine-needle aspiration (FNA) biopsy may expedite the diagnosis if an enlarged lymph node is found.

Professional Considerations

There are no approved therapies for reversing or stabilizing leukoplakia or erythroplakia.

Practice Questions for Eyes, Ears, Nose, and Throat Review

1. Treatment of bacterial conjunctivitis in the setting of gonococcal infection includes

    (A) amoxicillin 500 mg TID x 14 days.
    (B) ceftriaxone 1 g IM.
    (C) clindamycin 100 mg BID x 21 days.
    (D) ceftriaxone IM plus azithromycin 1,000 mg po.
    (E) ceftriaxone 250 mg IM.

2. Corneal ulcers involve multiple layers of the cornea and may lead to loss of vision if not treated expeditiously and appropriately. Which of the following measures/treatments is contraindicated in management of corneal ulcers?

    (A) Fluoroquinolone antibiotic po
    (B) Topical antibiotics
    (C) Topical corticosteroids
    (D) Vancomycin
    (E) None of the above

3. Keratitis associated with contact lens use is most often caused by

    (A) *Staphylococcus aureus.*
    (B) Streptococci.
    (C) *Moraxella catarrhalis.*
    (D) *Pseudomonas aeruginosa.*
    (E) HSV.

4. You are examining a 3-year-old female with complaints (from mom) of chronic matting of her eyes with crusting. On examination, you note mild swelling over the lacrimal area and, when gently pressed, tears and mucopurulent drainage is expressed. The scerla is mildly injected; however, vision is unimpaired and there are no systemic symptoms. The findings are present in the right eye only. This presentation is consistent with a diagnosis of

    (A) viral conjunctivitis.
    (B) corneal ulcer.
    (C) bacterial conjunctivitis.
    (D) dacrocystitis.
    (E) keratitis.

5. You are examining a 26-year-old patient in the ED. She reports she completely and suddenly lost all vision in his left eye this morning. She reports pain when she moves her eyes. On examination, the optic disc appears normal. Some peripheral vision is retained; however, central vision loss in the affected eye is profound. Based on history and these findings, you suspect

    (A) giant cell arteritis.
    (B) optic neuritis.
    (C) Parkinson's disease
    (D) orbital cellulitis.
    (E) intracranial tumor.

6. Management for wet (neovascular, exudative) macular degeneration includes

   (A) long-term oral corticosteroid administration.
   (B) long-term broad spectrum antibiotic administration.
   (C) long-term antibiotics.
   (D) surgical resection of macular tissue.
   (E) long-term repeated intraocular injections.

7. You are seeing a 30-year-old male in the clinic with a chief complaint of "ringing in the ears," decreased hearing of the right ear, and foul-smelling drainage from the right ear. The patient states the problem has been going on for probably about a year with symptoms waxing and waning. He reports he has always had a lot of ear infections, beginning in childhood. On examination of the affected ear, you note a sac-like structure on the flaccid portion of the TM. The area appears to be filled with exudative material. Purulent drainage is seen in the ear canal. Findings are consistent with

   (A) acute otitis media.
   (B) tympanic membrane perforation.
   (C) mastoiditis.
   (D) cholesteatoma.
   (E) none of the above.

8. The most common cause of acute sinusitis is:

   (A) *Staphylococcus aureus.*
   (B) group B beta-hemolytic streptococci.
   (C) rhinovirus.
   (D) *Psuedomonas aeruginosa.*
   (E) *H. influenzae.*

9. You see a 19-year-old male in the ED who presents with complaints of severe sore throat with fever and difficulty swallowing. You note medial deviation toward the left of the soft palate and peritonsillar area and an abnormal muffled ("hot potato") voice. Your differential diagnoses includes

   (A) peritonsillar abscess.
   (B) mastoiditis.
   (C) necrotizing ulcerative gingitivitis.
   (D) glossitis.
   (E) infectious mononucleosis.

10. Treatment recommendations for management of sialadenitis includes

    (A) oral cephalexin.
    (B) oral augmentin.
    (C) IV nafcillin.
    (D) IV vancomycin.
    (E) oral clindamycin.

Answers Explained

1. **(D)** Conjunctivitis associated with gonococcal infection requires treatment with ceftriaxone and azithromycin together. Opthalmology evaluation is also recommended. (A, B, C, E) These options are not indicated as first-line treatment of gonococcal conjunctivitis.

2. **(C)** Topical corticosteroids are contraindicated in the treatment of corneal ulcers as these agents may worsen the ulcer or delay healing. All other options (A, B, D, E) are used in management of corneal ulcer based on presentation and severity.

3. **(D)** Keratitis in contact lens wearers is most often caused by infection with *Pseudomonas aeruginosa*. (A, B, C, E) These organisms have not been implicated as common causes of keratitis in this population.

4. **(D)** The history of PE findings are consistent with dacrocystitis, which presents with swelling over the lacrimal sac along with tearing, eyelash matting, and crusting. Because this condition is affecting only one eye, the likelihood of conjunctivitis is lessened. The most common organisms associated with dacrocystitis are *Staph aureus* and *Streptococcus*. *E. coli* may be cultured in some cases. Corneal ulcer is found on slit-lamp exam with staining, and the presentation includes pain of the affected eye with a "foreign-body" sensation, which is unilateral. (E) Keratitis does not present with the symptoms described in this scenario.

5. **(B)** Optic neuritis presents with unilateral vision loss and pain with movement of the eyes. This condition is associated with sardoidosis and systemic lupus erythematosus. In fact, optic neuritis is often the initial sign of SLE and should be suspected in patients who present with this condition. (A) Giant cell arteritis occurs mainly in individuals over age 50 and presents with headache, claudication of the jaw, and polymyalgia rheumatica. (C) PD is a progressive neurologic disorder presenting with tremor, rigidity, bradykinesia, and progressive postural instability. Vision loss is not associated with PD. (D) Orbital cellulitis is characterized by proptosis, restricted extraocular movements, fever, and swelling and erythema of the lids. Immediate treatment with IV antibiotics is needed to prevent loss of vision and spread of infection. (E) Brain tumors may present with vision changes and even vision loss depending on location. However, pain with movement of the eyes is not a characteristic finding.

6. **(E)** Management of exudative macular degeneration includes the use of vascular endothelial growth factors (VEGF), which may promote regression of disease and stabilization of vision loss to some extent. Long-term repeated intraocular injections are needed and are given several times per year or monthly based on presentation. (A, B, C, D) These options are not indicated in management of wet macular degneration.

7. **(D)** Cholesteatoma is a form of chronic otitis media caused by prolonged eustachian tube dysfunction and the creation of a squamous epithelium-lined sac, which often becomes impacted and infected. This chronic condition may lead to tinnitus, hearing loss, and purulent drainage. Management is surgical excision of the sac. (A) Acute otitis media presents with pain of the affected ear. On examination, the TM is often erythematous and perforations may be seen with purulent drainage. This infection is often accompanied by fever and, in infants, with poor feeding. (B) TM perforation presents as an acute decrease in hearing or may be asymptomatic. On examination, an open area is seen within the membrane itself. (C) Mastoiditis is inflammation of the mastoid bone behind the ear and may be a complication of severe or untreated acute otitis media. Patients experience postauricular pain and erythema along with a spiking fever. This condition requires IV antibitics initially and, if not improved, may require surgical mastoidectomy.

8. **(C)** Most causes of acute sinusitis are viruses. Patients present with headache, malaise, cough, and nasal drainage. The nasal mucosa is erythematous and engorged. Symptoms are usually self-limiting < 10 days. (A, B, D, E) Acute bacterial sinusitis is less common than viral sinusitis; however, the condition is common and may result from viral sinusitis. The most common pathogens include *Strep pneumoniae*, *H. influenzae*, *Staph aureus*, and *Moraxella catarrhalis*.

9. **(A)** Peritonsillar abscess occurs when bacterial infection penetrates the tonsillar capsule and surrounding tissues. Peritonsillar cellulitis is the result. Patients present with severe sore throat, odynophagia, trismus, medial deviation of the soft palate, and the classic "hot potato voice." IV or po antibiotics are recommended and, for some patients, tonsillectomy is required. (B) Mastoiditis is inflammation of the mastoid bone. Patients present with post-auricular pain and spiking fever. The mastoid bone is often red and tender. IV antibiotics are required to prevent meningitis. (C) Necrotizing ulcerative gingivitis is commonly seen in young adults undergoing stress (college exams, etc.). The infection is caused by spirochetes and fusiform bacilli. Patients present with painful, acute inflammation of the gingival tissue with bleeding often reported. On exam, halitosis is present often with cervical lymphadenopathy. (D) Glossitis is inflammation of the tongue and leads to a red, smooth-surfaced tongue. (E) IM often presents with some degree of pharyngitis; however, symptoms are not consistent with the above presentation.

10. **(C)** Treatment of sialadenitis with IV nafcillin along with measures such as warm compresses and lozenges to increase salivary flow are first-line recommendations. (A, B, D, E) These options are not recommended treatment for sialadenitis.

6

Gastrointestinal/Nutrition Review

Learning Objectives

In this chapter, you will review:

→ Biliary disorders
→ Colorectal disorders
→ Esophageal disorders
→ Gastric disorders
→ Hepatic disorders
→ Ingestion of toxic substances or foreign bodies
→ Metabolic disorders
→ Neoplasms
→ Pancreatic disorders
→ Small intestine disorders

Biliary Disorders

Cholelithiasis

Gallstones are associated with advancing age and obesity and occur twice as frequently in women than men and more frequently in Caucasian and Native American populations than in people of African descent. Cholesterol gallstones are more common in North America in > 75% of cases. Pigmented gallstones are associated with cirrhosis and hemolysis and in those of East Asian descent. Cholelithiasis can be asymptomatic in many patients. Gallstones may remain in the gall-bladder, obstruct the cystic duct, obstruct the common bile duct, obstruct the pancreatic duct, erode into adjacent bowel (i.e., gallstone ileus), or pass into the duodenum. It is also noted that patients can develop gallstones within the common bile duct years after a cholecystectomy, especially if decreased bile flow secondary to stenosis, extrinsic compression, or lesion.

Acute and Chronic Cholecystitis

Pathophysiology

Acute cholecystitis, or inflammation of the gallbladder, is usually caused by obstruction of the cystic duct by gallstones.

Clinical Presentation

Symptoms are usually RUQ abdominal pain, fever, and leukocytosis, but not always. Patients may awaken with RUQ abdominal pain, with radiation to the right infrascapular region in a crescendo-decrescendo pattern over 4–6 hours. Nausea and vomiting may also be associated in the classic presentation of biliary colic. However, acute cholecystitis may present as retrosternal chest pain with normal ECG, heartburn not relieved with antacids, or dyspepsia with nausea.

Diagnostic and Lab Studies

Leukocytosis, possible elevated aminotransferases especially if just passing a gallstone, or normal. There is increased bili. A sonogram usually shows gallstones, possible gallbladder wall thickening, and pericholecystic fluid. Radionuclide biliary scan may indicate lack of filling of the gallbladder, delayed passage of radiotracer to the duodenum.

Chronic cholecystitis is usually the result of repeated episodes of acute cholecystitis, often with chronic thickening/scarring of the gallbladder wall. Patients will often relate a history of repeated episodes of biliary colic but did not seek medical attention. Laboratory studies may indicate leukocytosis. A sonogram will usually indicate gallstones and gallbladder wall thickening. Radionuclide biliary scan, usually without obstruction of biliary tree, may have decreased gallbladder filling and ejection fraction.

Differential diagnosis of RUQ abdominal pain includes:

- Acid peptic disease
- Pancreatitis
- Gastroparesis

Health Maintenance and Patient Education

Usually weight loss, treat metabolic disorders (e.g., diabetes, hyperlipidemia).

Treatment (Pharmaceutical and Clinical Intervention)

- Cholecystectomy
- Conservative, NPO, IVF
- Antibiotics if indicated
- Pain control
- Avoid fatty foods

Professional Considerations

- Gastroenterology consult if not classic presentation
- Surgical consultation re: cholecystectomy

Cholangitis

Pathophysiology

Acute cholangitis is usually caused by bacterial infection with biliary obstruction and migration of bacteria from the duodenum. Procedural intervention (e.g., biliary sphincterotomy), occluded biliary stent, biliary strictures, retained biliary gallstones (choledocholithiais), and neoplasm are the most common causes. Primary sclerosing cholangitis (PSC) is typically seen on MRI/CT as "beading" of the intra- and extra-hepatic bile ducts from recurrent inflammation. It is an autoimmune disorder and often associated with inflammatory bowel disease, especially ulcerative or Crohn's colitis. Increased risk of cholangiocarcinoma in dominant strictures. Patients typically present with RUQ abdominal pain, fever, and jaundice (Charcot triad).

Diagnostics and Lab Studies

Elevated bilirubin, alkaline phosphatase, leuokocytosis, gamma GT, and possible aminotransferases can be seen through the following diagnostics.

Imaging

- *Sonogram*—good sensitivity for biliary ductal dilation but less sensitivity for retained stones, strictures
- *CT abdomen*—good sensitivity/specificity for biliary ductal dilation, extrinsic compression from pancreatic cancer but less sensitive for retained stones
- *MRI/MRCP*—best sensitivity/specificity for retained biliary stones, strictures, and pancreatic neoplasm
- Cholangiography

Differential Diagnosis

Hepatic abscess, perforated duodenal ulcer, pancreatitis, and colonic abscess/perforation.

Health Maintenance and Patient Education

Discuss potential risks/complications from endoscopic/surgical intervention of the biliary tree, and instruct patients to seek immediate medical care should symptoms occur/recur.

Treatment (Pharmaceutical and Clinical Intervention)

- Antibiotics
- ERCP
- Percutaneous cholangiogram (interventional radiology)
- Surgical bypass intervention of strictures, benign/malignant

Professional Considerations

Consultations with:

- Gastroenterology
- Biliary surgery
- Interventional radiology

Acute Hepatitis

Pathophysiology

Hepatitis is an inflammatory process of liver cells often with necrosis caused by a number of etiologies. Viral hepatitis includes hepatitis A (water/food-borne illness), with incubation before symptoms of ~4 weeks, and hepatitis B (from body fluids or blood from infected individuals), with incubation period before symptoms of 2–4 months. In East Asia and the western Pacific Islands, hepatitis B is often passed by vertical transmission at birth in areas with low vaccination rates. Hepatitis C (blood-borne) from blood transfusions, intravenous drug abuse (IVDA), and amateur tattoos is usually asymptomatic in > 80% of patients with virus detectable in blood by PCR

2 weeks after infection but HCV-Ab not detectable for 12–16 weeks. Of viral hepatitis, only B, C, and delta (super infection with B) have a chronic infection, indicated by elevated liver tests for over 6 months and detectable virus.

Toxins, including alcohol and drugs, may also induce an acute hepatitis (drug-induced liver injury, DILI).

Hepatitis may also be caused by autoimmune diseases including autoimmune hepatitis (AIH) with elevated aminotransferases; primary biliary colangitis (PBC), which presents with elevated alkaline phosphatase/GGT and at times elevated aminotransferases; and primary sclerosing cholangits (PSC), a disorder of the bile ducts with inflammatory strictures and often associated with inflammatory bowel disease, which can have elevated bilirubin, alkaline phosphatase, and at times aminotransferases. Metabolic disorders may cause acute and subsequent chronic hepatitis, including hereditary hemochromatosis (iron storage disease); Wilson's disease (copper storage disease); alpha 1 antitrypsin deficiency, which can cause advanced lung and liver injury; and nonalcoholic steatohepatitis (NASH), caused by the metabolic syndrome.

Clinical Presentation

Patients may present to the emergency department with fatigue, flu-like symptoms, and jaundice. Laboratory studies in acute hepatitis usually have aminotransferases (AST/ALT) in the hundreds to thousands and often with hyperbilirubinemia and jaundice.

Differential Diagnosis

Includes other acute viral infections:

- Epstein-Barr virus
- Gallbladder disease with cholangitis
- Pancreatic cancer/pancreatitis

Health Maintenance and Patient Education

Includes contact tracing for acute infectious hepatitis and appropriate vaccination against other liver diseases, including hepatitis A and B.

Professional Considerations

A consultation with gastroenterology/hepatology, if available.

Treatment (Pharmaceutical and Clinical Intervention)

Treatment is often supportive as most patients will recover from acute hepatitis A, B, and toxin exposure.

Autoimmune and metabolic disorders with chronicity may require specific immunosuppressant/modulating medications.

Chronic Hepatitis

Pathophysiology

Chronic hepatitis can be caused by hepatitis C or B, HEV—the autoimmune hepatitis disorders, and metabolic causes. Chronic inflammation may induce fibrosis by the hepatic stellate cells and ultimately develop cirrhosis. Complications of advanced fibrosis/cirrhosis can have significant morbidity and mortality.

Portal hypertension with development of esophageal/gastric varices can develop catastrophic bleeding; ascites and risk for spontaneous bacterial peritonitis with increased mortality; encephalopathy, which can range from mild sleep disturbances to coma, induced by high ammonia levels; and, with more decompensated disease, hepatorenal and hepatopulmonary syndromes. All patients with cirrhosis have increased risks for developing hepatocellular carcinoma, while patients with hemochromatosis and chronic hepatitis B may develop liver cancer in the absence of cirrhosis.

Clinical Presentation

Patients with chronic hepatitis may be asymptomatic or referred when elevated liver enzymes or jaundice occurs. Most patients can be diagnosed accurately with serologies and imaging but some may require liver biopsy for the appropriate diagnosis, e.g., autoimmune or metabolic liver disease.

Assessment of patients with chronic hepatitis includes the staging of the disease, i.e., the extent of fibrosis usually on a 1–4 scale with 1 as mild and 4 as cirrhosis. This can be done by transjugular, percutaneous, or laparoscopic liver biopsy. Indirect methods include Fibroscan, elastography, and MRI. Patients with cirrhosis and portal hypertension will often have splenomegaly, decreased platelets ($<$ 150 k), decreased albumin, elevated bilirubin, and elevated INR. A score is often used to determine the severity of cirrhosis with serum sodium, creatinine, total bilirubin, and INR/protime. A formula indicates a medical end stage liver disease (MELD) score, which can estimate risk of complications from anesthesia, abdominal surgery, or need for liver transplant evaluation.

Differential Diagnosis

Differential diagnosis includes the following malignancies:

- Pancreatic, metastatic colon
- Lymphoma
- Ischemia

Health Maintenance and Patient Education

Discuss with patients and their families the importance of routine labs, serial imaging to screen for liver cancer in patients with cirrhosis, endoscopy to screen for varices in patients with portal hypertension, and chronic management. Provide patient education for prevention of transmission.

Treatment (Pharmaceutical and Clinical Intervention)

Treatment of disease is specific, but some metabolic disorders have no specific treatment other than the contributing factors/diseases, e.g., obesity, diabetes, cardiovascular disease.

Professional Considerations

Consultation with hepatology, if available, or gastroenterology for guidance on treatment and surveillance strategies.

Colorectal Disorders

Inflammatory Bowel Disease (IBD)

Pathophysiology

Inflammatory bowel disease (IBD) is an umbrella term used to describe disorders causing chronic inflammation of the gastrointestinal tract. IBD includes two conditions:

- Crohn's disease (CD)
- Ulcerative colitis (UC)

Both are chronic, recurrent, inflammatory diseases characterized by periods of exacerbation (flares) and remission.

Crohn's disease (CD) involves mainly the terminal ileum and proximal ascending colon but can affect any segment of the gastrointestinal tract from the mouth to the anus. The rectum is spared.

- Most commonly on right side
- It is characterized by a patchy, noncontinuous presentation.
- The inflammation is transmural (it can involve the five layers of the GI tract); as a result, it can cause ulcerations, strictures, fistula development, and abscess formation.

Ulcerative colitis (UC) mainly involves the sigmoid colon and rectum.

- It is characterized by diffuse inflammation and frailty of the mucosa and/or submucosa (two outermost layers).
- It can extend proximally in a continuous fashion.

Clinical Presentation

Crohn's Disease Signs

- Crohn's disease can lead to transmural inflammation of all layers of the gut; therefore, ulceration, strictures, fistulas, perianal abscesses, skin tags, or anal fissures can develop. Fistulas can extend and penetrate adjacent structures in the abdomen or retroperitoneally. Fistulas extending to the abdomen can cause bacterial overgrowth.
- Fistulas extending to the urinary bladder can lead to recurrent UTIs, urine with feces, and painful urination. Those extending to the vagina can lead to malodorous discharge and issues with hygiene. Fistulas and abscess should be suspected if the patient presents with symptoms like the ones previously mentioned, or if fever, chills, and elevated white blood cell count is present.
- Patients can also present with cholelithiasis (gallstones) and/or nephrolithiasis (kidney stones) due to intestinal dysfunction and malabsorption of bile, urate, or calcium oxalate. Diarrhea in CD occurs due to malabsorption of bile salts (which are absorbed mainly in the ileum) or lactase deficiency (produced in the small intestine).

Crohn's Disease Symptoms

- Patients may complain of bouts of right lower quadrant (RLQ) or periumbilical abdominal pain, tenderness, cramping, or a mass. Why abdominal right lower quadrant (RLQ)? Because the most common area affected (≈50% of cases) is the terminal ileus (ileitis) extending to the proximal ascending colon (ileocolitis). Why "mass-like" areas? Due to loops of inflamed intestine that can also lead to narrowing of the lumen, spasms, and fibrotic stenosis.

- These changes can cause excessive postprandial bloating and loud rumbling noises related to movement of fluids and gasses in the intestines.
- Patients can also complain of excessive fatigue and intermittent non-bloody diarrhea (although unlikely, it can be bloody with fecal urgency like UC).
- Other symptoms may include:
  - Fevers
  - Chills
  - Malaise
  - Weight loss with nutritional deterioration

Ulcerative Colitis Signs

- Ulcerative colitis involves the mucosal and/or submucosal layers of the rectosigmoid area (proctosigmoiditis), but it can also extend proximally to the splenic flexure and beyond.
- Diffuse friability can cause erosions and bleeding.
- UC is more common in nonsmokers or former smokers. Surprisingly, for those smokers with active disease, exacerbations and severity may worsen if they quit smoking.

Ulcerative Colitis Symptoms

- Bloody diarrhea (Hematochezia) and fecal urgency are the hallmarks of this condition.
- Patients can also present with left lower quadrant (LLQ) abdominal pain (rectosigmoid area), cramps, and tenesmus.
- The recurrence of symptoms and frequency of episodes may help the provider determine the severity of the disease (mild, moderate, or severe).
- In severe cases, patients can also develop orthostatic hypotension, hypovolemia, severe anemia, and deterioration in nutritional status with hypoalbuminemia.

Diagnostic and Lab Studies

IBD diagnosis is based on clinical picture, supported by endoscopic, radiologic, histologic, and pathologic findings. There is no one specific test to make a CD or UC unequivocal diagnosis.

If Crohn's disease is suspected, colonoscopy and capsule imaging are useful procedures to evaluate the terminal ileum and colon. EGD is only considered in patients with upper GI signs and symptoms. Typical findings include ulcers, strictures, and asymmetric areas of granulomatous inflammation adjacent to areas of normal-appearing mucosa (patchy appearance). Colonic mucosa biopsies may report granulomas; however, they are present in only one-fourth of the cases.

- CT/MRI enterography uses contrast to identify areas of bowel wall thickening, vascularity, and mucosal changes, as well as fat stranding.
- Fat stranding, although nonspecific, is suggestive of infectious, inflammatory, malignant, or traumatic processes.
- Barium-based small bowel imaging can also help with identification of ulcers, strictures (string sign), and fistulas.
- It should be considered in patients with obstructive symptoms and, also, previous to video capsule endoscopy to decrease risk of capsule retention.

Ulcerative colitis mainly extends from the anal verge to the rectosigmoid junction. These changes are referred to as proctitis or UC Category I, and sigmoidoscopy is the preferred alternative for proper evaluation. Affected areas extending proximally may require alternative procedures. UC Category II or left-sided colitis (sigmoid to splenic flexure) and UC Category III or extensive colitis (beyond the splenic flexure) require colonoscopy. Symptoms or findings to suggest proximal GI involvement may require EGD or cross-sectional imaging; however, findings beyond the ileum are highly suggestive of Crohn's disease (CD) rather than UC.

Colonoscopy should be avoided in severe UC disease due to risk of perforation. Consider this option (instead of sigmoidoscopy) to assess the extent of UC colonic disease only in times of remission or when the patient demonstrates improvement with therapy. Edema, friability, mucopus (mucus + pus), erosions, and red blood on rectal examination are common findings in UC endoscopic evaluations. Plain radiographs are useful in severe UC given probability of significant colonic dilation. Contrast in the form of barium-based images and enemas should be avoided for severe UC evaluation given increased risk of toxic megacolon.

Laboratory findings in IBD are not specific; however, results are expected to reflect blood and fecal changes associated with mucosal damage such as bleeding, infection, intestinal protein loss, and malabsorption. Low hemoglobin, low hematocrit, leukocytosis, hypoalbuminemia, as well as iron (Fe), vitamin B12, and vitamin D deficiencies, are common findings. Fecal fat is also indicative of malabsorption.

Although not specific, changes in blood and fecal laboratory results can be used to assess disease severity and monitor response to treatment. Multiple blood and fecal inflammatory markers can be elevated in the setting of inflammation.

Some of the most common include:

- Serum C-reactive protein (CRP): It is an acute-phase reactant produced by the liver that goes up with inflammation seen in a subset of patients with CD. It has a short half-life of 19 hours. Because of its short half-life, serum concentrations decrease quickly, making CRP a useful marker to detect and monitor inflammation.
- Erythrocyte sedimentation rate (ESR): It is nonspecific and may be elevated in patients with Crohn's disease. It does not differentiate IBD patients from those with irritable bowel syndrome or healthy controls.
- Fecal calprotectin (fCal): It is a calcium-binding protein that is derived from neutrophils and plays a role in the regulation of inflammation. Fecal calprotectin is elevated in infectious and inflammatory colitis but not in noninflammatory causes of diarrhea such as irritable bowel syndrome; therefore, it is a helpful test to differentiate between IBD and IBS.
- Fecal lactoferrin (FL): It is an iron-binding protein found in secondary granules of neutrophils.

The two fecal-derived markers of intestinal inflammation, fecal lactoferrin (FL) and fecal calprotectin (fCal), are superior to serologic tests ESR and CRP. ESR and CRP usefulness is limited, given they can be normal in up to 40% of patients with inflammation. Fecal calprotectin and fecal lactoferrin measurements can also be useful in monitoring disease activity and differentiating IBD from IBS. IBD signs and symptoms can overlap with infectious enteritis and colitis. Stool studies become useful in ruling out common pathogens such as bacteria, ova, parasites, and *C. diff.*

Differential Diagnosis/Formulating the Most Likely Diagnosis

Distribution and depth of colonic mucosal involvement are key features to differentiate between UC and CD; however, when these affect only the colon, differentiation between the two, can be challenging. Testing for common pathogens helps rule out infectious etiologies. Undiagnosed AIDS, intestinal lymphoma, tuberculosis, and CMV infection can also present with fever, pain, weight loss, and radiographic similarities. *C. diff* and CMV infections can mimic disease recurrence. consider testing if there is concern. Fecal calprotectin is elevated in infectious and inflammatory colitis but not in noninflammatory causes of diarrhea, such as irritable bowel syndrome; therefore, it is a helpful test to differentiate between IBD and IBS. Celiac disease serologic testing can also be considered in patients with diarrhea.

Health Maintenance and Patient Education

Cigarette smoking is strongly associated with development, exacerbation, progression, and recurrence of CD; it also worsens resistance to medical therapy. Active smoking cessation programs are encouraged. NSAID avoidance is strongly recommended. Stress, depression, and anxiety should be addressed during evaluation of IBD patients because they can exacerbate flares, as well as lead to decreased quality of life and low adherence to treatment.

IBD patients have an increased risk of colon cancer; therefore, annual screening for dysplasia or cancer with EGD/colonoscopy is recommended for patients with a history of 8 or more years. Although rare, these patients have a higher risk of lymphoma and small bowel adenocarcinoma. As expected, many nutritional changes are recommended to avoid further irritation, exacerbated symptoms, and complications in IBD patients. Fried or greasy foods should be avoided, as well as lactose, nuts, popcorn, or coffee. Raw fruits or vegetables can exacerbate constipation and bloating. Good hydration is of essence, especially if the patient is complaining of diarrhea or experiencing hypotension symptoms. Malabsorption is common; therefore, intramuscular vit B12 and iron infusions may be necessary. In severe cases, supplemental enteral therapy is needed, especially in kids with growth retardation.

Treatment (Pharmaceutical and Clinical Intervention)

Overall treatment approach and maintenance of IBD patients is mainly directed towards terminating the acute symptomatic attacks, reducing the rate of disease progression, preventing recurrence of symptoms, and improving quality of life. Therapy is selected based on disease location, level of activity, extent of inflammation, severity, and prognostic factors. Pharmacologic agents are the same for UC and CD. They may include oral, topical (rectal), and systemic therapies, as well as surgery (resection). Treatment of IBD is usually divided into induction and maintenance therapy. The phases involve achieving control of inflammation relatively quickly (acute disease control with induction of remission—over 3 months or less) and then sustaining that control for prolonged periods of time (maintenance of remission—beyond 3 months). The ideal goal is to obtain and maintain a steroid-free remission.

Specific Drug Therapies
- 5-aminosalicylates (5-ASA): sulfasalazine, mesalamine
- Antibiotics: metronidazole, ciprofloxacin, rifaximin
- Corticosteroids: budesonide, prednisone
- Immunomodulators: azathioprine, mercaptopurine, methotrexate

Biologics
- Anti-TNF agents: infliximab, adalimumab, certolizumab pegol
- Agent targeting leukocyte trafficking: vedolizumab, natalizumab
- Anti-p40 (anti-IL-12/23) antibody: ustekinumab
- 5-ASA agents are used as initial treatment in the setting of acute mild-to-moderate active symptoms.
- Corticosteroids suppress acute severe symptoms dramatically.

Patients that require long-term corticosteroids should also be given an immunomodulatory drug. Corticosteroids are down titrated while the immunomodulatory drug is up titrated based on disease response. Agents are continuously adjusted until the goal of "steroid-free remission" is achieved.

The most recent data suggests that the "step-up maintenance therapy," which uses corticoids followed by azathioprine and subsequently Infliximab, is obsolete. Early use of anti-TNF agents in combination with an immunomodulator is preferred and reduces risk of antibody development against the anti-TNF agent. However, it may increase risk of complications such as non-Hodgkin lymphoma and opportunistic infections. Anti-TNF agents should be used to treat disease that is resistant to treatment with corticosteroids. Combination therapy of anti-TNF agents with immunomodulators is more effective than treatment with immunomodulators alone.

Symptomatic Medications

- Secretory diarrhea, due to reduced absorption caused by mucosal changes or resection, is responsive to cholestyramine, colestipol, and colesevelam. The medications bind to the malabsorbed bile salts.
- Diarrhea due to lactase deficiency may respond to loperamide.
- Enteral fistulas and impaired motility can lead to bacterial overgrowth, which sometimes presents as bloating. A course of broad-spectrum antibiotics may be beneficial in these cases.

Irritable Bowel Syndrome (IBS)

Pathophysiology

Irritable bowel syndrome (IBS) is a gut-brain interaction functional disorder characterized by chronic (more than 6 months) recurrent gastrointestinal symptoms, with no evident structural or biochemical abnormalities.

- Episodes usually present with abnormal motility (disordered defecation) related to abdominal pain (visceral hypersensitivity) or emotional stress (altered central nervous system processing: anxiety, depression, somatization).
- Syndrome can be classified into three categories based on the predominant bowel movement: IBS with diarrhea (IBS-D), IBS with constipation (IBS-C) or IBS with mixed constipation and diarrhea (IBS-M).

Clinical Presentation

Presentation includes abdominal pain or discomfort that has two of the three following features:

1. Relief with defecation
2. Change in frequency of stools
3. Change in form or appearance of stool (lumpy or hard, loose or watery)

Constipation may be reported as less than three bowel movements a week. Diarrhea may be reported as more than three bowel movements a day. Mixed syndrome includes a firm stool in the morning, followed by multiple loose stools the rest of the day.

Additional Symptoms

- Distention or bloating
- Abnormal stool passage
- Straining
- Urgency

Signs

- Symptoms usually begin in late teens to early 20s, and two out of three patients are women.
- Hematochezia
- Fever
- Weight loss
- Severe diarrhea
- Severe constipation

New onset after 40 years old are features not compatible with IBS and warrant further evaluation.

Diagnostics and Lab Studies

IBS is a diagnosis of exclusion. In patients with IBS-D, serologic testing to rule out celiac disease (CD) is recommended.

- Fecal calprotectin (fCal) is a calcium-binding protein that is derived from neutrophils and plays a role in the regulation of inflammation. Fecal calprotectin is elevated in infectious and inflammatory colitis but not in noninflammatory causes of diarrhea such as irritable bowel syndrome. fCal is a helpful test to differentiate between IBD and IBS.
- Of the serologic testing available, CRP has the highest utility for distinguishing IBD from IBS. Serum C-reactive protein (CRP) is an acute-phase reactant produced by the liver that has a short half-life of 19 hours. Because of its short half-life, serum concentrations decrease quickly, making CRP a useful marker to detect and monitor inflammation.

Although not specific, the combination of CRP with fCal may provide even greater discrimination. Stool testing for enteric pathogens in patients with IBS is not recommended because treatment for bacterial and viral infections does not prevent development of IBS. The only exception is patients with high pretest probability and definite risk factors for Giardia exposure. Testing for food allergies or sensitivities is not recommended.

Differential Diagnosis/Formulating the Most Likely Diagnosis

Multiple disorders can present with similar symptoms including colon cancer, IBD, parasites, celiac disease, lactase deficiency, bacterial overgrowth, thyroid issues, and psychiatric disorders.

Consider evaluation for those conditions if the presumed IBS patient does not improve within 2–4 weeks of empiric treatment.

Health Maintenance and Patient Education

Emphasis of treatment is on finding better ways to cope with symptoms. Patients should be educated about the gut-mind interaction and exacerbation of symptoms by environmental, social, and psychological factors. Colonoscopy is not recommended for IBS patients younger than 45 years old.

A patient's lifestyle modifications may include smoking cessation, low fat foods, avoiding sorbitol-containing foods, and cruciferous vegetables

Treatment (Pharmaceutical and Clinical Intervention)

The elimination of dietary fermentable oligosaccharides, disaccharides, monosaccharides, and polyols (FODMAPs) is popular as an IBS treatment. FODMAPs lead to increased GI water secretion and increased fermentation in the colon, thus producing short-chain fatty acids and gases that can lead to luminal distension and the triggering of meal-related symptoms, such as bloating, flatulence, and diarrhea.

Some examples include fructose (corn, syrups, apples, pears, honey, watermelon, raisins), lactose, fructans (garlic, onions, leeks, asparagus, artichokes), wheat-based products (breads, pasta, cereals, cakes), sorbitol (stone fruits), and raffinose (legumes, lentils, brussel sprouts, soybeans, cabbage). Given the variety of IBS symptoms, no single pharmacologic agent is expected to provide relief and those should be considered only when patients do not respond to conservative management. Categorizing patients per IBS subtype improves patient therapy. Considerations for classification include: predominant stool consistency and number of days having abnormal movements. Evaluation should be made during a 2-week period while off treatment. Patterns include D, C, M, or undetermined. Currently, there are no approved medications for the treatment of IBS-M or IBS-U. When needed, medications are targeted towards the dominant symptom: pain, constipation, or diarrhea.

Global IBS
- Not recommended: antispasmodics, probiotics, fecal transplant
- Recommended: peppermint, TCAs, gut-directed psychotherapies

IBS-C
- Not recommended: polyethylene glycol (PEG) products, which are osmotic laxatives
- Recommended: chloride channel activators; guanylate cyclase activators; 5-HT4 agonist tegaserod in women younger than 65 years with number-one cardiovascular risk factors, who have not adequately responded to secretagogues

IBS-D
- Not recommended: bile acid sequestrants
- Recommend: rifaximin; alosetron in women with severe symptoms who have failed conventional therapy; mixed opioid agonists/antagonists

Professional Considerations

Although the true prevalence of anorectal dysfunction in IBS is unknown, the estimated rate is 40%, and it occurs in all subtypes of IBS (IBS-D, IBS-C, and IBS-M). Anorectal physiology testing is recommended for patients with IBS and symptoms suggestive of a pelvic floor disorder and/or refractory constipation not responsive to standard medical therapy.

Esophageal Disorders

Esophagitis

Pathophysiology

Esophagitis is the inflammation of the esophageal mucosa and can be caused by acid-peptic disease (i.e., gastroesophageal reflux disease), rarely bile reflux, infection, allergic reaction, or medications.

Clinical Presentation

Acid-peptic disease, associated with GERD as below, usually affects the distal esophagus, as does bile reflux esophagitis.

Allergy-associated esophagitis, eosinophilic esophagitis (EoE), can be associated with acid reflux or allergies, including environmental and food, and is more common in the atopic individual. Patients will often c/o dysphagia to solids and retrosternal discomfort.

Medication-induced esophagitis can cause erosions and deep ulcerations and is usually associated with odynophagia, painful retrosternal swallowing, with radiation to the back. Medications frequently associated with pill-induced esophagitis include tetracycline/doxycycline, slow release KCl tablets, alendronate and other bisphosphonates, and NSAIDs including ASA. The location of the inflammation/ulcer is frequently at the level of the bifurcation of the trachea/bronchi in the mid-upper third of the esophagus.

Infectious esophagitis is also seen in patients with recent antibiotic exposure, immunosuppression, and immune-incompetence. Frequent infections are Candida, which can be asymptomatic and herpetic infections, which are usually very painful and often prompt an ED visit.

Diagnosis

Diagnosed usually by endoscopy and biopsies, if needed.

Differential Diagnoses/Formulating the Most Likely Diagnosis

Differential diagnoses can include cardiac ischemia, pneumonia, dissecting ascending aortic, and aneurysm.

Health Maintenance and Patient Education

- Lifestyle modifications for GERD, drink plenty of water with medications, and stay upright for 30 min.
- Inform patients of potential issues with sustained-release medications, especially in the elderly.
- Avoid irritatnts such as smoking, EtOH, chocolate, caffeine, spicy foods, NSAIDs, beta-blockers, and calcium channel blockers.
- Weight loss, if obese
- Pregnancy can exacerbate symptoms.

Treatment (Pharmaceutical and Clinical Intervention)

- Acid suppression (H2 blockers, PPIs), sucralfate liquid, bile acid sequestrants, d/c of harmful mediations. EoE may respond to acid suppression in up to 50% of patients, but most need allergy testing and treatment with an inhaled but swallowed steroid, e.g., budesonide, fluticasone.

Professional Considerations

- Gastroenterology and, with suspected EoE, allergy/immunology consultations

Pancreatic Disorders

Acute Pancreatitis

Pathophysiology

Acute inflammation of the pancreas with alcohol toxicity and gallstones causing > 66% of cases. Other causes include:

- Hypertriglyceridemia (> 500)
- Drug toxicity, e.g., azathioprine, sulfonamides; genetic (familial, hereditary)
- Cigarette smoking and exacerbation of any of the above

Morbidity is 10–15% and mortality of 20–30% if Ranson criteria is met: hypotension, hypocalcemia, fall in hct > 10%, hypoxemia, hypoalbuminemia, and increased BUN after hydration within the first 48 hours.

Clinical Presentation

Patients usually present with upper abdominal pain (LUQ > RUQ) and Epigastric pain, with radiation to the back and associated with nausea and vomiting. Laboratory abnormalities include elevated pancreatic enzymes, lipase > specificity than amylase, aminotransferases (AST/ALT) if recent passage of gallstone, and radiographic cross-sectional imaging of pancreatic inflammation.

Differential Diagnosis

Includes peptic ulcer disease, diverticulitis, and cholangitis.

Treatment (Pharmaceutical and Clinical Intervention)

- IV fluid hydration, npo, monitor for worsening signs/labs, Ranson criteria.
- Antibiotics given if presence of necrotizing or infectious pancreatitis features

Health Maintenance and Patient Education

Avoid alcohol and cigarette smoking; weight loss is recommended if obese.

Professional Consideration

Gastroenterology and surgical consultations early in admission, especially if suspicion for gallstone-induced pancreatitis.

Chronic Pancreatitis

Pathophysiology

Commonly caused by chronic alcohol use disorder; severe acute necrotizing pancreatitis; cystic fibrosis, familial, repeated episodes of acute pancreatitis; and idiopathic.

Clinical Presentation

Patients usually present with chronic upper abdominal pain, usually LUQ and radiation to the back and a type of neuropathic pain. Nausea and vomiting frequently experienced with exacerbations. Associated conditions include exocrine pancreatic insufficiency with steatorrhea, fat soluble vitamin (A, D, E, and K) deficiencies, vit B12 deficiency, small intestinal bacterial overgrowth (SIBO), and insulin-dependent diabetes with significant loss of gland function, termed type 3.

Diagnosis

- Cross-sectional radiography with calcifications, dilation of main pancreatic duct
- Pancreatic enzymes, amylase/lipase may be normal during exacerbations
- Decreased serum trypsinogen and fecal pancreatic elastase can be reduced as well and an indicator of need for pancreatic enzyme supplementation.

Differential Diagnosis/Formulating the Most Likely Diagnosis

Other neuropathic pain syndromes, malabsorption syndromes, e.g., SIBO, and functional GI disorders, e.g., gastroparesis.

Health Maintenance and Patient Education

Patients should avoid all alcohol use and cigarette smoking.

Treatment (Pharmaceutical and Clinical Intervention)

Similar to treatments for neuropathic pains with non-narcotic analgesia, little indication for celiac plexus block unless carcinoma as not durable. Pancreatic enzyme and vitamin supplementation as indicated. Dietary modification with avoidance of fatty foods and large volume meals. Endoscopic therapy with ERCP for pancreatic duct strictures, obstructions by calculi in select patients. Surgical intervention helpful in some patients (e.g., Peustow or Frey procedures) to "filet" the pancreas and allow drainage into a jejunal limb.

Professional Consideration

Consultation with gastroenterology for complications and possible endoscopic therapy.

Surgical consultation for advanced chronic pancreatitis and pain. Pain management specialists helpful with use of non-narcotic analgesia and methods as used for other neuropathic pain syndromes.

Acute Hepatitis

Pathophysiology

Hepatitis is an inflammatory process of liver cells, often with necrosis. It can be caused by a number of etiologies.

Viral hepatitis includes hepatitis A (water/food-borne illness) with incubation before symptoms of ~4 weeks.

Hepatitis B is from body fluids or blood from infected individuals, with an incubation period before symptoms of 2–4 months. In East Asia and the western Pacific Islands it is often passed by vertical transmission at birth in areas with low vaccination rates.

Hepatitis C (blood-borne), from blood transfusions, IVDA, amateur tattoos, is usually asymptomatic in > 80% of patients with virus detectable in blood by PCR 2 weeks after infection but HCV-Ab not detectable for 12–16 weeks.

Clinical Presentation

Patients may present to the emergency department with fatigue, flu-like symptoms, and jaundice. Laboratory studies in acute hepatitis usually have aminotransferases (AST/ALT) in the hundreds to thousands and often with hyperbilirubinemia and jaundice.

Diagnosis

Of viral hepatitis only B, C, and delta (super infection with B) have a chronic infection, indicated by elevated liver tests for over 6 months and detectable virus. Toxins, including alcohol and drugs, may also induce an acute hepatitis (drug induced liver injury, DILI). Hepatitis may also be caused by autoimmune diseases, including autoimmune hepatitis (AIH) with elevated aminotransferases, primary biliary colangitis (PBC), which presents with elevated alkaline phosphatase/GGT and, at times, elevated aminotransferases.

- Primary sclerosing cholangits (PSC), a disorder of the bile ducts with inflammatory strictures and often associated with inflammatory bowel disease, which can have elevated bilirubin, alkaline phosphatase, and, at times, aminotransferases

- Metabolic disorders may cause acute and subsequent chronic hepatitis, including hereditary hemochromatosis (iron storage disease); Wilson's disease (copper storage disease); Alpha 1 antitrypsin deficiency, which can cause advanced lung and liver injury; and nonalcoholic steatohepatitis (NASH), caused by the metabolic syndrome.

Differential Diagnosis

Includes other acute viral infections, e.g., Epstein-Barr virus, gallbladder disease with cholangitis, and pancreatic cancer/pancreatitis.

Health Maintenance and Patient Education

Includes contact tracing for acute infectious hepatitis, appropriate vaccination against other liver diseases, including hepatitis A and B.

Professional Considerations

Consultation with gastroenterology/hepatology, if available.

Treatment (Pharmaceutical and Clinical Intervention)

Treatment of acute hepatitis is often supportive, as most patients will recover from acute hepatitis A, B, and toxin exposure. Autoimmune and metabolic disorders with chronicity may require specific immunosuppressant/modulating medications.

Chronic Hepatitis

Pathophysiology

Chronic hepatitis can be caused by chronic hepatitis C or B, the autoimmune hepatitis disorders, and metabolic causes. Chronic inflammation may induce fibrosis by the hepatic stellate cells and ultimately develop cirrhosis. Complications of advanced fibrosis/cirrhosis can have significant morbidity and mortality. Portal hypertension with development of esophageal/gastric varices can develop catastrophic bleeding; ascites and risk for spontaneous bacterial peritonitis with increased mortality; encephalopathy induced by high ammonia levels which can range from mild sleep disturbances to coma; and, with more decompensated disease, hepatorenal and hepato-pulmonary syndromes. All patients with cirrhosis have increased risks for developing hepatocellular carcinoma, while patients with hemochromatosis and chronic hepatitis B may develop liver cancer in the absence of cirrhosis.

Clinical Presentation

Patients with chronic hepatitis may be asymptomatic or referred when elevated liver enzymes or jaundice occurs. Most patients are diagnosed accurately with serologies and imaging, but some may require liver biopsy for the appropriate diagnosis, e.g., autoimmune or metabolic liver disease.

Diagnosis and Lab Studies

Assessment of patients with chronic hepatitis includes the staging of the disease, i.e., the extent of fibrosis, usually on a 1–4 scale with 1 as mild and 4 as cirrhosis. This can be done by transjugular, percutaneous, or laparoscopic liver biopsy. Indirect methods include Fibroscan, elastography, and MRI.

- Patients with cirrhosis and portal hypertension will often have splenomegaly, decreased platelets ($<$ 150 k), decreased albumin, elevated bilirubin, and elevated INR. A score is often used to determine the severity of cirrhosis with serum sodium, creatinine, total bilirubin, and INR/protime.
- A formula indicates a medical end-stage liver disease (MELD) score, which can estimate risk of complications from anesthesia, abdominal surgery, or need for liver transplant evaluation.

Differential Diagnosis

Includes malignancies, e.g., pancreatic, metastatic colon, lymphoma, or ischemia.

Health Maintenance and Patient Education

Discuss with patients and their families the importance of routine labs, serial imaging to screen for liver cancer in patients with cirrhosis, endoscopy to screen for varices in patients with portal hypertension, and chronic management.

Treatment (Pharmaceutical and Clinical Intervention)

Treatment is disease specific but some metabolic disorders have no specific treatment other than the contributing factors/diseases, e.g., obesity, diabetes, and cardiovascular disease.

Professional Considerations

Consultation with hepatology, if available, or gastroenterology for guidance on treatment and surveillance strategies.

Practice Questions for Gastrointestinal/Nutrition Review

1. Your patient is a 38-year-old male who presents to the ED with complaints of abdominal pain in his right upper quadrant, fever with chills, and nausea. He states the symptoms have been progressively getting worse over the past few days. He has had several episodes of pain over the past few months; however, this is his worst episode yet. On examination, you note significant jaundice. He rates his pain at a 9 out of 10 and has difficulty lying still on the bed. Based on this presentation, you suspect cholangitis. RUQ abdominal pain, jaundice, and fever with chills represents

   (A) Budd-Chiari syndrome.
   (B) Charcot triad.
   (C) alpha-1-antitrypsin abnormality.
   (D) gastrinoma triangle.
   (E) Murphy sign.

2. You see a patient who presents with severe pain in the right upper quadrant of the abdomen along with nausea and vomiting. The patient states she has experienced this before, usually after eating a big meal. She states the pain would usually subside if she vomited. On physical examination you find marked tenderness of the RUG of the abdomen with guarding and rebound tenderness. You note the patient "holds her breath" while you are palpating her upper abdominal area. This particular finding is called

   (A) Murphy sign.
   (B) Shawl sign.
   (C) Ranson criteria.
   (D) Ogilvie syndrome.
   (E) Mayer reflex.

3. Your patient is a 45-year-old male with a history of IV drug abuse. He presents with nausea, vomiting, poor appetite, and jaundice. In addition, he tells you that, although he has been a heavy cigarette smoker for several years, recently he finds he can't stand to be around cigarette smoke. Among your differential diagnoses is acute hepatitis B. You order lab studies and understand that the first biochemical finding in the presence of acute hepatitis B is

   (A) anti-HBs.
   (B) HBeAg.
   (C) anti-HBc.
   (D) HBsAg.
   (E) HBV DNA.

4. You are treating a patient in the ED with a known history of cirrhosis of the liver. The patient has been in and out of the hospital several times for paracentesis and blood transfusions due to coagulopathies. Today, the patient, a 34-year-old male, is experiencing severe shortness of breath that actually improves when the head of his bed is lowered. His pulse oximetry reading is 94% on room air. This also improves when he is lying down. Based on these findings, you suspect which of the following complications of cirrhosis?

   (A) Hepatopulmonary syndrome
   (B) Hepatic encephalopathy
   (C) Hepatorenal syndrome
   (D) Spontaneous bacterial peritonitis
   (E) Cardiorenal syndrome

5. Cholelithiasis, or gallstones, is seen more commonly in females, with highest rates in individuals over age 60 years. There is significantly increased incidence of gallstones in Pima and other American Indians. There is also an increased incidence of gallstones in persons with which diagnosis?

   (A) IBS (irritable bowel syndrome)
   (B) Appendicitis
   (C) Crohn's disease
   (D) Peptic ulcer disease
   (E) Pyogenic hepatic abscess

6. Your clinic patient is a 56-year-old male with a history of ulcerative colitis. Today, he presents with a chief complaint of severe left lower quadrant abdominal pain, bloody diarrhea, and fecal urgency. He also reports a low-grade fever for the past several days. In order to assess the severity of his disease, you consider all of the following studies, except

   (A) fecal lactoferrin level (FL).
   (B) fecal calprotectin (fCal) level.
   (C) colonoscopy.
   (D) abdominal CT.
   (E) MRI.

7. Management of mild-to-moderate symptoms of proctitis associated with ulcerative colitis may include the use of

   (A) alvimopan.
   (B) mesalamine.
   (C) adalimumab.
   (D) injection sclerotherapy.
   (E) cyclosporine.

8. Several medications have been implicated in the development of erosive esophagitis. All of the following agents may contribute to erosive esophagitis, except

   (A) slow-release potassium chloride (KCl).
   (B) doxycycline.
   (C) alendronate.
   (D) cephalexin.
   (E) celecoxib.

9. A large majority of cases of acute pancreatitis are caused by

   (A) alcohol toxicity.
   (B) decreased triglyceride levels.
   (C) elevated HDL cholesterol levels.
   (D) autoimmune disease.
   (E) cholelithiasis.

10. Your patient is a 68-year-old male with a history of chronic pancreatitis. He reports episodes of steatorrhea (fatty stools) and cramping LLQ abdominal pain. Exocrine pancreatic insufficiency is treated with

    (A) biologic immunomodulators.
    (B) lipase.
    (C) tramadol.
    (D) broad-spectrum antibiotics.
    (E) long-term corticosteroids.

Answer Explanations

1. **(B)** Charcot triad is the combination of jaundice, right upper quadrant abdominal pain, and fever with chills. This is a classic presentation of acute cholangitis. (A) Budd-Chiari syndrome is a disorder involving venous obstruction of the hepatic system. (C) Alpha-1-antitrypsin clearance serves as a diagnostic marker for gut disorders associated with protein loss and malabsorption. (D) The gastrinoma triangle is an anatomical area consisting of the porta hepatis, the neck of the pancreas, and the third portion of the duodenum. This area is the site of approximately 80% primary gastrinoma development, often associated with Zollinger-Ellison syndrome. (E) Murphy sign is a test for gallbladder disease. Patients are asked to inhale and experience pain on abdominal palpation.

2. **(A)** Murphy sign is inhibition of inspiration because of pain upon abdominal palpation of the right upper quadrant. (B) The Shawl sign is a characteristic rash covering the face, neck, shoulder, upper chest, and back in patients with immune-mediated myopathic disease. (C) Ranson criteria is a method used to assess the severity of acute pancreatitis. (D) Ogilvie syndrome is acute colonic pseudo-obstruction, which occurs in patients postoperatively or with severe medical illness. There is severe abdominal distention with absent or very mild abdominal pain. On imaging, massive dilation of the cecum or right colon is seen. (E) Mayer reflex is elicited by grasping the ring finger and flexing it at the MTP joint. Normal reponses are adduction and apposition of the thumb. This test may be used to assess for disease of the pyramidal system.

3. **(D)** The appearance of the hepatitis B surface antigen (HBsAg) is the first sign of infection and often occurs even before there is evidence of liver disease. This antigen persists in the serum throughout the clinical course of the illness. If HBsAg persists in the serum longer than 6 months, consider chronic hepatitis B. (A) Anti-HBs is the specific antibody made by the body to fight HBsAg. This is seen in the serum after clearance of HBsAg and after successful vaccination against hepatitis B. The appearance of anti-HBs and disappearance of HBsAg indicates recovery from HBV infection. This also indicates the person is noninfective and immune to the the hepatitis B virus. (B) HBeAg is a secretory form of the hepatitis B HBcAg (hepatitis B core antigen) that is seen in the serum during the incubation period of the disease and shortly after the appearance of HBsAg. (C) Anti-HBc is an IgM antibody that appears shortly after HBsAg. This indicates a diagnosis of acute hepatitis B. Rarely, patients may completely clear HBsAg before detectable antibodies are seen. The anti-HBc finding helps in the diagnosis in these patients. This serum marker may reappear during flares of chronic disease. IgG anti-HBc is also seen during acute disease and persists indefinitely, whether the patient recovers or chronic hepatitis B develops. Knowing the timing of the appearance of these serum markers is helpful in determining stage of disease and any history of hepatitis B. (E) HBV DNA usually paralells the presence of HBeAg and may be present in chronic disease, as well as acute hepatitis.

4. **(A)** Hepatopulmonary syndrome presents with a classic triad of chronic liver disease, intrapulmonary vascular dilatations resulting in a right-to-left intrapulmonary shunt, and an increased alveolar-arterial gradient while the patient is breathing room air. This syndrome occurs in about 5–30% of patients with cirrhosis. Many patients who develop this syndrome require long-term oxygen therapy. (B) Hepatic encephalopathy results from failure of the liver to detoxify noxious agents arising from the gut. The central nervous system becomes disordered and patients may experience a wide range of neurocognitive symptoms. They may become unable to differentiate night from day or may demonstrate cognitive decline or

psychomotor problems. Patients with hepatic encephalopathy have more motor vehicle accidents, and the encephalopathy may be found incidentally when the patient is treated in the ED following an accident. (C) Hepatorenal syndrome results from renal function loss as cirrhosis becomes more pronounced. Findings include increased serum creatinine (azotemia) of greater than 0.3 mg/dL within 48 hours, or an increase by 50% or more within the past 7 days, or a significantly decreased urine output. Typical findings are oliguria, hyponatremia, and low urinary sodium level. (D) Spontaneous bacterial peritonitis is a complication of cirrhosis and presents as abdominal pain, increasing ascites, fever, and progressive encephalopathy. Surprisingly, symptoms are usually mild. Risk factors include gastroesophageal varices with bleeding and the use of proton-pump inhibitors (PPIs). (E) Cardiorenal syndrome may be seen with acute or chronic heart failure, ischemic injury, acute or chronic kidney disease, and arrhythmias.

5. **(C)** Approximately 33% of individuals with inflammatory disease of the terminal ileum also have gallstones. This is thought to be due to a disruption in salt absorption from the intestine resulting in decreased solubility of bile. (A) Irritable bowel syndrome is a chronic functional disorder of the GI tract often presenting in the late teen years. Symptoms include abdominal pain with alterations in bowel habits. IBS is not associated with an increased risk of gallstones. (B) Appendicitis is an inflammatory process of the vermiform appendix. It is the most common abdominal surgical emergency and is seen most often in individuals between the ages of 10 and 30 years. (D) Peptic ulcer disease occurs when there is a break in the mucosa of the gastrum or duodenum. Patients usually report a long history of dyspepsia and heartburn. Ulcers are often caused by long-term NSAID use, particularly in elderly individuals. There is no significant association between PUD and cholelithiasis. (E) Pyogenic hepatic abscess presents with fever, right upper quadrant pain, and jaundice. Although this condition may occur in individuals with gallstones, there is no specific association between the conditions.

6. **(C)** During acute episodes of UC, colonoscopy should be avoided due to the risk for intestinal perforation or rupture. (A) Fecal lactoferrin and (B) fecal calprotectin are fecal derived markers of intestinal inflammation. These levels are elevated with inflammatory bowel disease and can be used to differentiate IBD from IBS. (D, E) Abdominal imaging via radiographs or CT are indicated in severe UC to assess for severe colonic dilatation.

7. **(B)** Mesalamine, administered topically, is the drug of choice for management of patients with mild-to-moderate symptoms of diarrhea. It is administered as a 1,000 mg suppository once a day at bedtime for proctitis. Hydrocortisone enema or foam are alternative treatments for proctitis. (A) Alvimopan is a peripherally-acting mu-opioid receptor antagonist used to reverse opioid-induced intestinal motility inhibition. (C) Adalimumab is an anti-TNF antibody used in the treatment of moderate to severe colitis. (D) Injection sclerotherapy is used in the treatment of patients with severe hemorrhoids who have recurrent bleeding despite conservative treatment. (E) Cyclosporine administration is reserved for patients with severe UC.

8. **(D)** Cephalexin is a cephalosporin antibiotic. This class of antibiotics has been associated with acute tubular necrosis and insterstitial nephritis. Cephalexin has not been seen as a causative factor in the development of erosive esophagitis. The other medications (A) slow-release KCL, (B) doxycycline, and (C) alendronate have been implicated as contributing to erosive esophagitis. NSAIDs are another class of medications associated with the development of this condition. (E) Celecoxib has been associated with development of erosive gastritis.

9. **(A)** Over 60% of cases of acute pancreatitis are associated with alcohol toxicity or gallstones. Other risk factors include triglyceride levels over 500 mg/dL, drug toxicity, and smoking. (B) Decreased triglyceride levels are not associated with development of acute pancreatitis. (C) Elevated HDL cholesterol levels are a protective factor in the development of cardiovascular disease but do not increase risk for pancreatitis. (D) Autoimmune disease has been implicated in some cases of acute pancreatitis; however, these do not represent the majority of patients with pancreatitis. (E) Cholelithiasis has not been associated with a majority of cases of acute pancreatitis.

10. **(B)** Pancreatic enzyme replacement therapy is used to treat pancreatic insufficiency. Lipase capsules, 40,000 units are administered with each meal. (A) Biologic immunomodulators are not indicated in the treatment of chronic pancreatitis. (C) Tramadol may be used for pain associated with chronic pancreatitis. Other preferred agents include acetaminophen and NSAIDs. (D) Broad-spectrum antibiotics may be indicated for acute pancreatitis, based on etiology. (E) Corticosteroids are not recommended for pancreatic insufficiency.

7

Genitourinary (Male and Female)

Learning Objectives

In this chapter, you will review:

→ Penile disorders

→ Urethral disorders

Penile Disorders

Erectile Dysfunction

Pathophysiology

A normal erection is dependent on autonomic and somatic nerve stimulation, arterial blood flow, hormonal and psychological stimulation, and venous resistance. Erectile dysfunction (ED) can result from organic (neurogenic, arterial, venous, hormonal) or psychogenic (generalized or situational) causes. The most common cause of ED is compromised arterial flow as a result of progressive vascular disease.

Clinical Presentation

Erectile dysfunction (ED) is the consistent inability to attain or maintain a penile erection for sexual intercourse. Initial presentation of endothelial dysfunction may present as preserved ability to attain an erection but inability to maintain an erection. Normal nocturnal or morning erections can suggest situational ED (partner or performance related).

Diagnostic and Lab Studies

Obtaining a thorough history and physical exam can guide evaluation. Past medical history should include dyslipidemia, hypertension, depression, neurologic disease, diabetes mellitus, kidney disease, endocrine disorders, and cardiac or peripheral vascular disease.

- History of pelvic trauma, surgery, or irradiation increases the possibility of ED.
- Medications should be reviewed, and the use of alcohol, tobacco, and recreational drugs can increase the risk of sexual dysfunction.
- Physical exam should evaluate for any deformities of the penis or abnormalities of either testicle.
- Laboratory evaluation should be based on history and physical exam and can include lipid profile, glucose, testosterone, thyroid function, and other hormones.
- Duplex doppler ultrasound can help assess vascular function and structural anatomy.

Differential Diagnosis

Erectile dysfunction should be distinguished from penile deformities such as Peyronie disease, premature ejaculation, and hypoactive sexual desire disorder.

Health Maintenance and Patient Education

Lifestyle modification aimed to reduce cardiovascular risk factors is important. Therapy or counseling can help with psychogenic components of ED.

Treatment (Pharmaceutical and Clinical Intervention)

- Oral treatment includes phosphodiesterase type 5 (PDE-5) inhibitors such as sildenafil, vardenafil, and tadalafil.
- Injectable prostaglandin E2 at the base and lateral aspect of the penis into the corpora cavernosa
- A vacuum erection device can draw blood into the corpora cavernosa, and an elastic band is placed to maintain erection.
- A semi-rigid or inflatable penile prostheses can be implanted.

Professional Considerations

The concomitant use of PDE-5 inhibitors and nitroglycerin or nitrates are contraindicated due to risk of hypotension and syncope. Patients being evaluated for acute chest pain should be asked about the use of PDE-5 inhibitors prior to the administration of nitroglycerin.

Hypospadias

Pathophysiology

Hypospadias results when fusion of the urethral folds is incomplete during urethral development at 8–15 weeks gestation. Hypospadias occurs in 1 in every 300 male children. Estrogen and progestins administered during pregnancy can increase the incidence of hypospadias.

Clinical Presentation

In hypospadias, the urethral meatus is displaced on the ventral penis and proximal to the tip of the glans. Classification of hypospadias is based on location: glandular (proximal glans), coronal (coronal sulcus), penile shaft, penoscrotal, and perineal.

Signs and Symptoms
- Difficulty directing the urine stream
- Ventral curvature of the penile shaft
- Decreased or absent ventral foreskin
- Increased incidence of undescended testicles

Diagnostic and Lab Studies

Karyotyping to help establish genetic sex is indicated in penoscrotal and perineal hypospadias, since it may often present as a bifid scrotum and ambiguous genitalia. Urethrocystoscopy can be useful in evaluating for normal development of internal sex organs, and excretory urography can evaluate for congenital abnormalities of the upper urinary tract.

Differential Diagnosis

Hypospadias is an expression of feminization, and thus patients should be evaluated for adreno-genital syndromes and disorders (differences) of sex development.

Health Maintenance and Patient Education

The most proximal forms of hypospadias can cause infertility due to inability to deposit semen into the vagina. Cosmetic outcomes and prevention of fistula formations are challenges of corrective surgery.

Treatment (Pharmaceutical and Clinical Intervention)

Corrective surgery is performed to straighten the penis and reconstruct/advance the urethra.

Professional Considerations

Circumcision should not be performed in newborns with hypospadias in order to preserve the preputial skin for future reconstruction.

Epispadias

Pathophysiology

The exact cause of epispadias is unclear but may be related to abnormalities of the cloacal membrane. Epispadias occurs in approximately 1 in 120,000 males and 1 in 450,000 females.

Clinical Presentation

In epispadias, the urethral meatus is displaced dorsally and urinary incontinence is common due to maldevelopment of the urinary sphincters. In males, classification of epispadias is based on location:

- Glandular (dorsum of the glans)
- Penile (between the pubic symphysis and coronal sulcus)
- Penopubic (penopubic junction)

A distal groove is present and usually extends from the meatus through the glans. Females with epispadias will have a bifid clitoris and separation of the labia.

Diagnostic and Lab Studies

Diagnosis of epispadias is clinical. Following diagnosis, an X-ray should be performed to evaluate for pubic diastasis and associated congenital abnormalities of the upper urinary tract.

Differential Diagnosis

Epispadias must be differentiated from bladder exstrophy, cloacal exstrophy, and urogenital sinus. Isolated epispadias can be identified from these diseases based on clinical examination.

Health Maintenance and Patient Education

Despite corrective surgery, the continence rate after surgery ranges from 50%–85%.

Treatment (Pharmaceutical and Clinical Intervention)

Surgical reconstruction of the genitalia and urethra is indicated for treatment for epispadias.

Professional Considerations

A pediatric surgeon/urologist should be consulted immediately after birth.

Paraphimosis/Phimosis

Pathophysiology

Paraphimosis is a result of chronic inflammation under the foreskin and formation of a tight ring when the foreskin is retracted behind the glans. The ring causes venous congestion resulting in edema and enlargement of the glans. Phimosis is most commonly caused by chronic infection due to poor local hygiene.

Clinical Presentation

Paraphimosis presents with significant pain, edema, and erythema of the glans with the inability to replace the foreskin to its normal position. With phimosis, the foreskin cannot be retracted over the glans. There can be edema, erythema, and tenderness of the prepuce with purulent discharge.

Diagnostic and Lab Studies

Diagnosis is based on physical exam.

Differential Diagnosis

Paraphimosis and phimosis should be differentiated from each other. Other conditions such as balanoposthitis can also cause inflammation of the foreskin and glans.

Health Maintenance and Patient Education

- To help prevent **paraphimosis**, the patient should always replace the foreskin after urinating or cleansing.
- To help prevent **phimosis**, the patient should be instructed on proper hygiene. The foreskin should be retracted to cleanse and then returned to normal position.

Treatment (Pharmaceutical and Clinical Intervention)

Paraphimosis should initially be treated with manual reduction by squeezing the glans for 5 minutes to reduce edema and then bringing the foreskin forward over the glans. Phimosis should be treated with a broad spectrum antibiotic if infection is present and a dorsal slit can be performed if needed.

Professional Considerations

In cases of paraphimosis, where the foreskin cannot be replaced manually, emergent urologic consultation is required to incise the constricting ring, otherwise the arterial occlusion and necrosis of the glans may occur. The foreskin should always be replaced after the placement of a foley catheter to prevent risk of paraphimosis. The foreskin should also not be forcibly retracted to insert a foley catheter. Phimosis can occur at any age; however, children under the age of 2 rarely have true phimosis. Their preputial opening is relatively narrow and widens gradually to allow for normal retraction with time.

Practice Questions for Genitourinary Review

1. Treatment of benign prostatic hypertrophy may include use of 5-alpha-reductase inhibitors. These medications block conversion of testosterone to dihydrotestosterone, resulting in reducing the size of the prostate gland. Medications in this class include finasteride and dutasteride. These medications demonstrate maximal effectiveness after adminstration for

   (A) 12 months.
   (B) 2 months.
   (C) 3 months.
   (D) 30 days.
   (E) 6 months.

2. Urinary stone disease is a common condition that presents with severe flank pain, nausea, and vomiting. Stones may be identifed by CT. The most common types of stones are those composed of phosphate or

   (A) struvite.
   (B) calcium oxalate.
   (C) uric acid.
   (D) cystine.
   (E) magnesium ammonium phosphate.

3. You are examining a 45-year-old female in the clinic who presents with urinary urgency and frequency, along with pain with bladder filling, which is relieved by emptying the bladder. She also reports getting up several times during the night to urinate. Urinalysis is normal with no evidence of bacterial infection or hematuria. This presentation, in the setting of normal lab studies, is characteristic of

   (A) interstitial cystitis.
   (B) chronic pelvic pain syndrome.
   (C) acute cystitis.
   (D) acute pyelonephritis.
   (E) bladder cancer.

4. Recommended outpatient treatment for stable patients with a diagnosis of chronic bacterial prostatitis includes

   (A) oral corticosteroid administration for 14 days.
   (B) oral trimethoprim-sulfamethoxaozle (TMP-SMZ) for 4–6 weeks.
   (C) long-term oral finasteride.
   (D) outpatient prostate resection.
   (E) oral augmentin for 6 weeks.

5. Patients who present with erectile dysfunction should be evaluated for

   (A) sexually transmitted infection.
   (B) bladder cancer.
   (C) cardiovascular disease.
   (D) kidney disease.
   (E) Peyronie disease.

6. Surgical indications for management of benign prostatic hypertrophy include all of the following, except

   (A) recurrent urinary tract infections.
   (B) refractory urinary retention.
   (C) bladder stones.
   (D) presence of weak urinary stream.
   (E) gross hematuria with symptoms.

7. Acute treatment for epididymitis includes

   (A) increased fluid intake.
   (B) oral corticosteroids.
   (C) bed rest, ice, and scrotal elevation.
   (D) IV antibiotics.
   (E) opioid analgesia.

8. To reduce the risk of urinary stone formation in patients who have vitamin D deficiency, recommended daily supplementation of vitamin D3 should not exceed

   (A) 1,000 IU.
   (B) 2,000 IU.
   (C) 3,000 IU.
   (D) 4,000 IU.
   (E) 5,000 IU.

9. The most common cause of microscopic hematuria in males is

   (A) urethral stricture.
   (B) bladder cancer.
   (C) benign prostatic hypertrophy (BPH).
   (D) renal stones.
   (E) strenuous excercise.

10. The most common causes of acute bacterial prostatitis include *E. coli* and

   (A) pseudomonas.
   (B) staphylococcus.
   (C) streptococci.
   (D) enterococci.
   (E) lactobacilli.

Answer Explanations

1. **(E)** 5-alpha-reductase inhibitors are limited because maximal effectiveness is not seen until at least 6 months of continous therapy. (A, B, C, D) These time frames are not associated with this class of medication.

2. **(B)** Most urinary stones are composed of phosphate or calcium oxalate. The five major types of stones include these two along with struvite, cystine, and uric acid.

3. **(A)** Interstitial cystitis is also called "painful bladder syndrome" and presents with pain with bladder filling relieved by emptying the bladder. Associated symptoms include urgency, frequency, and nocturia. There is no cure for IC; however, amitriptylline has proven beneficial at 10–75 mg daily. (B) Chronic pelvic pain syndrome is poorly understood and presents with symptoms of irritative voiding and perineal or suprapubic discomfort. (C) Acute cystitis presents with irritative voiding symptoms and a positive urine culture. (D) Acute pyelnephritis presents with fever, flank pain, irritative voiding symptoms, and a positive urine culture. (E) Bladder cancer most often presents with painless hematuria.

4. **(B)** Gram-negative rods are most often implicated in the causation of chronic bacterial prostatis. If the patient is medically stable, outpatient treatment with TMP-SMZ (or based on prostatic culture) is recommended. (A, C, D, E) These options are not recommended for management of this condition.

5. **(C)** Erectile dysfunction may be an early sign of cardiovascular disease. (A, B, D, E) ED is not associated with these conditions.

6. **(D)** Absolute indications for surgery include recurrent urinary tract infection, refractor urinary retention, bladder stones, problematic gross hematuria, or obstructive nephropathy. The presence of a weak urinary stream may be reported; however, this finding, on its own, is not an absolute indication for surgery.

7. **(C)** Initial treatment includes bed rest, ice, and scrotal elevation. Pharmacotherapy is based on etiology. Sexually transmitted epididymitis may be treated with ceftriaxone 250 mg IM pluse oral doxycycline for 10 days. Nonsexually transmitted infection is treated with a fluoroquinolone for 10 days. (A, B, D, E) These options are not indicated for management of epididymitis.

8. **(B)** Recommendations for vitamin D supplementation in individuals at risk for, or who have a prior history of, urinary stones include no more than 2,000 IU daily.

9. **(C)** BPH remains the most common cause of microscopic hematuria in males, causing approximately 13% of cases. Other causes include kidney stones, strictures of the urethra, and bladder cancer.

10. **(A)** *E. coli* and pseudomonas species are the most common pathogens associated with acute bacterial prostatis. Less commonly, enterococci (D) are implicated.

8

Hematologic Review

Learning Objectives

In this chapter, you will review:

→ Types of leukemia

→ Multiple myeloma

→ Lymphoma

→ Hodgkin/non-Hodgkin

→ Chemotherapy, radiation, and stem cells

Leukemia

Acute Lymphocytic Leukemia

Pathophysiology

Lymphoid stem cells produce a malignant clonal population of immature B or T lymphocytes from the bone marrow. These cells multiply and infiltrate the bone marrow with nonfunctioning clonal lymphoblasts.

Leads to:

- Anemia
- Thrombocytopenia
- Typically leukocytosis
- Sometimes leukopenia, due to the white blood cells' inability to leave the bone marrow

Lymphoblasts can be found in the periphery.

- CNS
- Lymph nodes
- Testicles, ovaries
- Liver
- Spleen

Clinical Presentation

ALL is the most common leukemia in children. The peak incidence is between 3 and 4 years of age. The 5-year survival rate for children is 91% and 75% for adolescents. ALL can occur in adults but happens less frequently. The 5-year survival rate for ALL for adults aged 20 and older is 36% with standard chemotherapy alone. With the addition of allogeneic stem cell transplantation, there is wider variation with outcomes showing survival rates of 26–60%.

Symptoms—Primarily Constitutional

- Fever
- Fatigue
- Joint pain
- Bone pain
- Easy bruising
- Easy bleeding
- Dyspnea
- Early satiety
- Meningeal signs
- Headache
- Altered mental status

Signs

- Ecchymosis
- Petechiae
- Splenomegaly
- Lymphadenopathy
- Hepatomegaly
- Fever
- Weight loss

Diagnostic and Lab Studies

History—1–2 week history of the presenting signs and symptoms:

- Lymphadenopathy
- Pallor
- Splenomegaly
- Hepatomegaly

CBC with differential—typically, pancytopenia:

- White blood cell count can be elevated, normal, or decreased.
- Sometimes there are circulating lymphoblasts.
- Bone marrow biopsy and aspirate—hypercellular marrow with 20% lymphoblasts or greater

The solid tissue sample is evaluated for leukemia cells and the aspirate is utilized for cytogenetics to evaluate the chromosomal abnormalities of the leukemia. Flow cytometry can be performed on bone marrow aspirate or peripheral blood. It helps to identify cellular structure and type to diagnose the subtype of leukemia. Cytogenetics—FISH and PCR used to determine the cellular mutation of the leukemia and direct treatment and outcome. Lumbar puncture needs to be done on all patients with ALL to evaluate for CNS involvement. Most chemotherapy regimens for ALL include CNS therapy. Use a chest radiograph to evaluate for any chest masses, especially in T cell ALL.

Differential Diagnosis/Formulating the Most Likely Diagnosis

AML

- Typically will have myeloblasts on the peripheral smear
- AML tends to be a leukemia of older patients (but not always), while ALL tends to be a leukemia of younger patients (but not always).

CLL

- Look for mature (not immature) lymphocytes on the peripheral smear.
- Smudge cells are correlated with CLL.
- CLL is almost always a disease of older patients.

Health Maintenance and Patient Education

Ensure patients know the adverse effects of their chemotherapy.

Chemotherapy will induce neutropenia. Neutropenic precautions include avoiding raw foods, avoiding crowds, monitoring for fever, and wearing a mask if you must go out.

- Educate the patient on who they should call should an emergency arise.
- Discuss support options and counseling.
- Ensure patients know when and how to take all medications, including chemotherapy and prophylactic antibiotics, if indicated (neutropenia).

Treatment (Pharmaceutical and Clinical Intervention)

Induction/intensification chemotherapy. Use a multi-drug regimen over the course of 6–12 months. If there is CNS involvement, intrathecal chemotherapy is given several times throughout the course of the therapy. Typical drugs include dexamethasone, vincristine, and L-asparaginase. For patients with high risk ALL, an anthracycline chemotherapeutic is often added, such as daunorubicin. If a patient's cytogenetics reveal the Philadelphia chromosome, a tyrosine kinase inhibitor may be added.

Consolidation/Intensification

- Following remission, consolidation chemotherapy is given for several months to decrease the tumor burden.
- This regimen typically has multiple drugs to prevent the leukemia cells from developing resistance.
- Intrathecal chemotherapy is continued during this phase.
- Typical drugs include methotrexate, 6-mercaptopurine, L-asparaginase, vincristine, and prednisone.
- For patients with high risk ALL based on cytogenetics etoposide, cyclophosphamide, cytarabine, and doxorubicin are often used.
- Tyrosine kinase inhibitors are continued in patients with the Philadelphia chromosome.
- Often there is a second round of consolidation chemotherapy, known as delayed intensification.

Maintenance

- Maintenance begins when patients finish the consolidation/intensification and induction/intensification rounds of chemotherapy and continue to be in remission.
- This phase lasts approximately 2 years.
- Typical drugs include 6-mercaptopurine, methotrexate, vincristine, and prednisone.

Radiation

- Radiation is utilized sparingly in ALL.
- Occasionally, it is used to treat extramedullary disease in the CNS and gonads, especially if it relapses after chemotherapy.

Stem Cell Transplant

- Stem cell transplant is used in some patients with high risk ALL, including Philadelphia chromosome positive ALL.
- Immunotherapy

CAR T-Cell Therapy

- The patient's own T cells are manipulated in a lab to attach to leukemia cells and destroy them.
- This is FDA approved for B-cell precursor ALL in people up to 25 years of age who have already received traditional chemotherapy.
- CAR T-cell therapy carries a risk for cytokine release syndrome in which patients develop hypotension, fever, and mild to severe CNS symptoms. Typically, these effects occur early in treatment, within the first few days, however, severe neurotoxicity may persist.
- Monoclonal antibodies—specific antigens on the leukemic cells—can be targeted by antibodies in an attempt to treat the disease.
- CNS-directed therapy

Intrathecal Chemotherapy

- Given to prevent the spread of leukemia to the brain or spinal cord. If there is CNS involvement, or a CNS prophylaxis, intrathecal chemotherapy is given throughout the course of the therapy through a lumbar puncture or Ommaya catheter.

Professional Considerations

Side Effects

- Watch absolute neutrophil; count for profound neutropenia.
- Will require frequent monitoring of blood counts and electrolytes.
- Nausea/vomiting prophylaxis

Tumor Lysis Syndrome

- Caused by the lysis of tumor cells as the result of initiation of chemotherapy on a large tumor burden. This results in the emptying of the contents of the cells into the bloodstream. The clinical result is increased uric acid, phosphorus, and potassium. Calcium levels in the blood are decreased.
- Patients with tumor lysis syndrome can rapidly develop renal failure and death if untreated.

- Treatment includes frequent monitoring of electrolytes, copious IV fluids, allopurinol, rasburicase, and dialysis in extreme cases.
- Fertility preservation—if there is time, consider consulting with a reproductive endocrinologist for options for fertility preservation in children and younger adults.

Secondary Cancers
- Myelodysplastic syndrome
- Acute myelogenous leukemia (AML)

Health Issues Due to Chemotherapy and/or Radiation
- Heart disease
- Stroke
- Learning difficulties
- Growth delays
- Infertility
- Osteoporosis
- Social/emotional issues and depression

Risk Factors for ALL
- Genetic conditions
- Down syndrome
- Neurofibromatosis type 1
- Fanconi anemia
- Klinefelter's syndrome
- Ataxia-telangiectasia
- Ionizing radiation
- Exposure to benzenes
- Prior therapy for malignancies
- Human T-cell lymphotropic virus type 1 (HTLV-1) can cause a rare type of ALL, adult T-cell leukemia
- Primarily in Japan and the Caribbean
- Presumptively has and needs an oncologist soon

Acute Myeloblastic Leukemia

Pathophysiology

Myeloid stem cells produce a malignant clonal population of immature cells from the bone marrow. These cells multiply and infiltrate the bone marrow with nonfunctioning clonal myeloblasts.

Causes
- Anemia
- Thrombocytopenia
- Typically leukocytosis
- Sometimes leukopenia, due to the white blood cells' inability to leave the bone marrow

AML is often idiopathic, typically arising from genetic point mutations.

NOTE

ALL is the most common acute leukemia in adults. The median incidence is 67 years of age. AML is an aggressive disease. The 5-year survival rate is 27%.

Clinical Presentation

Patients who present with acute myeloblastic leukemia may present in a range of ways, but primarily they have constitutional complaints. They complain often of fever, fatigue, joint pain, easy bruising, dyspnea, and sometimes early satiety due to splenomegaly.

Symptoms
- Fatigue
- Pallor
- Easy bruising or bleeding
- Dyspnea
- Infection
- Bone and joint pain
- +/− Meningeal signs
- Headache
- Altered mental status

Signs
- Ecchymosis
- Petechiae
- Splenomegaly
- Lymphadenopathy
- Hepatomegaly
- Fever
- Weight loss

Diagnostic and Lab Studies

History—less than 3 month history of the presenting signs and symptoms

Physical exam—evaluate for lymphadenopathy, pallor, splenomegaly, hepatomegaly

CBC with differential, and peripheral blood smear—typically pancytopenia, occasionally leukocytosis, but can be normal or decreased. Occasionally, circulating lymphoblasts. Auer rods are pathognomonic of AML if seen.

Bone Marrow Biopsy and Aspirate
- Hypercellular marrow with 20% myeloblasts or greater. The solid tissue sample is evaluated for leukemia cells.
- The aspirate is utilized for cytogenetics to evaluate the chromosomal abnormalities of the leukemia.

Flow Cytometry
- Can be performed on bone marrow aspirate or peripheral blood
- Identifies cellular structure and type to diagnose the subtype of leukemia
- Typically the WHO staging system is used to classify AML

Cytogenetics and Genetic Rearrangements

FISH and PCR are used to determine the cellular mutation of the leukemia and direct treatment and outcome.

- Favorable risk
  - Gene mutations: CEBPA, NPM1
  - Cytogenetics: inv(16) (p33;q23), t(8,21), t(15,17)
- Intermediate risk
  - Normal cytogenetics
  - Cytogenetics: +8, t(9,11)
- Adverse risk
  - Gene mutation: FLT3
  - Cytogenetics: -5, 5q-, -7, 7q-, 11q23 other than t(9,11), inv(3, t(3,5), t(6,9), t(9,22)
  - Complex findings (greater than 3 clonal chromosomal abnormalities)

Lumbar Puncture

- A lumbar puncture needs to be done on any patient with AML who presents with CNS complaints to evaluate for CNS involvement.
- If they have CNS involvement, or certain subtypes of AML, they will need CNS treatment or prophylaxis.

Differential Diagnosis/Formulating the Most Likely Diagnosis

- ALL
- CML
- Mononucleosis

Health Maintenance and Patient Education

- Will require frequent clinic visits.
- Ensure patients know the adverse effects of their chemotherapy.
- Chemotherapy will induce neutropenia. (Neutropenic precautions include avoiding raw foods, avoiding crowds, monitoring for fever, and wearing a mask if you must go out.)
- Educate them on who they should call should an emergency arise.
- Discuss support options and counseling.
- Ensure patients know when and how to take all medications, including chemotherapy and prophylactic antibiotics, if indicated (neutropenia).

Treatment (Pharmaceutical and Clinical Intervention)

Induction Chemotherapy

Induction chemotherapy is used to induce remission. The drugs used in this regimen are based on the patient's age, cytogenetics, and performance score. The typical drugs include daunorubicin or idarubicin and cytarabine. For older patients, the same drugs are typically used, but at lower doses. In patients with FLT3 gene rearrangement, midostaurin may be included. Allogeneic transplantation is recommended in CR1 for patients with FLT3 positivity. In patients with acute promyelocytic leukemia (APL), which is AML subtype M3, the addition of tretinoin (ATRA) and arsenic is the foundation of treatment. Induction chemotherapy can be dangerous for this subgroup, resulting in DIC or APL syndrome. In APL syndrome, the patient develops fever, dyspnea, chest pain, pleural infiltrates, and hypoxemia due to tumor cells attaching to the pulmonary vasculature.

Consolidation Chemotherapy

Consolidation chemotherapy is used to further reduce the tumor burden that is not detectable by current studies. It follows induction chemotherapy, and the typical drugs include intermediate to high dose cytarabine for two to four cycles.

Allogeneic Stem Cell Transplant

Allogenic stem cell transplants are for patients with intermediate to high-risk disease. They must first be in complete remission, be less than 75 years of age, and have an HLA-matched donor.

Professional Considerations

Prior therapy for cancer is a strong risk factor for AML.

Genetic Conditions at Risk for AML
- Fanconi anemia
- Diamond-Blackfan disorder
- Down syndrome
- Ataxia-telangiectasia

Other Risk Factors
- Ionizing radiation
- Exposure to benzenes
- Require frequent monitoring of CBC and electrolytes
- Watch absolute neutrophil count for profound neutropenia
- Will require prophylaxis against opportunistic infection

Side Effects of Chemotherapy
- Nausea/vomiting prophylaxis
- Tumor lysis syndrome
- Caused by the lysis of tumor cells as the result of initiation of chemotherapy on a large tumor burden
- Results in the emptying of the contents of the cells into the bloodstream
- The clinical result is increased uric acid, phosphorus, and potassium. Calcium levels in the blood are decreased.
- Patients with tumor lysis syndrome can rapidly develop renal failure and death if untreated.
- Treatment includes frequent monitoring of electrolytes, copious IV fluids, allopurinol, rasburicase, and dialysis in extreme cases.

Fertility Preservation
- Consult reproductive endocrinologist if timing of chemotherapy permits
- Often in acute leukemia, timing does not permit in female patients, as emergent chemotherapy is required for life preservation

Secondary Cancers
- Myelodysplastic syndrome
- Other neoplasms due to therapy

Health Issues Due to Chemotherapy and/or Radiation

- Heart disease
- Stroke
- Learning difficulties
- Growth delays
- Infertility
- Osteoporosis
- Social/emotional issues and depression

Chronic Myeloblastic Leukemia

Pathophysiology

Chronic myeloblastic leukemia is an uncontrolled production of mature and maturing granulocytes, and reciprocal translocation of chromosomes 9 and 22 t(9;222)(q34;q11) creates an oncogene BCR-ABL1. The oncogene encodes for the oncoprotein BCR ABL. This oncogene has uninhibited tyrosine kinase activity and is responsible for myeloid hyperproliferation.

Clinical Presentation

There are three phases to this condition:

1. Chronic phase
2. Accelerated/transformation phase
   - Leukocytosis
   - Increasing constitutional symptoms
   - Increased blasts and basophils on the peripheral blood smear

Criteria

- 10–19% blasts in the blood and bone marrow
- 20% or more peripheral basophils
- Cytogenetic clonal evolution
- Thrombocytopenia less than 100 thousand per liter

3. Blastic phase/blast crisis (one or more of the following)
   - 30% or more peripheral or marrow blasts
   - Sheets of blasts in extramedullary disease
   - 70% of people have myeloid blasts in blast crisis.
   - 30% of people have lymphoid blasts in blast crisis.
   - Often diagnosed in chronic phase on routine blood tests and patients are asymptomatic
   - The median age at diagnosis is 55–65 years of age.
   - Uncommon in children
   - CML occurs in males more frequently than females (1.6:1).

Symptoms

- Often minimal at presentation
- Fatigue

Signs

- Often minimal at presentation
- Splenomegaly, hepatomegaly, lymphadenopathy, weight loss

Rarely Hyperviscosity Related Issues

- Priapism
- Myocardial infarction
- CVA

Diagnostic and Lab Studies

Diagnostic labs include CBC with peripheral blood smear.

Chronic Phase

- WBC: 10–500 3 109/L
- Thrombocytosis

Left Shift

- Bands
- Blasts
- Neutrophils
- Myelocytes
- Occasional anemia

Bone Marrow Biopsy

- Hypercellular with myeloid hyperplasia. Myeloid to erythroid ratio of 15–20:1. Blasts less than 5% (if greater than or equal to 15% then has transformed to accelerated phase). Increased reticulin fibrosis by silver stain.

Cytogenetics and Flow Cytometry

- FISH/PCR for BCR/ABL1 + − translocation of 9 and 22 - Philadelphia chromosome
- FISH for quantity
- PCR to look for variants

Differential Diagnosis/Formulating the Most Likely Diagnosis

Essential Thrombocythemia

- Elevated platelets
- Bone marrow biopsy shows megakaryocytic proliferation
- Large megakaryocytes
- No Philadelphia chromosome +JAK2 mutation

Acute Myelogenous Leukemia

- Acute onset (vs. insidious onset of CML)
- More mature blasts seen on peripheral blood smear
- AML has more blasts on the bone marrow biopsy (greater than or equal to 20%).

Health Maintenance and Patient Education

- Will require routine clinic visits
- Ensure patients know the adverse effects of their chemotherapy.
- Educate them on who they should call should an emergency arise.

NOTE

Women of childbearing age must be aware and utilize effective birth control methods. If pregnancy occurs, TKI therapy must be discontinued. Ionizing radiation is a risk factor for CML.

- Discuss support options and counseling.
- TKI therapy is teratogenic.

Treatment (Pharmaceutical and Clinical Intervention)

Prior to the year 2000, the 10-year survival rate was 30%. In 2000, tyrosine kinase inhibitors (TKI) were introduced, which vastly improved remission and survival rates for patients with this disease. Currently the 10-year survival rate is 85%. Treat with tyrosine kinase inhibitors. Currently there are six drugs approved by the FDA.

First-Generation TKI

- Imatinib

Second-Generation TKI

- Dasatinib
- Nilotinib
- Bosutinib

Third-Generation TKI

- Ponatinib

Chronic Phase

First or Second Generation TKI

- Imatinib
- Nilotinib
- Dasatinib
- Bosutinib

All are approved by the FDA for chronic phase.

Transformation/Accelerated Phase

If on a first-generation TKI, move to a second-generation TKI.

- +/– Traditional chemotherapy
- If in transformation without evidence of blast phase, may consider low-dose regimens with drugs such as cytarabine, idarubicin, decitabine, or hydroxyurea.

Blast Phase

If on a first-generation TKI, move to a second-generation TKI. Can consider a third-generation TKI for appropriate patients (T315l mutations):

- +/– Traditional chemotherapy
- If in lymphoid blastic phase, the traditional chemotherapy plan resembles ALL chemotherapy.
- If in myeloid blastic phase, the traditional chemotherapy plan resembles AML chemotherapy.

Allogeneic Stem Cell Transplant

Once considered first-line treatment, but now it is used with TKI therapy:

- After TKI failure
- In patients who present in blast crisis

Professional Considerations

TKI therapy is very expensive. Many treatment failures are due to nonadherence.

Myeloma

Plasma Cell Myeloma (Multiple Myeloma)

This type of myeloma has had a recent name change and happens in a rare form of Down syndrome, where the chromosomes 21 translocate instead of trisomy.

Pathophysiology

A monoclonal proliferation of plasma cells. These abnormal cells secrete varying amounts of abnormal immunoglobulins, termed M proteins. The increase in M protein is a monoclonal gammopathy. The neoplastic plasma cells cause a reduction in normal immunoglobulin levels. Also, can cause excess light chans that deposit in the kidney causing renal failure. These are Bence Jones proteins.

Clinical Presentation

- Occurs twice as frequently in men than women
- Median age at diagnosis is 65
- Sometimes is an incidental finding

Symptoms
- Anemia
- Hypercalcemia
- Weakness
- Fatigue
- Bone pain

Due to Lytic Lesions
- Back pain
- Paralysis (cord compression by plasmacytoma (tumor of monoclonal plasma cells))
- Frequent infections

Signs
- Weight loss
- Pallor
- Compression fracture
- Renal failure

Diagnostic and Lab Studies

A helpful mnemonic is:

Patients with plasma cell/multiple myeloma have **CRAB** (Hyper**C**alcemia, **R**enal failure, **A**nemia, **B**one lesions).

Serum Protein Electrophoresis
- Determines the monoclonal protein spike
- Diagnostic criteria:
    - IgG > 3.5 g/dL or IgA > 2.0 g/dL

Urine Protein Electrophoresis

- 24-hour urine collection
- Diagnostic criteria:

  ○ Kappa or lambda light-chain excretion > 1.0 g/d on 24-h urine protein electrophoresis

Serum Immunofixation

- Confirms clonality
- Specifies type of monoclonal protein

CBC with Differential

- Normocytic anemia
- Pancytopenia
- May see rouleaux formation (stacked coins)

Chemistry Panel

- Renal failure
- Elevated calcium
- Elevated LDH
- Quantitative immunoglobulins

Diagnostic Criteria

- IgM < 50 mg/dL
- IgA < 100 mg/dL
- IgG < 600 mg/dL

Serum-Free Light Chains

- To evaluate for light chain myeloma

Beta 2 Microglobulin

- For staging

Bone Marrow Biopsy and Aspirate

- Greater than 30% plasma cells
- Sheets of plasma cells

Differential Diagnosis/Formulating the Most Likely Diagnosis

MGUS

- Does not have CRAB (hypercalcemia, renal failure, anemia, or bone lesions)
- Less than 10% bone marrow plasma cells
- Less than 3 g/dL M protein

Solitary Plasmacytoma

- A solitary plasmacytoma is a single bone lesion.
- May have an M spike
- No bone marrow involvement
- No CRAB (hypercalcemia, renal failure, anemia, or bone lesions)

> **NOTE**
>
> Due to excess immunoglobulin coated red blood cells clinging together.

Health Maintenance and Patient Education

- Ensure patients know the adverse effects of their chemotherapy.
- Educate them on who they should call should an emergency arise.
- Discuss support options and counseling.
- Ensure patients know when and how to take all medications including chemotherapy.

Treatment (Pharmaceutical and Clinical Intervention)

Stage 1

- Watchful waiting
- Observe at 3–6 month intervals

Stage 2/3

Symptomatic patients need treatment:

- Hypercalcemia
- Renal failure
- Cytopenias
- Bony lesions

Determine risk by cytogenetics:

- Steroids
- Thalidomide

Traditional Chemotherapy

Typical drugs include:

- Melphalan
- Cyclophosphamide
- Adriamycin
- Etoposide
- Bisphophonates
- Lenalidomide
- Bortezomib

Radiotherapy:

- To plasmacytoma
- To any spinal cord impingement lesions

Professional Considerations

Chemotherapy can cause severe pancytopenia, and alkylating drugs can reduce the ability to collect stem cells for autologous stem cell transplant.

- Lenalidomide is associated with risk for DVT (needs anticoagulation).
- Bortezomib is associated with VZV reactivation (can be controlled with acyclovir).
- Bisphophonates (avoid in renally impaired patients, and can cause osteonecrosis with long-term use)

Diagnostic criteria is split into major and minor.

Major Criteria

- Plasmacytomas on tissue biopsy
- More than 30% plasma cell on bone marrow biopsy
- Monoclonal immunoglobulin spike on serum electrophoresis:
  - IgG > 3.5 g/dL (most common)
  - IgA > 2.0 g/dL
  - Kappa or lambda light-chain excretion > 1.0 g/d on 24-h urine protein electrophoresis

Minor Criteria

- 10–30% plasma cells on bone marrow biopsy
- Minor elevations in the level of monoclonal immunoglobulins
- Lytic bone lesions
- Low levels of antibodies in the blood
  - IgM < 50 mg/dL
  - IgA < 100 mg/dL
  - IgG < 600 mg/dL

Guidelines

- Any two major criteria
- Major criterion 1 plus minor criterion b, c, or d
- Major criterion 3 plus minor criterion a or c
- Minor criteria a, b, and c, or d

Lymphoma

Hodgkin Lymphoma

Pathophysiology

A lymphoma is a monoclonal proliferative disorder of mature B Lymphocytes (Reed Sternberg cells). It is associated with Epstein-Barr virus in 30% of cases and is typically based within the lymph nodes.

Non-Hodgkin Lymphoma

Pathophysiology

- A monoclonal proliferative disorder of mature B, T, and NK lymphocytes
- Can be associated with immunodeficiency
- Typically based within the lymph nodes
- Associated with genetic mutations and chromosomal translocations
- The exact pathophysiology is unknown.

Clinical Presentation

Symptoms
- Fever
- Weight loss
- Night sweats
- Confer poorer prognosis

Signs

- Painless lymphadenopathy
- Lymphadenopathy that is attached to underlying structures
- Pruritus
- Symptoms are often dependent on the area of involvement
- Hodgkin disease

A mediastinal mass is common on presentation with Hodgkin Disease (HD).

- Causes shortness of breath, cough, and chest pain
- Some patients complain of pain in their lymph nodes after drinking alcohol

NHL

- Less likely to have mediastinal involvement than HD
- More likely to have peripheral involvement of the bone marrow, skin, or CNS than HD

Diagnostic and Lab Studies

Review Patient History

- Determine the progression of symptoms
- Determine if the lymphoma is indolent or aggressive

Physical Exam

Hodgkin lymphoma:

- Cervical lymphadenopathy
- Typically mediastinal lymphadenopathy (can't palpate)
- Splenomegaly in 20% of patients
- LDH may be elevated
- CBC may be abnormal
- Anemia
- Leukocytosis
- Lymphopenia
- Eosinophilia
- Thrombocytopenia
- Hypoalbuminemia

Diagnosis can only be made on excisional biopsy. Morphology and flow cytometry are used to distinguish the specific subtype of lymphoma.

Hodgkin Lymphoma

- Reed Sternberg cells

Non-Hodgkin Lymphoma

- CD20—B cells
- CD3—T cells

Many more cell surface markers to differentiate between Burkitt's lymphoma: follicular, diffuse, mantle cell, cutaneous T cell, small lymphocytic, etc.

Evaluate for further disease:

- CT scan, PET scan, lumbar puncture
- Evaluate for CNS disease if suspected staging
- Use International Prognostic Index

Risk factors:

- Age greater than 60
- Serum LDH greater than normal
- ECOG performance status less than or equal to 2
- Number of involved extranodal sites more than 1

Differential Diagnosis/Formulating the Most Likely Diagnosis

Cat-Scratch Disease

- Tender swollen lymph nodes, usually near the site of a scratch or bite

May develop systemic symptoms like:

- Fatigue
- Headache
- Chills
- Muscular pain
- Joint pain
- Back pain
- Abdominal pain

Acute Lymphocytic Leukemia

- These two diseases live on the same spectrum of disease.
- ALL is primarily in the bone marrow, while lymphoma is primarily in the lymph nodes.

Burkitt's Lymphoma

- Very rare lymphoma that happens primarily in children
- Very rapidly growing lymphoma

Can present as:

- Jaw or facial mass
- African endemic form

- Abdominal mass
- Nonendemic form

- Immunodeficiency related
- Classic "starry sky" appearance of the mass by microscopy

Health Maintenance and Patient Education

- Ensure patients know the adverse effects of their chemotherapy.
- Educate them on who they should call should an emergency arise.
- Discuss support options and counseling.
- Ensure patients know when and how to take all medications, including chemotherapy.

> **NOTE**
>
> May take 7–60 days for the lymphadenopathy to appear following the scratch or bite.

Treatment (Pharmaceutical and Clinical Intervention)

Treatment varies depending on the type of lymphoma.

Indolent

- Not indicated unless symptomatic
- If symptomatic/advanced, typically an anthracycline or purine analog-based therapy when treated
- Use rituximab whenever possible
- Not curable with chemotherapy
- No role for stem cell transplant in indolent lymphoma unless relapsed

Aggressive

- Treat on diagnosis
- Typically an anthracycline-based chemotherapy
- Use rituximab whenever possible
- Considered curable with chemotherapy
- No role for stem cell transplant unless relapsed

Hodgkin Lymphoma

- Treatment typically involves chemotherapy +/– radiation.
- Typical drugs include Adriamycin, bleomycin, vinblastine, dacarbazine

Professional Considerations

Hodgkin's disease has an 85% survival rate.

Consider long term complications in these patients and secondary cancers:

- Myelodysplastic syndrome
- Acute myelogenous leukemia (AML)
- Carcinoma
- Screening mammograms important

Consider health issues due to chemotherapy and/or radiation, especially if radiation was included in therapy:

- Heart disease
- Stroke
- Thyroid disease
- Infertility
- Osteoporosis
- Social/emotional issues and depression

Myelodysplasia

Pathophysiology

Myelodysplasia is a clonal hematopoietic stem cell disorder, typically related to age, in which the bone marrow has ineffective hematopoiesis leading to pancytopenia.

- Significant risk of transformation to AML

- Typically idiopathic
- Can be a result of chromosome and genetic instability
- Similar mutations as AML

Risk factor: exposure to prior chemotherapy or radiotherapy

Clinical Presentation

- The median age is 70–75 years old.
- Risk increases with age.
- Incidence higher in males than females

Symptoms
- Often asymptomatic
- Found on routine blood testing

Signs
- Hepatosplenomegaly
- Pallor

Diagnostic and Lab Studies

CBC
- Anemia
- MCV normal or increased
- May see macro-ovalocytes
- WBC usually normal or low
- Sometimes neutropenic

Platelets Normal or Low
- Reticulocyte count reduced
- Need to eliminate other causes of bone marrow failure
- Prognosis correlates with the proportion of marrow blasts

Assigns a risk and median survival based on:

- Bone marrow blasts
- Karyotype
- Cytopenias

Differential Diagnosis/Formulating the Most Likely Diagnosis

Nutritional Deficiency (B12, Folate, Copper)

- Can look very similar to MDS
- Check B12, folate, and copper
- Correlate with clinical history

HIV

- Check HIV status
- Correlate with clinical history

Medication-Induced Bone Marrow Suppression

- Methotrexate, azathioprine, chemotherapy
- Correlate with clinical history
- Chronic alcohol use
- Can cause marrow suppression
- Correlate with clinical history

AML

- On bone marrow biopsy, AML will have greater than 20% blasts.

Parvovirus B19 Infection

- Can cause transient bone marrow suppression
- Correlate with clinical history

Health Maintenance and Patient Education

Will require frequent clinic visits, and ensure patients know the adverse effects of their chemotherapy. Patients may already be neutropenic.

Neutropenic precautions include:

- Avoiding raw foods
- Avoiding crowds
- Monitoring for fever
- Wearing a mask if you must go out

Educate them on who they should call should an emergency arise. Discuss support options and counseling, and ensure patients know when and how to take all medications, including chemotherapy and prophylactic antibiotics, if indicated (neutropenia).

Treatment (Pharmaceutical and Clinical Intervention)

Supportive Care

- For patients with low-risk disease, this is the mainstay of treatment.
- Hematopoietic growth factor support
- Immune suppression
- Antithymocyte globulin
- Calcineurin inhibitor

Allogeneic Stem Cell Transplant

- For higher risk disease
- Only cure for MDS
- Age is a barrier, as often these patients are older.
- Most patients with MDS do not go to transplant for this reason.

Chemotherapy

- For higher risk disease
- Must balance therapy with drug toxicity
- MDS is fairly refractory to chemotherapy.

Common drugs used include:

- Azacitidine—improved blood counts and survival

Side effect—bone marrow suppression.

- Decitabine—similar to azacitidine but more potent

Professional Considerations

- Patients often rapidly progress to AML.
- Need frequent follow-up and lab checks
- Many patients die, most often from transformation to AML or pancytopenia.

Practice Questions for Hematologic Review

1. The most commonly occurring leukemia in children is

   (A) acute lymphocytic leukemia (ALL).
   (B) acute myelocytic leukemia (AML).
   (C) plasma cell myeloma.
   (D) lymphoma.
   (E) chronic lymphocytic leukemia (CLL).

2. Iron deficiency anemia is characterized by a serum ferritin level of

   (A) < 10 ng/mL.
   (B) < 12 ng/mL.
   (C) < 15 ng/mL.
   (D) < 20 ng/mL.
   (E) < 25 mg/mL.

3. Patients with glucose-6-phosphate dehydrogenase (G6PD) deficiency develop episodes of hemolysis in response to infection or

   (A) cold temperatures.
   (B) high altitudes.
   (C) oxidant drugs.
   (D) trauma.
   (E) none of the above.

4. The hallmark laboratory finding of aplastic anemia is

   (A) markedly elevated WBCs.
   (B) markedly decreased hemoglobin and hematocrit levels.
   (C) pancytopenia.
   (D) markedly increased inflammatory markers.
   (E) decreased WBCs.

5. A 23-year-old male presents to the clinic with a complaint of "swollen lymph nodes." He denies fever, recent infections, or exposures to toxins. He does report recent onset of night sweats and weight loss. On examination, diffuse lymphadenopathy is noted. This presentation is consistent with

   (A) acute myelocytic leukemia.
   (B) non-Hodgkin lymphoma.
   (C) hairy cell leukemia.
   (D) chronic lymphocytic leukemia.
   (E) plasma cell myeloma.

6. You are evaluating a 68-year-old male with a complaint of bone pain in his back, hips, and ribs. He states this is fairly recent onset and taking ibuprofen has not helped. He is having some increased difficulty and pain with walking because of his hip pain. You include myeloma in your differential diagnoses. Initial imaging should include

   (A) bone radiographs.
   (B) CT of the axial skeleton.
   (C) MRI of the long bones.
   (D) radionuclide imaging.
   (E) PET scan.

7. Your patient is a 72-year-old female who is seen for a regular annual exam. Her CBC reveals elevated platelets (> 500,000). The rest of her labs are normal, and her PE is unremarkable. You consider a diagnosis of essential thrombocytosis and the increased risk of

   (A) thrombosis.
   (B) hemolytic anemia.
   (C) rheumatoid arthritis.
   (D) chronic myeloblastic leukemia.
   (E) acute myelocytic leukemia.

8. You are managing the care of a patient with iron deficiency anemia. Expected return to normal hematocrit level with consistent administration of ferrous sulfate is

   (A) 1 month.
   (B) 2 months.
   (C) 3 months.
   (D) 6 months.
   (E) 9 months.

9. Beta-thalassemia primarily affects individuals of

   (A) Southeast Asian origin.
   (B) Chinese origin.
   (C) Mediterranean origin.
   (D) African origin.
   (E) Hispanic origin.

10. Most patients with vitamin B12 deficiency have serum levels less than

    (A) 200 pg/mL.
    (B) 400 pg/mL.
    (C) 600 pg/mL.
    (D) 1000 pg/mL.
    (E) 1500 pg/mL.

Answers Explained

1. **(A)** ALL is the most common leukemia in children and occurs most often in children between the ages of 3–4 years.

2. **(B)** A serum ferritin level of less than 12 ng/mL is characteristic of iron deficiency anemia. IDA is caused by bleeding, unless it is ruled out.

3. **(C)** G6PD is a hereditary condition that causes episodes of hemolysis in response to infection or exposure to oxidant drugs such as nitrofurantoin, quinolones, dapsone, methylene blue, and trimethoprim-sulfamethoxazole, among others. The other factors included are not implicated in hemolytic episodes in G6PD deficiency.

4. **(C)** Pancytopenia is characteristic of aplastic anemia and represents bone marrow failure. Patients often present for care with complaints of severe weakness and fatigue.

5. **(B)** Non-Hodgkin lymphoma often presents as painless lymphadenopathy. Patients may also report systemic symptoms such as night sweats, fever, and weight loss. On exam, the lymphadenopathy may be localized or diffuse. Tissue biopsy is required for diagnosis. (A) AML presents wtih short duration of fatigue, fever, and bleeding. (C) Hairy cell leukemia often presents with massive splenomegaly. (D) CLL occurs most often in older patients and presents as fatigue or lymphadenopathy. Liver or spleen enlargement may or may not be present. (E) Bone pain is often the first symptom of plasma cell myeloma. Pain is reported in the spine, ribs, or proximal portions of the long bones.

6. **(A)** Bone radiographs are useful in evaluating for myeloma, as lytic lesions may be identified on the axial skeleton, spine, skull, proximal long bones, and the ribs. Other studies mentioned may be indicated later in the management process; however, radiographs are key for diagnostic clarity.

7. **(A)** Essential thrombocytosis is characterized by the presence of elevated platelets without other abnormal findings. Patients may present with thrombosis and may occur in unusual sites, such as the hepatic vein. Splenomegaly is present frequently. (B, C, D, E) These conditions may co-exist but are not associated with essential thrombocytosis.

8. **(B)** The hematocrit should begin to rebound within weeks of starting therapy and should be halfway to normal within 3 weeks. After 2 months, the hematocrit should return to normal levels.

9. **(C)** Beta-thalassemia is seen primarily in persons of Mediterranean origin. It is seen less often in those with Asian or African origin.

10. **(A)** At diagnosis, most patients with vitamin B12 deficiency have levels lower than 200 pg/mL. However, symptomatic patients may present with levels below 100 pg/mL.

9

Infectious Disease Review

Learning Objectives

In this chapter, you will review:

→ Viral exanthems and diseases
→ Measles
→ Hand-foot-mouth disease
→ Fifth disease

Viral Exanthems

Measles (Rubeola)

Pathophysiology

Measles is a part of the paramyxovirus family of viruses. It is highly contagious with greater than 90% of contacts developing infection and is spread through direct contact and airborne transmission. Measles is more common in resource-limited areas due to low vaccination rates or communities with declining vaccine uptake. Susceptible individuals include those who have never been or only been partially vaccinated and children too young for vaccination.

Clinical Presentation

There are three stages of clinical presentation:

Stage 1: Incubation
Lasts 10–14 days during which time patients are typically asymptomatic.

Stage 2: Prodrome
Characterized by onset of fever and the classic triad of cough, coryza, and conjunctivitis. During this phase, severity of symptoms tends to increase and lasts 5–7 days. Koplik spots, white-gray dots with surrounding erythema on the buccal mucosa, appear 48 hours prior to rash and are considered pathognomonic of measles.

Stage 3: Exanthem
Erythematous maculopapular rash, which starts on forehead, hairline, or behind ears and spreads in cephalocaudad progression to trunk and extremities, including the palms and soles. A rash becomes confluent and lasts 3–7 days and fades in the same manner it appeared.

Diagnosis and Lab Studies

High clinical suspicion should be maintained in patients with cough, coryza, conjunctivitis, and a febrile rash who have not completed measles vaccination. All cases of measles should be reported to the local health department.

Diagnosis is confirmed via:

- PCR testing via oropharyngeal swab or urine
  (can be detected up to 5 days before symptoms)
- Serologic anti-measles IgM antibodies
  (typically not detected until 3 days after exanthem appears)
- Four-fold increase between acute and convalescent serologic anti-measles IgG antibodies

Treatment (Pharmaceutical and Clinical Intervention)

Treatment is largely supportive, including rest and antipyretics. Recovery occurs 7–10 days after the onset of symptoms. Patients should be isolated through 4 days after onset of rash. Complications include upper and lower respiratory bacterial superinfection, encephalitis, and hemorrhagic measles. Complications are more common in immunosuppressed, pregnant, or malnourished patients.

Health Maintenance and Patient Education

Measles is vaccine-preventable via 2 dose immunization series. Two formulations of combination vaccine are available in the United States. Both vaccines are live-attenuated and vaccination typically begins at 12 months of age.

- Measles-mumps-rubella (MMR)
- Measles-mumps-rubella-varicella (MMRV)

Hand-Foot-Mouth Disease (HFMD)

Pathophysiology

Hand-foot-mouth disease (HFMD) is caused by coxsackie, a virus, part of the enterovirus family. It is most common in children less than 10 years old with peak presentation in summer and fall. HFMD is highly contagious, and outbreaks are common in daycare or school settings.
The majority of transmission is fecal-oral route and has a relatively short incubation period of 4–6 days, viral shedding.

Clinical Presentation

- Nonspecific 1–2 day prodrome of fever and malaise followed by development of sore throat
- Characteristic exanthem is vesicular rash on palms and soles.
- Lesions may be tender.
- Classically associated with enanthem of oral lesions on tongue, which can be painful leading to decreased oral intake and dehydration
- Over two-thirds of patients have both the characteristic exanthem and oral enanthem.
- Lesions resolve in 1–2 weeks.
- Complications are rare with the most common being aseptic meningitis.

Diagnostic and Lab Studies

Diagnosis of HFMD is based on clinical appearance. The lesions appear on the buccal mucosa, hands, and feet beginning as vesicles, forming bullae, and then ulcerating. The lesions are highly contagious.

Differential Diagnosis

Differential diagnosis includes vesicular eruptions, such as herpes simplex virus and varicella. For patients with lesions limited to the mouth, consider aphthous ulcers.

Treatment (Pharmaceutical and Clinical Intervention)

Treatment is supportive care with particular attention to avoiding dehydration.

Erythema Infectiosum (Fifth Disease)

Pathophysiology

Erythema infectiousum is caused by parvovirus B19 and most commonly affects school-aged children. Infection is thought to confer lifelong immunity. Transmission is typically via respiratory route, through vertical transmission is an important consideration as congenital infection is associated with poor fetal outcome. Contagious period is only until onset of generalized rash.

Clinical Presentation

After approximately 1 week incubation period:

A nonspecific prodrome of fever is followed by appearance of a bright red facial rash, described as "slapped cheeks." Within 1–2 days, a lacy reticular rash appears and spreads distally on trunk and extensor surfaces of extremities. The palms and soles are typically spared. The rash may persist for 2–3 weeks before slowly fading.

Diagnosis and Lab Studies

Diagnosis in children is often based on clinical appearance, though specific IgM antibody tests are available. Pregnant women with known exposure to a patient with parvovirus B19 infection should have IgG, IgM, and PCR for DNA testing to determine susceptibility and/or infection.

Treatment (Pharmaceutical and Clinical Intervention)

No specific treatment is available for erythema infectiosum; most illnesses are benign. Fetal infection with parvovirus B19 can result in hydrops fetalis and fetal death.

Practice Questions for Infectious Disease Review

1. The classic symptom triad characterizing measles includes cough, conjunctivitis, and

   (A) fever.
   (B) coryza.
   (C) diarrhea.
   (D) rash.
   (E) vomiting.

2. Hand-foot-mouth disease is caused by

   (A) herpes simplex virus.
   (B) coxsackie virus.
   (C) Epstien-Barr virus.
   (D) paramyxovirus.
   (E) adenovirus.

3. Erythema infectiousum (fifth disease) is a common childhood illness characterized by a bright red rash on the cheeks ("slapped cheek") and circumoral pallor which progresses to a lacy, maculopapular rash with fever. The rash usually affects the arms, legs, and torso. This infection is caused by

   (A) Epstien-Barr virus.
   (B) paramyxovirus.
   (C) parvovirus B19.
   (D) coxsackie virus.
   (E) rhinovirus.

4. You are evaluating a 17-year-old male who presents with complaints of a "rash" on his trunk, arms, and legs. On exam, you note pearly-appearing, raised, umbilicated nodules on the limbs and torso. The palms and soles are unaffected. This dermatologic presentation is consistent with

   (A) variola infection.
   (B) varicella infection.
   (C) molluscum contagiosum.
   (D) paravaccinia.
   (E) infectious mononucleosis.

5. Severe Acute Respiratory Syndrome (SARS-CoV-1) is a respiratory illness first seen in China in 2002. The illness may range in severity from mild to severe; however, there is a high mortality rate associated with SARS. Patients usually present with dry cough, dyspnea, and fever. The disease continues to be endemic in many areas of Asia. The natural host/reservoir of SARS is

   (A) cattle.
   (B) the horseshoe bat.
   (C) monkeys.
   (D) sheep.
   (E) dogs.

6. Respiratory syncytial virus (RSV) is a paramyxovirus that causes annual outbreaks of respiratory illness with most cases seen

   (A) between late January and early March.
   (B) between early March and May.
   (C) during the summer months.
   (D) between mid-October and early January.
   (E) year-round.

7. Seasonal influenza is caused by types A, B, and C viruses. Types A and B may cause more serious illness presentation, whereas type C usually produces a milder illness. Treatment is supportive along with antiviral therapy for lab-confirmed illness. The CDC recommends which of the following as first-line pharmacotherapy for all age groups for seasonal influenza?

   (A) Baloxavir
   (B) Inhaled zanamivir
   (C) IV peramivir
   (D) Oral oseltamivir
   (E) Oral amoxicillin

8. Rabies is a severe disease with 100% mortality if untreated. The disease is caused by

   (A) paramyxovirus.
   (B) rhabdovirus.
   (C) parvovirus.
   (D) arbovirus.
   (E) enterovirus.

9. Rubella is a common childhood illness caused by a togavirus. Transmission is via

   (A) oral-fecal route.
   (B) exposure to body fluids such as saliva.
   (C) inhalation of respiratory droplets.
   (D) direct skin-to-skin contact.
   (E) exposure to contaminated water.

10. Measles is a highly contagious disease presenting as a bright red, maculopapular rash along with Koplik spots, coryza, cough, fever, conjunctivitis, malaise, and photophobia. The first dose of the measles vaccine is given at

    (A) 2 months of age.
    (B) 6 months of age.
    (C) age 4 years.
    (D) 18–24 months of age.
    (E) 12–15 months of age.

Answer Explanations

1. **(B)** Measles is caused by a paramyxovirus and is highly contagious. The classic symptom triad includes cough, coryza, and conjunctivitis. Other symptoms may be present; however, they are not included in the classic triad.

2. **(B)** HFMD is caused by coxsackie and is seen most commonly in children under age 10. The disorder is highly contagious and spread is usually by the fecal-oral route.

3. **(C)** Parvovirus B19 is the underlying etiology for EI.

4. **(C)** Molluscum contagiosum presents with pearly-appearing, umbilicated nodules on the torso and limbs, sparing the palms of the hands and soles of the feet. Patients may develop keratoconjunctivitis; therefore, ocular exam should be performed. Molluscum contagiosum is spread sexually or through close personal contact. (A) Variola/vaccinia is smallpox infection, which is highly contagious associated with high mortality rates. The lesions in smallpox develop and resolve synchronously, which helps differentiate the disease from varicella infection. (B) Varicella is chickenpox, another highly contagious disorder that is seen less often in the US since the advent of widespread vaccination. (D) Paravaccinia (milker's nodules) is an occupational disease spread through contact with cattle or sheep/goats.

5. **(B)** The horseshoe bat is considered to be the reservoir for SARS, which is spread through the fecal-oral route. The other animals mentioned are not considered host carriers of SARS CoV-1.

6. **(D)** RSV cases are seen annually starting in mid-October and extending through early January. Treatment is supportive and most patients recover without sequelae; however, the disease may be serious in young neonates/infants.

7. **(D)** Oral oseltamivir is dosed at 75 mg BID for 5 days in the presence of confirmed influenza. Maximum benefits are seen when the drug is started within 48 hours of symptom onset. The CDC recommends this as first-line treatment for all ages and includes women who are pregnant and patients who are hospitalized. (A) Baloxavir is given orally with the dosing based on weight. Effects and efficacy for patients younger than age 12 and older than 65 years have not been established. (B) Inhaled zanamivir is given as 2 inhalations of 10 mg twice daily for 5 days with indications for patients 7 years and older. The medication has a relative contraindication in patients with asthma because of the risk for bronchospasm. (C) Peramivir is given as a single IV dose of 600 mg in patients aged 18 years and older. This medication is reserved for individuals in whom there may be inadequate absorption of oral medication.

8. **(B)** Rabies is caused by a rhabdovirus, producing a severe encephalitis. The disease is transmitted through the saliva of an infected animal, usually through a bite. In the United States, bats, skunks, and racoons make up 82% of rabid animals found. Other animals known to carry and transmit the disease include dogs, cats, foxes, and cattle. Presentation often includes a history of a known bite from an animal; however, bat bites may be imperceptible. Postexposure prophylactic treatment is almost 100% effective in preventing disease if given before symptoms develop.

9. **(C)** Rubella is transmitted through inhalation of respiratory droplets. This very common illness is usually mild with symptoms of fever, coryza, malaise, and rash. The primary concern with rubella, however, is exposure of a fetus. The disease has severe consequences on the unborn fetus. Fetal death, especially if exposed during the first trimester, is common. Exposure during the second trimester causes deafness. Congenital malformations, preterm delivery, and congenital rubella are among the devastating effects of rubella on the developing fetus.

10. **(E)** The first dose of the measles vaccine is given between 12–15 months with the second dose between 4–6 years of age.

10
Musculoskeletal Review

Learning Objectives

In this chapter, you will review:

→ Chest/rib disorders
→ Compartment syndrome
→ Degenerative disorders
→ Infectious disorders
→ Lower extremity disorders
→ Upper extremity disorders
→ Neoplasms
→ Rheumatologic disorders
→ Spinal disorders

Chest/Rib Disorders

Sternum Fractures

Pathophysiology

Fractures of the sternum may occur as direct fractures resulting from a force applied to the sternum, usually from a body blow affecting the lower part of the bone. Indirect fractures result from a flexion-compression injury of the cervico-thoracic spine, which causes the upper two ribs to force the manubrium down. This type of injury may be exacerbated by the chin being forced down, hitting the manubrium, and always involves the upper two parts of the sternum. Stress fractures of the sternum may occur as a result of repetitive motion of chest muscles, ribs, and clavicles. This type of repetitive motion occurs when playing golf, wrestling, and weight lifting. Muscular fractures occur from violent muscle spasms through opposing muscle groups, such as occurs with tetanus. This type of fracture is extremely rare. In adults, most sternal fractures are a result of motor vehicle accidents.

Clinical Presentation

Symptoms

- Usually a history of injury or an incident in which the fracture occurs
- Pain with inspiration
- Transient dyspnea

Signs

- Localized tenderness over fracture site, usually readily reducible
- Bruising
- Swelling
- Palpable or visible "step-off" deformity with displaced fracture
- Palpable crepitus
- Edema, bruising

Diagnostic and Lab Studies

A chest PA and lateral radiograph is gold standard for diagnosis. Fractures are missed in over 80% of AP views.

- X-rays of cervical, thoracic, and lumbar spines to look for other injuries
- Consider echocardiogram, CT, etc., if underlying injury suspected

Differential Diagnoses

Differential diagnoses may include:

- Costochondral dislocation
- Sternal contusion
- Costochondritis
- Rib fracture/dislocation
- Cardiac causes including laceration, ischemia, myocarditis, contusion
- Aortic dissection
- Pleurisy
- Sickle cell crisis
- Osteomyelitis

Health Maintenance and Patient Education

Advise patients that sternal pain may last for up to 12 weeks and to try to avoid activities that cause pain. Also advise patients to avoid pulling or pushing with arms when moving in bed or getting up, and teach them to brace the chest with a pillow when coughing or sneezing.

Treatment (Pharmaceutical and Clinical Intervention)

Pharmaceutical

- NSAIDs for analgesia

Clinical

- Evaluate for life-threatening injuries when patient presents with sternum fracture
- Consider 24-hour observation in the setting of possible underlying injuries

Displaced fractures may be reduced by having the patient lie supine and lift the head and lower extremities at the same time. This separates the upper and lower parts of the sternum and will allow reduction by applying firm pressure on the displaced fragment. Local anesthetic should be injected prior to this maneuver.

- Open reduction internal fixation indicated with respiratory limitation due to pain or flail chest injury
- Immobilization usually not needed for non-displaced fractures

Professional Considerations

Patient should not return to contact sports until symptoms fully subside, usually 6–12 weeks. Although mortality from isolated sternal fractures is low, the high energy force required to fracture the sternum is usually associated with other, more severe injuries, and these injuries have a 25–45% mortality rate.

Compartment Syndrome

Pathophysiology

Compartment syndrome may be acute or chronic and affects hands, feet, arms, and legs. Acute compartment syndrome (ACS) may develop following injury such as a fracture, surgical procedures, or placement of a too-tight cast or bandage. The compartments of the leg and forearm are composed of muscles, bones, nerves, and ligaments and are encapsulated by fascia and skin, producing a closed space or compartment. Following injury, pressure builds up within the compartment, as a result of bleeding, fluids, and response of tissues to the injury itself. When the swelling continues to increase in this closed space, blood vessels and other tissues within the compartment become compromised. When tissue swelling, or pressure, rises to the level of the diastolic pressure, microcirculation is compromised, even though the peripheral pulse is unchanged. Nerve damage begins within 30 minutes. After 12 hours, irreversible loss of function occurs if the pressure is not relieved. Muscles require a large blood supply. When microcirculation is severely diminished, muscles become ischemic, and necrosis begins within 2–4 hours. After 12 hours, if the pressure is not relieved, this necrosis becomes irreversible. The overall pathophysiology of acute compartment syndrome is cellular anoxia due to ischemic changes within the affected compartment.

Compartment syndromes are sometimes seen following fractures of the forearm and tibia (Volkmann's ischemia). Volkmann's ischemia is often seen with supracondylar fractures of the humerus in children. Fracture of the tibia may result in anterior compartment syndrome.

Clinical Presentation

Symptoms of ACS

- Severe pain in the affected extremity, out of proportion to the injury
- A burning, aching pain deep in the muscles of the extremity that does not resolve
- Numbness, tingling, or paresthesia of the extremity (onset within 30 minutes to 2 hours of injury)
- Anterior compartment syndrome: pain of the anterior aspect of the tibia
- Loss of sensation between the great toe and the second toe
- Weakness and/or dorsiflexion of the foot on the affected side
- Volkmann's ischemia: pain, often referred to the palmar area

Signs of ACS

- Tense, "wood-like" finding on examination of compartmental area
- Pain with dorsiflexion of the toes
- Pain with passive extension of the toes
- Weakened toe flexion
- Swelling and blistering of the skin
- Marked redness or discoloration of skin
- Limited range of motion and/or mobility of affected extremity
- Paralysis of extremity, foot drop, contractures, gangrene (late findings)

> **Five classic signs of arterial insufficiency (may or may not be present);**
> **5 P's: pain, pallor, pulselessness, paresthesias, poikilothermia.**

Diagnostic and Lab Studies

Diagnosis usually based on clinical findings in conjunction with the following measures:

- Measurement of compartment pressures: ACS delta pressure = diastolic BP-measured compartment pressure
- ACS delta pressure < 20–30 mmHg indicates need for fasciotomy
- Continuous compartment pressure monitoring
- Lab findings are abnormal in late stages: increased serum creatine kinase (CK), myoglobinuria within 4 hours of onset

Differential Diagnoses

Rapid progression of symptoms and signs over a few hours is highly suggestive of ACS, especially when combined with multiple examination findings consistent with the diagnosis.

Health Maintenance and Patient Education

ACS

- Advise patients who sustain limb fractures or undergo casting or surgery on an extremity and to report pain that is worse than expected; burning pain or deep aching that does not go away; or numbness, tingling, or loss of feeling in an extremity.
- Clearly explain the need for emergent evaluation and treatment.
- Complications may include loss of function and/or limb; mortality is high for patients who require fasciotomy, especially if treatment is delayed.

Treatment (Pharmaceutical and Clinical Intervention)

ACS

Pharmaceutical
- Supplemental oxygen
- Analgesics
- Hypotonic IV saline boluses may be administered to treat hypotension, which further reduces tissue perfusion.

Clinical
- Immediate measures include the removal of all external sources of pressure on the compartment.
- Keep the limb level with the torso, not elevated or lowered.
- Continuous or serial measurements of compartment pressure
- Surgical fasciotomy to fully decompress affected compartments remains the definitive treatment.

Professional Considerations

High index of suspicion should be held for diagnosis in the setting of injury to limb. Consider that ACS may develop without injury or trauma.

Osteoarthritis (Degenerative Diseases)

Pathophysiology

Osteoarthritis (OA) is also known as degenerative joint disease (DJD). This condition is associated with aging, degeneration of joint cartilage, and hypertrophy of articular bone. There does seem to be a genetic component involved in development of DJD. Mechanical overuse of joints also predisposes individuals to DJD. The disease is also divided into primary and secondary types. Primary DJD affects the DIP and PIP joints of the fingers, MTP joint of the big toe, carpometa-carpal joint of the thumb, as well as the cervical and lumbar spine. Secondary DJD occurs as a sequelae to joint injury and may occur in any joint.

Clinical Presentation

Symptoms
- Insidious onset of joint stiffness, usually resolving within 15 minutes
- Pain in the joint made worse by activity and relieved by rest

Signs
- Flexion contractures or varus deformity of the knee on exam
- Bony enlargements of DIP (Heberden's nodes) and PIP (Bouchard nodes)
- Limited range of motion of affected joints
- Crepitus over the joint
- Mild joint effusion
- No systemic manifestations found

Diagnostic and Lab Studies

- No elevation of ESR or WBC
- Synovial fluid aspiration is noninflammatory.
- Radiographs may demonstrate joint space narrowing, presence of osteophytes, thickened subchondral bone, and bone cysts.

Differential Diagnoses

Differential diagnoses may include:

- Rheumatoid arthritis: presents with systemic signs; distribution of affected joints helps distinguish DJD from RA
- Skeletal symptoms of DJD may co-exist with metastatic neoplasia, osteoporosis, myeloma, or other bone diseases.
- Gout, pseudogout
- Peripheral vascular disease
- Neuropathy
- Infective arthritis
- Soft tissue injury
- Giant cell arteritis
- Osteopenia

Health Maintenance and Patient Education

- Nonpharmacologic measures: weight loss, physical therapy and exercise, online support groups
- Medications for arthritis include NSAIDs, topical therapies, acetaminophen, and joint injections
- Surgery reserved for severe disease

Treatment (Pharmaceutical and Clinical Intervention)

Pharmaceutical

- Oral NSAIDs
- Topical NSAIDs
- Acetaminophen and opioids
- Duloxetine
- Intra-articular injections

Clinical

- Assistive devices
- Weight loss
- Occupational and physical therapy
- Surgery for severe disease may include joint replacement.

Professional Considerations

Consider multidisciplinary care for severe cases, especially with functional impairment present.

Osteomyelitis (Infectious Diseases)

Pathophysiology

Osteomyelitis is an acute or chronic infection of bone as a result of hematogenous dissemination of bacteria, invasion of bone from a contiguous source of infection, direct inoculation of bacteria into intact bone via trauma or surgery, or skin breakdown associated with vascular insufficiency. Acute osteomyelitis involves a suppurative infectious process with associated edema and vascular compromise. Acute infection leads to development of sections of bony necrosis, which may include pus. Chronic osteomyelitis occurs in the setting of necrotic bony tissue or recurrence of a previous infection. Hematogenous osteomyelitis is usually caused by *Staphylococcus aureus*, coagulase-negative staphylococci and aerobic gram-negative bacteria, *Pseudomonas aeruginosa* (often seen with IV drug abuse), *Salmonella sp.* (sickle cell disease), and fungi (usually seen in immunocompromised individuals or endemic areas). Contiguous focus osteomyelitis usually involves several different organisms and is seen in patients with diabetes mellitus, those with a sacral decubitus ulcer, or those who have sustained a puncture wound through a shoe (e.g., stepping on a nail). Internal prosthetic devices may be associated with coagulase-negative staph and *S. aureus* infections.

Clinical Presentation

Symptoms

- Fever
- Chills
- Redness, swelling of affected area

Signs

- Limited range of motion
- Fever
- Tenderness, signs of localized infection
- Presence of exposed bone
- Finding of large decubitus ulcer
- Positive probe to bone test
- Presence of diabetes mellitus may mask classic symptoms and signs.

Diagnostic and Lab Studies

- CRP: usually elevated but is nonspecific
- WBC may be elevated or normal
- ESR usually high
- Elevated procalcitonin
- X-ray is first-line imaging: classic triad for osteomyelitis is demineralization, periosteal reaction, and bone destruction
- Bone scan indicated after X-ray, if prosthesis-related infection suspected
- Radionuclide scanning for ambiguous diagnosis
- MRI for suspected septic arthritis, spinal infection; indicated for associated soft-tissue involvement
- CT, if indicated, to assess for bony fragments and sequestration
- Vertebral disc aspiration, if indicated
- Blood culture
- Bone biopsy, if indicated

Differential Diagnoses

Differential diagnoses may include:

- Aseptic bone infarction
- Gout
- Fractures/trauma
- Systemic infection from another source
- Tumor
- Neuropathic joint disease (Charcot foot)
- Brodie abscess (subacute osteomyelitis)

Health Maintenance and Patient Education

Patients recommended to keep diabetes under control. Patients should also be mindful of foot care.

Treatment (Pharmaceutical and Clinical Intervention)

Pharmaceutical

- Antibiotics based on pathogen; if patient clinically stable, avoid starting antibiotics until culture results available
- If patient is unstable, start empiric antibiotic therapy based on probable organism
- Optimal antibiotic concentrations at infection site is critical; consider vascular perfusion

Treatment

- Is usually 4–6 weeks; consider longer for MRSA or chronic osteomyelitis

Clinical

- Surgical removal of prosthetic device, if indicated as source of infection
- Maintain adequate nutrition, hydration, and glycemic control
- Wound debridement, if indicated

Professional Considerations

Multidisciplinary care team required for optimal management and follow-up.

Septic Arthritis (Infectious Disease)

Pathophysiology

Nongonococcal acute bacterial (septic) arthritis usually results from hematogenous spread of bacteria into a joint. Rarely direct penetrating injury of a joint may be the cause. *Staphylococcus aureus* is the most common pathogen.

Clinical Presentation

Symptoms

- Acute onset of pain, swelling, and warmth of affected joint; pain worsens over the next few hours
- Knee is most commonly involved joint; others include the wrist, shoulder, hip, and ankle
- Chills and fever are common
- Infection of hip joint may cause increased pain with walking

Signs

- Joint effusions common
- 15% involve more than one joint
- Decreased range of motion due to pain

Diagnostics and Lab Studies

- Synovial fluid aspiration critical for diagnosis; always inflammatory
- Gram stain of synovial fluid
- Blood cultures: usually positive
- Imaging usually not indicated, especially early in the infectious process

Differential Diagnoses

Differential diagnoses may include:

- Gout and pseudogout
- Chronic Lyme disease
- Acute rheumatic fever

Health Maintenance and Patient Education

American Academy of Orthopedic Surgeons recommends prescribing antibiotic prophylaxis for any patient with a prosthetic joint replacement who is undergoing a procedure that could potentially cause bacteremia.

Treatment (Pharmaceutical and Clinical Intervention)

Pharmaceutical

- Appropriate antibiotic therapy based on culture of synovial fluid
- Empiric treatment recommendation is IV vancomycin plus a third-generation cephalosporin
- Duration of antibiotic therapy usually 4–6 weeks

Clinical

- Early orthopedic consultation indicated
- Drainage of affected joints via arthroscopic lavage and debridement
- Prosthetic removal may be indicated

Professional Considerations

Multidisciplinary team required for optimal management.

Lower Extremity Disorders

Avascular Necrosis of Bone

Pathophysiology

Avascular necrosis of bone is also known as osteonecrosis and is a complication of corticosteroid use, trauma, SLE, gout, sickle cell disease, alcoholism, pancreatitis, dysbaric syndrome, knee meniscectomy, and infiltrative disorders such as Gaucher disease. Sites most commonly affected include the proximal and distal femoral heads, which causes knee or hip pain. Other sites affected include the shoulder, ankle, and elbow. Osteonecrosis of the jaw has been associated with bisphosphonate therapy. Avascular necrosis is, essentially, death and architectural collapse of bone resulting from ischemia or injury. This bone collapse can lead to cartilage breakdown and arthritis.

Clinical Presentation

Symptoms

- May be asymptomatic in early disease
- Most common symptom is pain; pain in the groin and buttock are associated with AVN of the femoral head
- Pain with joint movement or weight-bearing
- Most patients report pain in the joint at rest; about one-third of patients report pain at night.

Signs

- Exam often nonspecific
- May find limited range of motion of affected joint
- Pain with internal rotation of leg
- Joint swelling may be present in advanced disease

Diagnostic and Lab Studies

Lab tests usually not useful for diagnosis; however, ESR and CRP elevated. Imaging determines stage of disease.

- Stages I and II: X-rays may be normal
- Stages III and IV: may reveal sclerosis of bone and areas of bone death
- MRI: gold standard to diagnose AVN
- Bone scans can reveal disease but are not useful in staging.

Differential Diagnoses

Differential diagnoses may include:

- Fracture
- Infection
- Arthritis/bursitis
- Tumor

Health Maintenance and Patient Education

Avoid or limit use of corticosteroids.

Treatment (Pharmaceutical and Clinical Intervention)

Pharmaceutical

- NSAIDs; acetaminophen for pain
- Potential benefit from high-dose HMG-CoA reductase inhibitors

Clinical

- Core decompression
- Stem cell transplant
- Bone grafting
- Osteotomy
- Arthroplasty or total joint replacement

Professional Considerations

Early orthopedic consult advised.

Development Dysplasia of the Hip (DDH)

Pathophysiology

Developmental dysplasia of the hip (DDH) involves complete or partial dislocation of the head of the femur from the acetabulum. DDH may occur any time, from conception until the skeleton has fully matured. Instability of the hip joint may be identified on newborn examination, and there are degrees of dysplasia including complete dislocation, a hip joint that is subluxable, as well as insufficient bony development of the acetabulum.

Clinical Presentation

Symptoms

Infants may cry with manipulation of the affected hip joint; there may be limited voluntary movement of the affected leg.

Signs

Exam findings with DDH may include asymmetrical inguinal or gluteal folds, unequal leg length, limited abduction of the hip joint, and unequal knee heights when the infant is supine with hips and knees flexed and feet side-by-side on the exam table (positive Galeazzi's sign). Positive Ortolani's sign (useful between the ages of 1 month and 3 months) and positive Barlow's sign. In toddlers and older children, limping, a waddling gait, toe-walking, leg length discrepancy, and lumbar lordosis may be seen.

Diagnostic and Lab Studies

- Positive Barlow and/or Ortolani tests on exam
- Positive Galeazzi sign on exam
- Pelvic ultrasound in neonates
- Anterior/posterior and Lauenstein X-rays after age 3 months
- MRI, tomography, and arthrography for difficult-to-diagnose cases
- Disruption of Shenton line (line drawn from the medial aspect of the femoral neck to the inferior border of the pubic rami)
- Measures of acetabular development (indices)

Differential Diagnoses

Differential diagnoses may include:

- Nonpathologic hip clicks may occur on newborn examination.
- Gait disturbances in older children may be due to neurologic pathology or injury/trauma to the lower extremity.
- Neoplasms of the bone may cause gait disturbances and pain in affected extremity.

Health Maintenance and Patient Education

Parental education about reporting symptoms of hip or extremity pain or discomfort; hip clicks or instability during diaper changes; delays in walking; reporting problems or concerns about gait in the ambulatory child.

Treatment (Pharmaceutical and Clinical Intervention)

Early treatment improves outcomes and reduces complication and need for more aggressive interventions.

- Abduction orthoses for 1–2 months: Pavlik harness or Frejka splint
- After age 6 months, surgical closed reduction
- After age 18 months, open reduction with osteotomy required

Professional Considerations

All well-child visits should include assessment for hip dysplasia. Possible complications include permanent dislocation of the femoral head with limited mobility. Aseptic and avascular necrosis of the femoral head may occur.

Hip Fracture

Pathophysiology

Hip fractures may be intracapsular or extracapsular, and 90% are caused by a twisting injury of a planted foot or a low-impact fall. Hip fractures occur predominantly in individuals 60 years or older. Most (80%) of hip fractures occur in women, although hip fractures in men are associated with higher mortality. Increased resorption of bone increases risk for osteoporosis and hip fracture. Primary causes include osteoporosis, direct blunt force trauma, avascular necrosis, pathologic disease (e.g., bone cancer), or overtraining leading to stress fractures.

Clinical Presentation

Symptoms

- Mechanism of injury important as falls to the side or high energy falls increase the risk of hip fracture
- Groin pain: if severe, displaced fracture likely
- Referred pain to the knee or distal femur
- Unable to walk

Signs

- When patient is lying supine, affected leg will be held in external rotation and abduction
- Affected extremity may be shortened
- Pain elicited with log roll maneuver
- Patient demonstrates inability to bear weight or perform straight leg raise

Diagnostic and Lab Studies

Radiographs are 90–95% sensitive. Views include:

- Cross-table lateral and AP
- Femoral shaft (include knee)
- Avoid frog-leg view, as this results in severe pain and may cause or worsen displacement.
- Obtain X-rays of other painful areas, as associated fractures are likely.
- MRI if hip fracture suspected but not seen on X-ray
- Preop labs based on patients general medical condition
- For patients over age 75, type and cross-match blood

Differential Diagnoses

Differential diagnoses may include:

- Pelvic fracture
- Osteoarthritis
- Pathologic fracture
- Rheumatoid arthritis
- Septic arthritis of hip
- Trochanteric bursitis
- Hip dislocation

Health Maintenance and Patient Education

Provide patient with treatment options early.

Treatment (Pharmaceutical and Clinical Intervention)

Pharmaceutical

- Local anesthetics for control of perioperative pain
- Opioids may be used for moderate pain; use shortest course feasible
- NSAIDs are not recommended.

Clinical Intervention

Urgent surgical repair, if indicated. Outcomes are better if surgery is performed within 24–48 hours of injury. Oxygen therapy as needed.

Professional Considerations

Initial care should be focused on control of pain and orthopedic consultation. Patients who were wheelchair confined prior to injury, or those who are poor surgical risk, may need conservative therapy only.

Osgood-Schlatter Disease (OSD)

Pathophysiology

Inflammation of the apophysis occurs due to repetitive strain to the tibial tuberosity. Commonly seen in adolescent boys and girls, especially those who participate in competitive sports. Etiology is unknown; however, association with exercise is clear. Sports that require jumping and pivoting place the highest strain on the tibial tubercle. Repetitive trauma to this area is likely the precipitating factor. Some evidence suggests association with tight hip flexors. Early specialization in sports is associated with a 4-fold risk for OSD.

Clinical Presentation

Symptoms

- Knee pain with crouching or squatting

Signs

- Absence of effusion or tenderness over the condyle
- Tenderness and swelling over tibial tuberosity
- Increased pain elicited with resisted knee extension or kneeling
- Redness over tibial tuberosity
- Single-leg squat (SLS; functional testing) and standing broad jump produces pain

Diagnostic and Lab Studies

Generally clinical diagnosis. No tests indicated. Radiographs may show heterotrophic calcification of the patellar tendon but are not needed for diagnosis.

Differential Diagnoses

Differential diagnoses may include:

- Proximal tibial stress fracture
- Osteomyelitis of proximal tibia
- Tumor
- Quadriceps tendon avulsion
- Infrapatellar tendinitis
- Tibial tuberosity fracture
- Iliotibial band syndrome
- Patellar fracture or stress fracture
- Osteochondritis dissecans

Health Maintenance and Patient Education

Patients should avoid any type of jumping sports or reduce activities that increase swelling and pain. Patients may safely return to play with mild pain. Quadriceps stretching and strengthening are important for patients to include in their daily routine. Reassure patients and family that symptoms will improve with time and rest.

Treatment (Pharmaceutical and Clinical Intervention)

Pharmaceutical

- NSAIDs as needed for pain

Clinical

- Ice applications 2–3 times per day for 20 minutes
- Rest and activity modification
- Physical therapy for hamstring strengthening and stretching
- Orthotics may help if patient has marked pronation
- Knee brace

Professional Considerations

Consider surgical referral if symptoms persist into adulthood.

Soft Tissue Injuries

Pathophysiology

Soft tissue injuries affecting the lower extremities include lacerations, abrasions, hematomas, and burns. Injuries are more commonly seen in children and adolescents who play competitive sports. Because of peripheral neuropathy associated with diabetes mellitus, adults may incur injury without being aware of it.

Clinical Presentation

Symptoms

- Symptoms should be consistent with history of event
- Localized pain may be present
- Active or slowed bleeding
- Limited use of extremity due to discomfort

Signs

- Physical exam findings should be consistent with history of injury
- No systemic findings present

Diagnostic and Lab Studies

None indicated for uncomplicated soft-tissue injury; however, if deeper injury or foreign matter is suspected, X-rays of area may be appropriate.

Differential Diagnoses

Differential diagnoses may include:

- Systemic disease such as rheumatoid arthritis
- SLE
- Abuse

Health Maintenance and Patient Education

Educate patient about first aid measures and signs of complications. Advise them to avoid activities that predispose them to further injury.

Treatment (Pharmaceutical and Clinical Intervention)

Pharmaceutical
Usually no medication is indicated for uncomplicated soft-tissue injuries.

Clinical Intervention
- Appropriate first aid management
- Recommend ice application
- Wound cleansing and debridement if appropriate

Professional Consideration

Soft tissue injuries may mask the presence of more serious deeper tissue disruption.

Ewing Sarcoma (Neoplasms)

Pathophysiology

Ewing sarcoma represents a family of cancers with shared etiology and treatment. Ewing sarcoma may affect the bone, soft tissues adjacent to bone, and chest wall. Most common sites for primary disease are pelvic bones, femur, and chest wall. Median age at diagnosis is 15 years; however, it can occur at any age. Most cases are sporadic with no association with familial cancers.

Clinical Presentation

Symptoms
- Pain most common symptom
- Pain often attributed to minor injuries
- Palpable mass
- Fever
- Limp
- Systemic symptoms of fever and weight loss (more common with metastatic disease)

Signs
- Palpable mass
- Local tenderness
- Pain with joint movement
- Fever
- Regional lymphadenopathy

Diagnostic and Lab Studies

- CBC to screen for bone marrow involvement
- LDH often elevated
- Liver function test
- Renal function tests
- Plain radiographs
- CT/MRI
- Biopsy

Differential Diagnoses

Differential diagnoses may include:

- Osteosarcoma
- Neuroblastoma
- Non-Hodgkin lymphoma
- Osteomyelitis
- Tendonitis
- Trauma
- Benign bone tumor

Health Maintenance and Patient Education

Five-year survival rate is around 60%.

Treatment (Pharmaceutical and Clinical Intervention)

Pharmaceutical

- Chemotherapy

Clinical Intervention

- Surgery
- Radiation therapy

Professional Considerations

Refer to physical therapy after surgery. Reproductive endocrinology referral should be indicated prior to treatment.

Rheumatologic Disorders

Fibromyalgia

Pathophysiology

Fibromyalgia is a disorder of central pain processing, and the etiology is unknown. Alterations in neuroendocrine, neurotransmitter, neuromodulation, and neuroreceptor function are present. Most frequently diagnosed in women aged 20–50.

Clinical Presentation

Symptoms

- Chronic widespread musculoskeletal pain
- Fatigue, headaches, and numbness
- Chronic generalized pain and aching stiffness
- Sleep disorders
- Irritable bowel syndrome
- Even minor exertion causes pain

Signs

- Physical exam normal with exception of tender "trigger points" produced on palpation

Diagnostic and Lab Studies

- Thyroid function tests
- Antinuclear antibody test

Differential Diagnoses

Differential diagnoses may include:

- Diagnosis of exclusion
- Rheumatoid arthritis

SLE

- Hypothyroidism
- Polymyalgia rheumatica
- Cancer: oncogenic osteomalacia

Health Maintenance and Patient Education

Course is typically fluctuating; however, around 30% may experience remission after 2 years of treatment.

Treatment (Pharmaceutical and Clinical Intervention)

Pharmaceutical

- FDA-approved medications: duloxetine, milnacipran, and pregabalin.
- Others are used off-label.

Clinical

- Educate about diagnosis, signs, symptoms, and treatment options
- Cognitive behavioral therapy improves mood, energy level, pain, and functional status.
- Aerobic exercise
- Strength training
- Weight loss
- Sleep hygiene

Professional Considerations

Patients with fibromyalgia are often prescribed multiple medications. Monitor for side effects and drug interactions at each visit.

Juvenile Idiopathic Arthritis (JIA)

Pathophysiology

JIA is a chronic inflammation of the synovial tissue, and the etiology is unknown. The diagnosis requires inflammation in at least one joint for at least 6 weeks. Age of onset is below 16 years. There are seven different subtypes of JIA:

Oligoarticular arthritis affects less than five joints during the first 6 months of diagnosis. Larger joints are most often affected, especially the knee. Usually occurs between 1 and 6 years. Most are ANA positive.

Juvenile psoriatic arthritis (JPsA) presents with sausage fingers or toes and nail pitting or splitting. It is a close relative with psoriasis; undifferentiated JIA inflammation in one or more joints and does not fit into other categories of JIA.

Polyarticular JIA affects five or more joints and may occur at any age. Patients with rheumatoid factor negative polyarticular JIA test negative for rheumatoid factor (RF); patients with rheumatoid factor positive polyarticular JIA test positive for RF on two occasions three months apart.

Systemic-onset disease presents with high spiking fevers and a pink/salmon-colored rash. Arthritis may not appear until several weeks following development of fever and rash.

Enthesitis-related arthritis (ERA) involves arthritis occurring at sites of attachment between ligaments or tendons and bone. Usually affects boys in late childhood or adolescence.

Clinical Presentation

Symptoms

- Morning stiffness that improves after a warm bath or shower
- Young children may not complain of pain but may walk with a limp or refuse to walk down a set of stairs in the morning.
- Joints often become painful again in the evening.
- Patients do not complain of severe pain; however, they avoid using affected joints.
- In systemic JIA, the patient has spikes of fever but is completely afebrile between episodes.

Signs

- Enthesitis and sacroiliac tenderness may be present.
- Rash, if present, suggests systemic disease.
- Lymphadenopathy and hepatosplenomegaly may be found in systemic disease.

Diagnostic and Lab Studies

There are no lab findings diagnostic for JIA.

- Patients with systemic disease may have elevated sed rates and anemia.
- ANA is useful in classifying disease type and assessing risk for uveitis.
- RF is positive in 15–20% of patients with polyarticular JIA, and this usually indicates a more aggressive disease presentation.
- Radiography is usually normal in early disease.

Differential Diagnoses

Differential diagnoses may include:

- Septic arthritis
- Trauma

- Lyme disease
- Acute rheumatic fever
- Malignancies
- Viral or postviral illness
- Inflammatory bowel disease
- SLE

Health Maintenance and Patient Education

The patient goal is to maintain range of motion and function of joints.

Treatment (Pharmaceutical and Clinical Intervention)

Pharmaceutical

- Glucocorticoids first line
- Intra-articular injections when only one or two joints are affected
- NSAIDs first line for mild JIA
- DMARDs
- Biologic agents

Clinical

- Treatment response varies widely
- Physical and occupational therapy
- Goal is to maintain function, range of motion, and muscle strength

Professional Considerations

Complications include joint degeneration, contractures, leg length discrepancy, growth retardation, uveitis, pericarditis, and cervical spine dislocation.

Polyarteritis Nodosa (PAN)

Pathophysiology

Polyarteritis nodosa is a segmental necrotizing inflammatory disorder affecting the medium and small arteries of the muscles. Intimal proliferation, thrombosis, and end-organ tissue damage are involved with this disorder. Most cases are idiopathic; however, about 20% are related to hepatitis B or C infection. Hepatitis B PAN causes direct injury to blood vessels as a result of viral replication and/or deposition of immune complexes with activation of complement and inflammatory responses. Classic triad of upper and lower respiratory tract disease with glomerulonephritis.

Clinical Presentation

Upper Respiratory Symptoms

- Nasal congestion, sinusitis, otitis, mastoiditis, stridor, gingivitis

Lower Respiratory Symptoms

- Dyspnea, cough, hemoptysis
- Migratory pain of the joints
- Red, irritated eyes
- Fever, malaise, weight loss

Signs

- Congestion, crusting, ulceration, bleeding of nasal septum
- "Saddle nose deformity" occurs late in disease
- Otitis media, proptosis, scleritis, episcleritis, conjunctivitis
- New hypertension
- Venous thrombosis

Diagnostic and Lab Studies

- Serum ANCA
- CBC with diff
- CMP
- Acute phase reactant levels
- Tissue biopsy for diagnosis confirmation
- Chest CT may show infiltrates, nodules, masses, and lung cavities
- Radiographs may prompt evaluation for cancer
- Sinus imaging may show extensive, severe sinusitis with sinus erosions

Differential Diagnoses

Differential diagnoses may include:

- Acute sinusitis
- Acute otitis media
- Rheumatoid arthritis
- Lung cancer

SLE

- Basement membrane disease
- Cocaine use

Health Maintenance and Patient Education

Patients are advised to follow a low salt diet, add a vitamin D supplementation, and are referred to a national support website for patients with PAN.

Treatment (Pharmaceutical and Clinical Intervention)

Two phases: induction of remission and maintenance of remission.

Pharmaceutical

- Rituximab with prednisone (induction)
- Cyclophosphamide with prednisone (induction)
- Azathioprine, methotrexate, or rituximab (maintenance)

Clinical

- Aggressive management of hypertension to prevent MI, stroke, renal failure

Professional Considerations

PAN requires multidisciplinary care.

Polymyalgia Rheumatica

Pathophysiology

Etiology is unknown. Pathology involves an interplay of multiple genetic and environmental factors. There is histologic evidence of GCA and parvovirus B19 in temporal artery DNA samples.

Clinical Presentation

Symptoms

- Pain and stiffness of shoulders and hips lasting for several weeks with no other cause determined
- Fever, malaise, and weight loss

Patients report problems combing their hair, putting on a coat, or rising from a chair. Symptoms may be unilateral at first but become symmetrical.

Signs

- Decreased range of motion of shoulders, hips, and neck
- Normal muscle strength
- Muscle tenderness to palpation
- Disuse atrophy
- Coexisting carpal tunnel syndrome
- Synovitis of small joints

Diagnostic and Lab Studies

Diagnostic tests and lab studies show:

- ESR: usually elevated
- CRP: elevated
- CBC with diff: normochromic anemia
- Anti-CCP antibodies: usually negative
- Rheumatoid factor: usually negative
- Liver function tests: mild elevation
- EMG: normal
- Muscle biopsy: normal histology
- CK: always normal

Differential Diagnoses

Differential diagnoses may include:

- Rheumatoid arthritis
- Thyroid disease
- Osteoarthritis
- Parathyroid disease
- Polymyositis-dermatomyositis

SLE

- Sjogren syndrome; fibromyalgia
- Psoriatic arthritis

- Ankylosing spondylitis
- Occult infection or malignancy
- Rotator cuff syndrome

Health Maintenance and Patient Education

Review side effects of corticosteroid use and discuss symptoms of giant cell arteritis (which commonly co-occurs)—headache, visual loss, diplopia. Advise to seek care immediately if these occur. Patients should not abruptly stop steroids. Ensure patients have adequate calcium and vitamin D intake.

Treatment (Pharmaceutical and Clinical Intervention)

Pharmaceutical

Initial prednisone therapy for 2–4 weeks with slow taper. Dramatic improvement should be noted within 72 hours. If this is not seen, consider diagnosis. Most patients require prednisone for a minimum of 1 year.

Clinical

- Address risk of steroid-induced bone loss
- Recommend daily calcium and vitamin D
- Physical therapy for strength training

Professional Considerations

Consider PMR in patients over 50 who present with shoulder and hip stiffness and pain.

Polymyositis: Reactive Arthritis

Pathophysiology

Polymyositis is one of a group of immune-related inflammatory myopathies. These diseases are characterized by progressive muscle weakness and demonstrate inflammatory infiltration of muscle tissue. Pathophysiology occurs as a result of an inflammatory process mediated by T cells and cytokine release. This causes damage to skeletal muscle cells. The etiology is unknown but viral component may be involved.

Clinical Presentation

Symptoms

- Progressive muscle weakness occurring over weeks to months
- Weakness usually involves proximal muscle groups of the arms and legs, as well as the neck. Leg Weakness usually occurs before arm weakness.
- "Sticking sensation" below the sternum

Signs

Proximal muscle weakness involving:

- Shoulder muscles
- Hip girdle muscles
- Muscle swelling, stiffness, and induration

Rash over face may be present; also affects upper chest and dorsal hands.

- Periorbital edema
- Cardiac impairment, cardiac arrhythmia, cardiac failure

Diagnostic and Lab Studies

- Creatine kinase (CK) and/or aldolase elevation
- Abnormal EMG
- Muscle biopsy

Differential Diagnoses

Differential diagnoses may include:

- Vasculitis
- SLE
- RA
- Sarcoidosis
- ALS
- Muscular dystrophy
- Lambert-Eaton syndrome
- Thyroid disorders
- Cushing syndrome
- Drug-induced myopathies
- Infectious myositis

Health Maintenance and Patient Education

Limit physical activity in early phases.

Treatment (Pharmaceutical and Clinical Intervention)

Pharmaceutical

- Oral prednisone 40–60 mg daily initially
- Adjust dose downward while monitoring muscle strength and serum CK levels
- Immunosuppressive drugs are often prescribed to decrease overall corticosteroid exposure.

Clinical

Patients should be monitored closely for signs of disease extension or development of complications of long-term corticosteroid use.

Professional Considerations

All patients with myositis should receive a rheumatology and/or neurology referral. Patients should be monitored for signs of rhabdomyolysis.

Scleroderma

Pathophysiology

Scleroderma is a systemic disease that is characterized by development of diffuse fibrosis of the skin and visceral organs, along with vascular dysfunction. The disease may range from mild to severe based on systems affected. Diffuse disease involves thickening of the skin of the distal and proximal extremities, while limited disease is restricted to the hands, fingers, and face. Limited disease is characterized by CREST syndrome: calcinosis, Raynaud phenomenon, esophageal dysmotility, sclerodactyly, and telangiectasia.

Clinical Presentation

Symptoms

- Coldness and pallor of hands (Raynaud phenomenon)
- Thickening of the skin
- Puffy hands
- Itching
- Gastrointestinal reflux

Signs

- Digital pitting or ulcerations
- Tightness and swelling of skin on the fingers and toes
- Hypo or hyperpigmentation of skin
- Narrowing of the oral aperture
- Telangiectasia
- Joint stiffness
- Polyarthralgia
- Proximal muscle weakness
- Dysphagia
- Hypertension
- Dry crackles heard at lung bases
- Neuropathy

Cardiac conduction abnormalities:

- cardiomyopathy

Diagnostic and Lab Studies

- Nail fold capillary microscopy: characteristic finding is drop out
- CBC
- Creatinine
- Urinalysis: may show albuminuria, hematuria
- ANA: positive in > 90% of patients
- Anti-Scl-70 antibody: highly specific for systemic disease
- Chest X-ray: may show diffuse reticular pattern and/or bilateral pulmonary fibrosis in bases
- Hand X-ray: soft tissue atrophy
- ECG: may show conduction abnormalities
- Echocardiograph: may show pulmonary hypertension or cardiomyopathy
- High resolution CT: alveolitis or fibrosis

Follow-up testing for patients should include pulmonary function testing.

Differential Diagnoses

Differential diagnoses may include:

- Scleroderma
- Nephrogenic systemic fibrosis
- Mixed connective tissue disease
- Eosinophilia-myalgia syndrome

Health Maintenance and Patient Education

Patients should be encouraged to increase fluid intake and stay as active as possible while avoiding overexertion.

Treatment (Pharmaceutical and clinical intervention)

Pharmaceutical

ACE inhibitors first line to preserve renal blood flow and treat hypertensive renal crisis.

- Corticosteroids
- NSAIDs
- Antibiotics: for secondary infection
- PPIs, antacids for gastric reflux
- Metoclopramide: for intestinal dysfunction
- Hydrophilic skin ointments to improve hydration
- Immunosuppressants recommended for life-threatening or crippling symptoms
- PDE5 antagonists, fluoxetine, nitrates for Raynaud phenomenon

Clinical

- Avoid caffeine
- Physical therapy to maintain function
- Lung transplant may be needed for pulmonary hypertension and ILD
- Stem cell transplant for rapidly progressing disease

Professional Considerations

Overall prognosis is poor, especially if renal, pulmonary, or cardiac abnormalities develop early. Complications include renal failure, respiratory failure, flexion contractures, disability, megacolon, pulmonary hypertension, and possible association with lung and other cancers. It is possible to achieve some improvements in symptoms.

Spinal Disorders

Ankylosing Spondylitis

Pathophysiology

Ankylosing spondylitis is an inflammatory disorder characterized by sacroiliitis seen on X-ray. The disease affects the musculoskeletal, pulmonary, neurologic, cardiac, and optic systems. Onset is usually in the early 20s. Etiology is autoinflammation at sites of bacterial exposure, such as the intestines. Inflammation occurs at the insertion sites of tendons, fascia, and ligaments and causes erosion, remodeling, and new bone growth to occur.

Clinical Presentation

Symptoms

- Insidious onset of back pain with morning stiffness lasting longer than 1 hour
- Hip/buttock pain
- Weight loss, fatigue, low-grade fever
- Chest pain with inspiration
- Dactylitis, vision changes, painful red eyes

Signs

- SI joint tenderness
- Loss of lumbar lordosis
- Rotation of cervical spine
- Decreased spinal range of motion
- Tenderness at Achilles insertion site

Diagnostic and Lab Studies

- Individuals with genetic profiles containing HLA-B27 positivity
- ESR and CRP: normal or mildly elevated
- Rheumatoid factor: negative
- CBC: mild normochromic anemia
- X-rays of SI joints: oblique projection
- MRI is more sensitive in identifying early changes

Differential Diagnoses

Differential diagnoses may include:

- Osteoarthritis
- Vertebral compression fracture
- Infectious arthritis
- Diffuse idiopathic skeletal hyperostosis (DISH)

Health Maintenance and Patient Education

Advise patient to remain physically active and maintain good posture. Discuss fall prevention and the need for regular monitoring of CRP and/or ESR. Recommend DEXA screening for osteoporosis.

Treatment (Pharmaceutical and Clinical Intervention)

Pharmaceutical

- NSAIDs first line for pain and stiffness
- Injection of intra-articular corticosteroids provides temporary relief.
- Biologic agents are second line
- DMARDs are ineffective for axial disease.

Clinical

Primary treatment goals:

- Symptom management
- Maintaining spinal flexibility and normal posture
- Reducing functional limitations and prevention of complications
- Aggressive physical therapy is a critical component in management.

Professional Considerations

Complications include restrictive lung disease, cardiac conduction defects, osteoporosis, spinal fusion causing kyphosis.

Lumbar Disc Disease

Pathophysiology

Many disease processes may alter the normal anatomy of the discs located between spinal vertebrae. Alterations cause musculoskeletal and neurologic symptoms. Pathologic etiologies are diverse and include disc space narrowing, disc desication, sclerosis of end plates and lumber spine abnormalities. Often, a disruption of the annulus fibrosis occurs, which allows the disc to herniate and may irritate the adjacent nerve root. The most common sites for herniation are paracentral, foraminal, and central. Different stages of herniation exist: protrusion, extrusion, and sequestration. The most common site of herniation is L5-S1.

Clinical Presentation

Symptoms

- Back pain, which may vary in severity and duration
- Accumulated episodes of back pain may precipitate disc herniation.
- Pain worsened by coughing or sneezing
- Severe pain with herniation may occur following an injury involving lifting or twisting.
- Sciatic pain

Red flag symptoms
- Fecal or bowel incontinence
- Loss of motor function
- Saddle anesthesia
- Unexplained fever or weight loss

Signs
Provocative tests include SLR, Crossed SLR, and Laseque sign, which are specific and sensitive for disc herniation with nerve root involvement.

- Decreased or complete loss of sensation
- Tendon reflex changes
- Weak knee extension or hip flexion (L4 involvement)
- Weak ankle plantar flexion (S1 involvement)

Diagnostic and Lab Studies

An MRI is first-line imaging modality. In the absence of red flag symptoms; however, recommended wait for a 6 week trial of conservative management before ordering MRI. X-rays or CT may help rule out bony abnormalities.

Differential Diagnoses

Differential diagnoses may include:

- Arthritis of the knee or hip
- Sacroiliitis
- Spinal stenosis
- Vascular insufficiency
- Infection/abscess

Health Maintenance and Patient Education

Discuss symptoms of cauda equina syndrome and need for emergent evaluation.

Treatment (Pharmaceutical and Clinical Intervention)

Pharmaceutical

- NSAIDs, acetaminophen, muscle relaxers
- Epidural steroid injections

Clinical

- Surgery: open discectomy or microdiscectomy
- Physical therapy

Professional Considerations

Risk factors include sedentary lifestyle and smoking.

Kyphosis and Scoliosis

Pathophysiology

Kyphosis and scoliosis are both conditions in where there exists abnormal spinal curvature. Kyphosis is an exaggerated AP curve of the thoracic spine, while scoliosis is an abnormal lateral curve of the spine (> 10 degrees by Cobb Angle) along with vertebral rotation. Both conditions present as fixed abnormalities. Kyphoscoliosis is a combination of both disorders.

Clinical Presentation

Symptoms

Painless curvature of the back; and any advanced disease may produce chronic, severe back pain with respiratory compromise and limited mobility.

Signs

- Kyphosis: hyperlordosis of lumbar spine, noticeable "hump" on back
- Scoliosis: noticeable lateral curve of spine with vertebral rotation
- Scoliosis: Adam forward bend test is often positive. Scoliometer measure angle of trunk rotation. An ATR of 7 degrees or more correlates with a clinically significant curve.

Diagnostic and Lab Studies

- Kyphosis: AP/lateral chest X-ray
- Scoliosis: standing PA and lateral radiographs of entire spine. Pelvic assessment to determine Risser score.
- MRI indicated for age < 10 years; rapid progression of curve; abnormal neurologic findings; atypical pain

Differential Diagnoses

Differential diagnoses may include:

- Congenital kyphosis
- Vertebral fractures/trauma
- Benign or malignant tumors
- Osteogenesis imperfecta type 2
- Achondroplasia

Health Maintenance and Patient Education

Screen for risk factors in all patients.

Treatment (Pharmaceutical and Clinical Intervention)

Pharmaceutical

- Treatment of concomitant osteoporosis

Clinical

- Serial observation for progression of disease
- Bracing
- Surgery
- Physical therapy

Professional Considerations

Refer to orthopedica/spine specialist the following:

- Worsening curvature despite bracing
- Curvature in infants and children less than 10 years
- Curvature-associated malignancy
- Nonbraceable curve of thoracic spine

Spinal Stenosis

Pathophysiology

Spinal stenosis is narrowing of the spinal canal and foramen. This condition often occurs with aging. May be congenital or acquired. Degenerative spondylosis is the most common form. Other causes include trauma, neoplasms, rheumatoid arthritis, ankylosing spondylitis, osteoporosis, and Paget's disease.

Clinical Presentation

Symptoms

- Slow onset of discomfort with standing, paresthesias, and bilateral weakness of extremities
- Symptoms worsen with prolonged standing, walking down hill, or going down stairs.
- Symptoms improve with sitting, leaning forward while walking, walking upstairs or uphill, and lying in a flexed position.
- Pain, numbness, and weakness of lower extremities may be reported.

Signs

- Loss of lumbar lordosis
- Decreased spinal range of motion
- Positive SLR test
- Pain elicited with extension of lumbar spine
- Reduced or absent Achilles reflex

Diagnostic and Lab Studies

Prescribe an MRI to determine severity.

Differential Diagnoses

Differential diagnoses may include:

- Disc herniation
- Cervical myelopathy
- Vascular claudication

Health Maintenance and Patient Education

Recommend activity as tolerated, and advise patients to present for care if they develop bowel/bladder incontinence or progressive motor weakness.

Treatment (Pharmaceutical and Clinical Intervention)

Pharmaceutical

- NSAIDs first line
- Tramadol second line

Clinical

- Physical therapy
- Weight management
- Surgery rarely indicated as benefits decrease over time

Professional Considerations

Discuss chronic nature of disorder with patients.

Sprains and Strains

Pathophysiology

Sprains and strains are common injuries involving tendons, ligaments, and soft tissue. Ankle sprains are frequently inversion injuries or eversion injuries. Inversion of the foot with plantar flexion occurs when the person falls or lands on an uneven surface and, in sports, when landing on an opponent's foot. Eversion sprains are considered "high" ankle sprains, and these occur when the foot is turned outward during a fall.

Sprains are classified according to extent of ligamental injury.

Grade 1: stretch injury with no evidence of ligamental laxity

Grade 2: partial ligamental tear with increased laxity; firm end point noted on exam

Grade 3: complete tear of ligament, increased laxity, no firm end point on exam

Strains are classified according to degree:

First degree: minimal damage to muscle, tendon, or the muscle-tendon unit

Second degree: partial tear of muscle, tendon, or muscle-tendon unit

Third degree: complete disruption of the muscle, tendon, or muscle-tendon unit

Clinical Presentation

Symptoms
- Pain and swelling over lateral or medial aspect of ankle
- History of a fall, or "turning the ankle," while walking or during sports
- May or may not be able to bear weight on ankle directly after injury
- Limping

Signs
- Tenderness over lateral malleolus
- Testing for inversion ankle injuries: anterior drawer test and subtalar tilt test
- Testing for eversion sprains: external rotation test

Diagnostic and Lab Studies

Radiographs of the ankle (views depend on mechanism of injury) work best.

Differential Diagnoses

A differential diagnosis includes fracture of ankle bones.

Health Maintenance and Patient Education

Advise patients that healing may take several months.

Treatment (Pharmaceutical and Clinical Intervention)

Pharmaceutical
- NSAIDs

Clinical

Inversion ankle sprain:

- MICE: modified activities, ice, compression, and elevation
- Protected weight bearing with crutches
- Ankle stabilizer brace
- Physical therapy or exercise program because early motion of the joint is essential

Eversion ankle sprain:

- Avoid early motion of joint
- Walking boot or cast for 4–6 weeks, then protected weight bearing with crutches until patient can ambulate without pain
- Physical therapy to regain range of motion and maintain strength

Professional Considerations

Persistent or worsening joint instability requires orthopedic evaluation.

Thoracic Outlet Syndrome (TOS)

Pathophysiology

Thoracic outlet syndrome is characterized by symptoms that affect the head, neck, shoulders, and upper extremities caused by nerve compression (brachial plexus and subclavian vessels) at the thoracic outlet. The specific areas affected include the area superior to the first rib and posterior to the clavicle. Three forms are recognized including neurogenic, vascular, and nonspecific (which includes traumatic causes and conditions secondary to provocative movements). Risk factors include trauma to the shoulder area, presence of a cervical rib, occupational factors such as computer use, playing music, and repetitive work involving the shoulders, arms, and hands. Young females with long necks and "drooping" shoulders are also at risk.

Clinical Presentation

Symptoms
- Paresthesia of the head, neck, face, mandible, chest, upper back, the outer arm and hand
- Pain also reported in these areas
- Occipital and orbital headache
- Pain and numbness of the axilla and inner arm; symptoms often occur at night

Signs
- Tenderness of supraclavicular area
- Symptoms get worse with elevation of the arms, raising the arms over the head, or extending arms forward.

Diagnostic and Lab Studies

- CBC, ESR, CRP
- Chest, C-spine, and shoulder X-rays
- Nerve conduction studies and EMG
- CT or MRI (MRI recommended when nerve compression suspected)
- Doppler and duplex US to rule out vascular obstruction

Differential Diagnoses

Differential diagnoses may include:

- Carpal tunnel syndrome
- Rotator cuff injury or tendinitis
- Cervical disc disorder
- Ulnar nerve compression
- MS
- Migraines

Health Maintenance and Patient Education

Ergonomic modifications at work may be necessary, and physical therapy is beneficial.

Treatment (Pharmaceutical and Clinical Intervention)

Pharmaceutical

- Ibuprofen
- Tricyclic antidepressants for neuropathic pain
- Muscle relaxants as needed

Clinical

- Conservative management to reduce/redistribute pressure and traction through the use of physiotherapy and/or prostheses
- Physical therapy
- Surgery required for vascular involvement

Professional Considerations

Multidisciplinary care needed for optimal management.

Torticollis

Pathophysiology

Torticollis is a painful spasm of the neck muscles that causes the head to tilt to one side. The episodes may be continuous or episodic and may lead to chronic neck pain, stiffness, and headaches. Torticollis may be present at birth and is called congenital torticollis. Chronic torticollis may cause damage to muscles and vasculature of the neck. Torticollis may be caused by a pulled muscle, infection, or injury to the neck, brain, or nerves.

Clinical Presentation

Symptoms

- Head tilted to one side
- Neck pain, stiffness, swelling of the area
- One shoulder may be higher than the other
- Headaches common

Signs

- Presentation consistent with history
- Neck muscles tight; head may be turned toward one side

Diagnostic and Lab Studies

- X-ray of neck to rule out spinal abnormalities or bony lesions
- EMG
- CT or MRI to rule out tumor

Differential Diagnoses

Differential diagnoses may include:

- C-spine abnormalities
- Abscess or infection

Health Maintenance and Patient Education

Advise patients that stretching and neck strengthening exercises are extremely helpful for part of a successful recovery.

Treatment (Pharmaceutical and Clinical Intervention)

Pharmaceutical

- Short-term muscle relaxants

Clinical

- Advise application of heating pad
- Physical therapy for recurrent symptoms

Professional Considerations

Torticollis is frequently seen in individuals between 40 and 70. Females are more frequently affected than males.

Thoracic Spine Injury

Pathophysiology

Injury to the thoracic spine may occur through a number of traumatic events. Because the thoracic spine is connected to the ribs, the costovertebral articulations provide added strength and stability. This makes the thoracic spine a more rigid and protected area. Greater force is required to cause significant injury; therefore, these cases may present as emergent situations involving multiple injuries. Fractures of the thoracic spine may be considered stable or unstable. Stable fractures may include compression fractures, disruption of the transverse process, or an isolated fracture. Unstable fractures include burst fractures, injury with significant dislocations present, trauma involving flexion and dislocation, or flexion with distraction. This latter type is seen with seatbelt injuries associated with motor vehicle accidents. Disc herniations may occur in the thoracic area; however, these are not common due to the intrinsic stability of the area. Other injury modalities include muscular contusions, juvenile kyphosis, and facet syndrome.

Clinical Presentation

Symptoms

- Pain at injury site
- May report upper extremity weakness and limited range of motion

Signs

- Diagnosis confirmed with imaging
- Areas of ecchymosis, disruption of the skin may be present
- With seatbelt injuries, there is usually a clearly identified "seatbelt" pattern seen across the chest area.

Diagnostic and Lab Studies

- X-rays
- MRI/CT

Differential Diagnoses

Differential diagnoses may include:

- Spinal tumors
- Rib fractures
- Cervical or lumbar spine injury

Health Maintenance and Patient Education

Although seatbelts may be associated with certain types of injury, their use has demonstrated benefit in decreasing morbidity and mortality.

Treatment (Pharmaceutical and Clinical Intervention)

Pharmaceutical

- Analgesia based on severity of injury

Clinical

- Surgery for most spinal fractures

Professional Considerations

Unstable fractures require emergent management. The vertebral spine is the most common site for bone metastases. Maintain a high index of suspicion in patients with a history of cancer.

Low Back Pain

Pathophysiology

Low back pain develops from multiple pathophysiologic processes and may involve nerve root impingement and significant disability. Pain is often diffuse and may radiate down the buttocks or legs.

Clinical Presentation

Symptoms

- Insidious or acute onset of diffuse pain across the lumbar spine area
- Pain may extend across buttocks and down the back of the leg
- Pain may be unilateral or symmetric
- May be accompanied by paresthesias, tingling, and numbness
- Limited ability to bend, turn, or rotate torso often reported

Signs

The physical exam is often unremarkable. Spinal radiographs may demonstrate osteogenic changes in the architecture of the spine; and pain that is predominantly noted in the leg, rather than the back, is often associated with nerve root impingement.

Alarm symptoms/signs include:

- Unexplained weight loss
- Failure to improve with conservative treatment
- Pain at night and during rest
- Severe pain persisting for more than 6 weeks

Diagnostic and Lab Studies

Imaging not needed in the absence of red flag symptoms within the first 6 weeks. For persistent pain following a trial of conservative therapy, AP and lateral lumbar spine X-rays are recommended. An MRI can be used to indicate for symptoms not responding to conservative treatment or in the presence of red flag symptoms. An EMG may be useful in assessing possible nerve root compression.

Differential Diagnoses

Differential diagnoses may include:

- Spinal stenosis
- Ankylosing spondylitis
- Disc herniation

Health Maintenance and Patient Education

Advise patients about symptoms of cauda equina syndrome.

Treatment (Pharmaceutical and Clinical Intervention)

Pharmaceutical

- NSAIDs
- Duloxetine

Clinical

- Exercise
- Weight loss
- Physical therapy

Professional Considerations

Low back pain is the leading cause of disability globally.

Upper Extremity Disorders

Fracture of Distal Radius

Pathophysiology

Fracture involves the distal portion of the radius being dorsally displaced and angulated. This is commonly called a Colles fracture. Other variations include the Dorsal Barton fracture, which involves displacement of carpus with a distal fragment; the Volvar Barton fracture, which involves volar displacement; and the Galeazzi fracture, which is a fracture of the distal third of the radius and is associated with dislocation of the radioulnar joint.

Clinical Presentation

Symptoms

Commonly sustained after a fall onto an outstretched hand with the wrist in extension.

Signs
- Tenderness of dorsal aspect of the wrist
- Paresthesia, weakness, or area is cool to the touch
- Gross visualization may reveal obvious dislocation and any open wounds at site

Diagnostic and Lab Studies

Bilateral X-rays to compare angulation of injury.

- AP/lateral views of wrist, forearm, and elbow
- CT/MRI to evaluate intra-articular involvement and plan for surgery

Differential Diagnoses

Differential diagnoses may include a carpal fracture and an ulnar fracture.

Health Maintenance and Patient Education

The prognosis is generally good; most patients regain full function of the wrist.

Treatment (Pharmaceutical and Clinical Intervention)

Pharmaceutical
- Analgesia with oral or IV narcotics
- Pediatric fractures: Ibuprofen is equal to Tylenol with Codeine.
- Hematoma blocks or IV regional anesthesia for closed reduction

Clinical
- Nondisplaced fractures: may be initially immobilized by splinting until follow-up
- Reduction of displaced fracture

Professional Considerations

Fracture management varies depending on site, extent of injury, and overall patient presentation.

Fracture, Humeral Head

Pathophysiology

This type of fracture involves fractures of the head of the humerus, the greater and lesser tuberosities, and the anatomic and surgical neck. Mechanisms of injury often include: fall onto an outstretched hand, high-energy trauma in younger patients, low-energy trauma in older adults with osteoporosis, electrical shock or seizure, pathologic fracture from metastatic disease, or over-rotation of the arm in an abducted position. Risk factors for this type of fracture include low bone mineral density, smoking, steroid use, and rheumatoid arthritis.

Clinical Presentation

Symptoms
- Pain, swelling, tenderness of the shoulder area
- Problems initiating active movement of the arm
- Patient often holds arm in adducted position

Signs
- Crepitus over injury
- Diminished peripheral pulses
- Evidence of disruption of deltoid and subachromial sulcus

Diagnostic and Lab Studies

Diagnostic and lab studies inlcude standard X-rays while wearing sling in AP; scapular, axillary, and Y views. CT if articular involvement is possible.

Differential Diagnoses

Differential diagnoses may include:

- Dislocation of shoulder
- Rotator cuff tear
- Pathologic fracture

Health Maintenance and Patient Education

Preoperative teaching for patients on diagnosis. Physical therapy and proper immobilization is important for correct alignment during healing.

Treatment (Pharmaceutical and Clinical Intervention)

Pharmaceutical
- Analgesia as needed

Clinical
- Initial immobilization
- Closed reduction
- Surgery

If closed reduction:
- ORIF
- Hemi or total arthroplasty
- Intramedullary nail

Professional Considerations

Initial stabilization should include ABCs and secondary survey for other injuries.

Practice Questions for Musculoskeletal Review

1. Bouchard nodes, characteristic findings in osteoarthritis, affect the

   (A) distal interphalangeal (DIP) joints.
   (B) metacarpophalangeal (MCP) joints.
   (C) proximal interphalangeal (PIP) joints.
   (D) metatarsophalangeal (MTP) joints.
   (E) elbow.

2. Acute pyogenic osteomyelitis presents with fever, pain, and tenderness of the affected bone. Infection may develop secondary to trauma, pressure ulcers, and prosthetic joint replacement. The most common pathogen causing this contiguous form of infection includes

   (A) *Pseudomonas aeruginosa.*
   (B) *Staphylococcus aureus.*
   (C) serratia species.
   (D) salmonellae.
   (E) streptococci.

3. Fibromyalgia is a disorder causing widespread musculoskeletal pain and tenderness at multiple joint insertion sites, among other locations. The diagnosis is one of exclusion. Fibromyalgia is most often diagnosed among patients

   (A) 20–50 years old.
   (B) 30–60 years old.
   (C) 50–70 years old.
   (D) over age 65.
   (E) in all age groups.

4. Your patient is a 50-year-old female with complaints of severe pain in her right shoulder. She denies recent injury but does report rotator cuff repair several months ago. Patient states she was recovering well from surgery and actually returned to work earlier than she had anticipated. She states she has difficulty brushing her hair and getting dressed. On examination you note limited active and passive range of motion of the affected shoulder. In particular, you note limited movement associated with external rotation. Based on the history and physical exam, you would like to "rule out" which of the following?

   (A) Shoulder dislocation
   (B) Adhesive capsulitis
   (C) Epicondylitis
   (D) Bursitis
   (E) Rheumatoid arthritis

5. The Lachman test is used in orthopedic examinations to evaluate for

   (A) anterior cruciate ligament tears.
   (B) rotational laxity of the knee.
   (C) medial collateral ligament injury.
   (D) meniscus injury.
   (E) Achilles tendon injury.

6. You are examining a patient with a history of recent ankle injury. Part of your physical exam includes performing the

   (A) Neer test.
   (B) valgus stress test.
   (C) anterior drawer test.
   (D) Thessaly test.
   (E) apprehension test.

7. You are performing a sports participation physical examination. Your patient is an 18-year-old male who plays baseball. His position is catcher. As part of the examination, you note the patient experiences knee pain with squatting, and there is joint line tenderness of the knee. To further evaluate for a meniscus inury in this patient you order

   (A) plain radiographs of the knee.
   (B) an MRI of the knee.
   (C) a CT of the knee.
   (D) an ultrasound of the knee.
   (E) all of the above.

8. Your patient is a 42-year-old male with a chief complaint of pain in his left shoulder when he reaches above his head. He also states that he is unable to sleep on his left side at night, as he experiences pain. On questioning, he denies numbness or radiation of the pain below the elbow. Passive range of motion is preserved and the Neer and Hawkins tests are positive. This presentation and PE findings are consistent with a diagnosis of

   (A) osteoarthritis of the shoulder.
   (B) adhesive capsulitis.
   (C) subacromial impingement syndrome.
   (D) scapular fracture.
   (E) fracture of humeral head.

9. You are seeing a patient for follow-up after a recent diagnosis of rheumatoid arthritis. The most effective class of medications in slowing progression and decreasing inflammation is

   (A) non-steroidal anti-inflammatory drugs (NSAIDs).
   (B) disease-modifying antirheumatic drugs (DMARDs).
   (C) corticosteroids.
   (D) opioid pain receptor blocking agents.
   (E) non-opioid analgesics.

10. Your patient is a 62-year-old male with a presentation, history, and physical exam findings consistent with gouty arthritis. The diagnosis is often made based on history and physical; however, when there is diagnostic doubt, which finding/testing is confirmatory?

   (A) Presence of urate crystals in synovial fluid
   (B) Radiographic imaging of affected joint(s)
   (C) Ultrasound of affected joint(s)
   (D) Elevated serum C-reactive protein (CRP) level
   (E) CT of affected joints

Answers Explained

1. **(C)** Osteoarthritis is the most common joint disorder and is strongly associated with aging. Joints most commonly affected by degenerative changes of OA include the distal interphalangeal (DIP), proximal interphalangeal (PIP), knee, hip, carpometacarpal joint of the thumb, the big toe, and the cervical and lumbar spine. Heberden nodes are seen at the DIP joints; whereas, Bouchard nodes are seen at the PIP joints.

2. **(B)** Contiguous spread of infection into bone from a nearby focus of infection, such as trauma or joint replacement, is most often caused by *Staph aureus* or *Staphylococcus epidermis*. With these types of infection, polymicrobial innoculation is rare. Osteomyelitis, resulting from infection of the blood, is often associated with multiple pathogens, including pseudomonas, serratia species, and salmonellae.

3. **(A)** Fibromyalgia is diagnosed most frequently between the ages of 20–50 years. Women are affected more often than men.

4. **(A)** Acute shoulder dislocations occur with some sort of trauma or hyperextension of the joint. Movement of the shoulder is severely limited and pain is severe. Physical examination of the joint is usually confirmatory. (B) Adhesive capsulitis represents a type of impingement syndrome affecting the shoulder and presents as severe pain with minimal or no trauma. Occasionally, the condition develops postoperatively and may be associated with early termination of physical therapy exercises. The condition presents in three phases: inflammation, freezing, and thawing. During the acute inflammatory and freezing phases, NSAIDs and physical therapy may help to maintain joint mobility. The joint slowly returns to improved motion; however, the process may take up to two years. (C) Epicondylitis represents a tendinitis affecting the epicondyle, producing tenderness and limited range of motion of the affected area. (D) Bursitis occurs frequently around bony prominences, such as the elbow. The area is acutely painful, and there is usually localized swelling present. (E) RA is a systemic disorder involving multiple joints in a symmetric pattern.

5. **(A)** A positive Lachman test indicates injury to the anterior cruciate ligament. (B) The Pivot shift maneuver is used to assess for rotational laxity of the knee. (C) The Valgus stress test evaluates for medial collateral ligament injury. (D) A positive McMurray test indicates a possible meniscal injury. (E) An Achilles tendon injury is diagnosed by the doctor manipulating the areas of the lower foot and ankle.

6. **(C)** When performing the anterior drawer test, the clinician is assessing for ATF ligament disruption associated with ankle injuries. (A) The Neer impingement test evaluates for shoulder impingment. (B) The Valgus stress test assesses for medial collateral ligament injury. (D) The Thessaly test is used to evaluate knee stability and assess for ligamental injuries. (E) The apprehension test assesses stability of the shoulder joint in the setting of dislocation injury.

7. **(B)** The most sensitive and specific test for evaluating for mensical injuries is an MRI and is recommended if you suspect a menscal tear. Radiographs may reveal joint space narrowing or early signs of OA; however, they will not reveal a meniscal tear, as this is a soft tissue injury. A CT scan is not the most sensitive and specific test for this type of injury. The tests in (A), (B), and (C) are not needed for diagnosis.

8. **(C)** Subacromial impingement syndrome presents with shoulder pain that occurs with overhead motions and at night with inability to sleep on the affected shoulder. The Neer and Hawkins tests assess for impingement of the shoulder. Patients may experience numbness and radiation of pain below the elbow if cervical spine disease is present. (A) Osteoarthritis may co-exist with impingement syndrome; however, the disease most often presents in the joints of the hands first, unless there is a history of shoulder trauma, which is not given in this case. (B) Adhesive capsulitis is an impingement syndrome characterized by progressive "freezing" of the joint with limited activity AND passive range of motion. (D) Scapular fracture is associated with a history of trauma and with other injuries. A history of trauma or known injury is not given in this scenario. (E) A fracture of the humeral head is usually associated with a history of an injury and presents with acute symptoms of pain, which is inconsistent with the presentation in this scenario.

9. **(B)** DMARDs should be initiated as soon after RA diagnosis as possible, as these agents have activity in suppressing disease, reducing inflammation, reducing pain, and preventing deformity. (A) NSAIDs do provide a measure of symptomatic relief of symptoms associated with RA; however, they do not slow or prevent disease progression. (C) Corticosteroids are frequently administered as 'bridge' agents while waiting for the therapeutic effects of DMARDs to begin. (D) Opioid pain medications are not generally recommended in the management of RA due to their high side effect profile and their inability to alter disease progression. (E) Non-opioid analgesics may provide pain relief but do not slow disease progression.

10. **(A)** Synovial aspiration with findings of urate crystals in joint fluid is confirmatory for gouty arthritis. (B) Radiographs may be normal, especially in early disease. (C) Ultrasound of affected joint(s) may be helpful in confirming the diagnosis, as this method may detect smaller deposits of urate crystals in the tissue and small tophi undetectable on physical exam. (D) CRP may or may not be elevated with gouty arthritis. This finding is non-specific, as many conditions may cause elevation of CRP. (E) CT is not indicated for diagnosis of gouty arthritis. Synovial fluid aspiration is the confirmatory procedure.

11

Neurology/ Psychiatry/ Behavioral Health Review

Learning Objectives

In this chapter, you will review:

→ Neurological responses
→ Post-traumatic stress disorder
→ Adjustment disorder
→ Anxiety disorders
→ Brain abnormalities
→ SSRIs and SNRIs

Post-Traumatic Stress Disorder

Pathophysiology

Poorly understood, though proposed models to include potential role of sensitization of neurobiological systems involved in stress response, insufficient cortical inhibition of limbic activity, poor regulation of hypothalamic-pituitary-adrenal axis, and sympathetic nervous system response to stress, amongst other areas under investigation.

Clinical Presentation

- Exposure to actual or threatened trauma plus symptoms of intrusion (e.g., nightmares), avoidance (e.g., avoiding people or places reminding of trauma)
- Negative alterations in cognition and mood (e.g., guilt and negative emotional mood)
- Alterations in arousal and reactivity (e.g., hypervigilant and/or exaggerated startle response)

Diagnosis and Lab Studies

Made clinically using criterion A-E after reporting exposure to trauma, one or more intrusion symptoms, one or more avoidance symptoms, two or more negative alterations in cognition and mood, and two or more alterations in arousal and reactivity. Criterion F-H must also be met, which include symptoms resulting in significant impairment in functioning, lasting more than 1 month, and not resulting from substance use or another medical condition. No evidence to support regular use of labs or imaging for diagnosis of PTSD.

Differential Diagnoses

Differential diagnoses may include:

- Acute stress disorder with similar trauma history and symptoms but lasting less than 30 days
- Adjustment disorder with similar symptoms but severity of stressor is often what differentiates from PTSD
- Mood, anxiety, and substance use disorders can exist simultaneously with PTSD

Health Maintenance and Patient Education

Inform of possible waxing and waning of symptoms, with potential for symptoms to worsen around stressful settings or times of year.

- Role of psychotherapy, pharmacologic intervention (or both)
- Patient to contact provider or emergency services immediately if experiencing any suicidal thinking

Treatment (Pharmaceutical and Clinical Intervention)

Initial treatment is a trauma-focused psychotherapy, such as cognitive behavior therapy (CBT), cognitive processing therapy, or prolonged exposure therapy.

- SSRIs first-line pharmacologic treatment should psychotherapies be declined by patient or found ineffective
- Evidence to support non-FDA approved venlafaxine (SNRI) as an alternative to an SSRI

Other commonly used, though non-FDA approved, medications may include:

- Prazosin (off-label for nightmares)
- Trazodone (hypnotic agent for sleep)
- Lesser extent antipsychotic agents due to efficacy questions and potential adverse effects

Professional Considerations

Primary care PAs are a significant, and at times the only, resource for patients who suffer with mental health concerns. May require a referral to specialty mental health services, though PAs should be aware of service limitations in their practice area.

Adjustment Disorder

Pathophysiology

Like PTSD, an adjustment disorder is poorly understood though likely a result of various neuro-biological factors. There is little known regarding the genetic predisposition to this condition.

Clinical Presentation

Some symptom overlap with PTSD, including potential anxiety, depression, irritability, guilt, and sleep disturbance in setting of an identifiable stressor (e.g., financial strain, job loss, marital discord, etc.). Symptoms start within 3 months of stressor and resolve within 6 months of stressor removal.

Diagnosis and Lab Studies

Made clinically but without the more rigid criterion that accompanies diagnosis of PTSD. Unique to adjustment disorder is that symptoms and/or functional impairment are out of proportion to the stressor. Symptoms do not meet threshold for another mental health condition such as MDD or GAD. No evidence to support regular use of labs or imaging for diagnosis of adjustment disorder.

Differential Diagnosis

Differs from PTSD in accordance with the extreme severity of the stressor.

Due to symptom overlap, ensure that patient does not meet full criteria for an anxiety or mood disorder.

Health Maintenance and Patient Education

Contact provider or emergency services immediately if experiencing any suicidal thinking.

Treatment (Pharmaceutical and Clinical Intervention)

Psychotherapy and supportive measures focusing on coping skills are the mainstay.

Though used widely, evidence to support pharmacologic measures is lacking unless another comorbid condition warrants use.

Professional Considerations

- Importance of suicide assessment in those with adjustment disorder
- Screening for substance use given prevalence of comorbid substance abuse

Generalized Anxiety Disorder (GAD)

Pathophysiology

May be associated with abnormalities in functioning of GABA receptor/benzodiazepine receptor/chloride channel complex, the noradrenergic nucleus locus coeruleus and related brainstem nuclei, and the serotonin system. There does appear to be a genetic predisposition to development of GAD.

Clinical Presentation

Excessive and uncontrollable worrying accompanied by muscle tension, restlessness, fatigue, irritability, concentration impairment, and/or sleep impairment.

Diagnosis and Lab Studies

- Made clinically, needing to experience excessive worry plus at least three of the six symptoms above (adult criteria) most days for at least six months
- Causes significant distress or impairment and not due to substances, medical condition, or other mental health disorders
- No evidence to support regular use of labs or imaging for diagnosis of GAD

Differential Diagnosis

Rule out other anxiety disorders and other conditions with prominent obsessions (OCD, somatoform disorders, eating disorders, personality disorders) and always assess for depression given high rate of comorbidity.

Health Maintenance and Patient Education

Chronic in nature, symptoms commonly wax and wane. Potential involvement of physical manifestations secondary to anxiety.

Treatment (Pharmaceutical and Clinical Intervention)

- SSRIs and SNRIs are first-line pharmacologic treatment options for GAD
- Benzodiazepines sometimes used as shorter term adjunct therapy but should be avoided as solitary agents
- Other pharmacologic agents including buspirone, gabapentin, and beta blockers (notably propranolol) sometimes used, though questions exist regarding onset timing and overall efficacy
- Behavioral therapy and CBT have been found efficacious in the treatment of GAD

Professional Considerations

Majority of patients with GAD seen in primary care settings (as opposed to specialty mental health practices).

Panic Disorder

Pathophysiology

Due to an increase in cortisol or likely result of both neurobiologic and cognitive factors. Studies suggest that a strong genetic component with panic disorder may be the cause as well.

Clinical Presentation

Panic attack may present as an abrupt surge of intense fear or discomfort accompanied by palpitations, diaphoresis, trembling, sensation of shortness of breath, feeling of choking, chest pain, nausea, dizziness or unsteadiness, chills or heat sensations, paresthesias, derealization, fear of loss of control, and/or fear of dying. May occur with or without agoraphobia (marked fear across a range of public situations).

Diagnosis and Lab Studies

- Diagnosis of panic disorder made clinically and consisting of recurrent unexpected panic attacks reaching peak within minutes and consisting of four or more of above symptoms
- At least one attack has been followed by at least 1 month of persistent worry about having repeat attack and/or significant maladaptive behavior change related to attack
- Symptoms not due to substance, medical, or another mental health condition
- No evidence to support regular use of labs or imaging for diagnosis of panic attack (other than to exclude other potential diagnoses for presenting symptoms)

Differential Diagnosis

Social avoidance and somatic fears present in many other mental health conditions but lacking the presence of acute panic attacks as in panic disorder. It is important to differentiate (often clinically) from medical conditions including hyperthyroidism, pulmonary embolism, and various cardiac events, amongst others.

Health Maintenance and Patient Education

Patient education regarding benzodiazepine indications and potential risks including adverse effects and risk of abuse and dependency.

Treatment (Pharmaceutical and Clinical Intervention)

May require cognitive or behavioral therapy alone (without pharmacologic intervention).

If pharmacologic intervention deemed necessary, SSRI agent of choice may require utilization of a benzodiazepine short term while awaiting SSRI effectiveness.

Professional Considerations

Early clinical recognition important as often diagnosed late resulting in delayed treatment.

The majority of diagnostic testing should be reserved for cases involving other presenting features that warrant concern and justify further testing.

Practice Questions for Neurology/Psychiatry/Behavioral Health Review

1. Your patient is a 45-year-old female who reports a recent increase in anxiety and sadness since her youngest daughter moved away to college 2 months ago. She reports feeling weepy and worried every day. She is able to go to work every day and is performing her job functions, although she is experiencing increased fatigue. She denies thoughts of self-harm or suicide. The patient denies previous episodes of depression or severe anxiety. This presentation is consistent with a diagnosis of

   (A) generalized anxiety disorder (GAD).
   (B) major depressive disorder (MDD).
   (C) adjustment disorder.
   (D) post-traumatic stress disorder (PTSD).
   (E) social anxiety disorder.

2. First-line treatment for anxiety disorders includes management with

   (A) benzodiazepines.
   (B) selective serotonin reuptake inhibitors (SSRIs).
   (C) tricyclic antidepressants (TCAs).
   (D) monoamine oxidase inhibitors (MAOIs).
   (E) selective norepinephrine reuptake inhibitors (SNRIs).

3. Several medications have been associated with development of depressive symptoms. All of the following medications have been implicated, except

   (A) methyldopa.
   (B) retinoids.
   (C) interferon.
   (D) combined oral contraceptives.
   (E) metroprolol.

4. Which of the following medications carries a warning of QT prolongation and should be used with caution in older individuals and those with known cardiac disease?

   (A) Fluoxetine
   (B) Luvoxamine
   (C) Citalopram
   (D) Sertraline
   (E) Duloxetine

5. The most effective treatment for severe depression is

   (A) cognitive behavioral therapy (CBT).
   (B) electroconvulsive therapy (ECT).
   (C) transcranial magnetic stimulation (TMS) therapy.
   (D) selective serotonin reuptake inhibitors (SSRIs).
   (E) selective norepinepherine reuptake inhibitors (SNRIs).

6. Cardinal features of parkinsonism include bradykinesia, tremor, rigidity, and

    (A) cognitive decline.
    (B) dementia.
    (C) positive Myerson sign.
    (D) postural instability.
    (E) dysphagia.

7. Your patient is a 30-year-old female who presents with symptoms of optic neuritis. Management is directed at evaluation and management of this condition. Presentation of optic neuritis in a young adult should raise suspicion for

    (A) fibromyalgia.
    (B) brain tumor.
    (C) multiple sclerosis.
    (D) Lyme disease.
    (E) encephalitis.

8. Symmetric, proximal limb weakness beginning in the legs (without other explanation) should raise suspicion for a diagnosis of

    (A) systemic lupus erythematosis (SLE).
    (B) acute idiopathic polyneuropathy (Guillain-Barré syndrome).
    (C) muscular dystrophy (MD).
    (D) parkinson diesease (PD).
    (E) Lyme disease.

9. Treatment of Bell's palsy may include

    (A) long-term NSAID administration to decrease inflammation.
    (B) corticosteroid bolus and taper.
    (C) antiviral agents.
    (D) nerve block.
    (E) antibiotic administration.

10. Syringomyelia is a neurological condition characterized by destruction of white and gray matter adjacent to the spinal cord. This leads to accumulation of fluid and cavitation within the spinal cord itself. Although the exact pathogenesis has not been identified, many cases are associated with:

    (A) Charcot deformities.
    (B) Arnold-Chiari malformation.
    (C) demyelinating disease.
    (D) upper motor neuron disease.
    (E) cervical spondylosis.

Answers Explained

1. **(C)** Adjustment disorder is characterized by symptoms of anxiety and/or depression in the setting of a relatively recent life change or stressor. Symptoms are out of proportion to the causative event. Symptoms of depression are not severe enough to warrant a diagnosis of major depressive disorder and have not been present long enough to meet criteria for generalized anxiety disorder. (A) GAD is characterized by the presence of worry, fear, dread, difficulty concentrating, irritability, and/or insomnia. These symptoms have been present on most days for at least 6 months. (B) MDD consists of symptoms involving mood, cognitive, and physical components. Patients experience anhedonia, anxiety, disordered sleep, and changes in appetite, among others. Thoughts about dying or death are frequently reported. (D) PTSD is now classified as a trauma and stressor-related disorder instead of an anxiety disorder. Characteristics include exposure to a traumatic or life-threatening event. Patients report flashbacks, nightmares, intrusive images and thoughts, along with hypervigilance. (E) Social anxiety presents as symptoms of anxiety occurring with specific triggering events, such as going out to dinner with other people.

2. **(B)** SSRIs are first-line treatment for anxiety disorders. These medications include fluoxetine, escitalopram, and sertraline, among many others. (A) Benzodiazepines may be used for short-term adjunctive management of anxiety symptoms as SSRIs are being started. These medications have the disadvantage of causing physiologic dependency. Long-term use of certain benzodiazepines has been associated with development of dementia symptoms. (C) TCAs may be useful in management of anxiety symptoms after failure of first-line agents. TCAs are associated with a higher side effect profile than the SSRIs. (D) MOAIs may be used in management of mood disorders in treatment-resistant patients. This class of medications has a high side effect profile. (E) SNRIs may be helpful in managing anxiety disorders but are not recommended as first-line agents.

3. **(E)** Mood changes are seen with several medications including guanethidine, methyldopa, clonidine, digitalis, retinoids, and levodopa. Beta-blockers, such as metoprolol, have NOT demonstrated evidence for causing depressive symptoms.

4. **(C)** Citalopram carries a risk warning for QT prolongation, particularly at doses of 40 mg or above. Patients over age 60 who respond well to citalopram should be prescribed a dose no higher than 20 mg, and ECG monitoring may be indicated. (A, B, D, E) These agents have not been associated with QT prolongation.

5. **(B)** ECT remains the most effective treatment for severe depression with remission rates ranging between 45% and 85%. (A) CBT is recommended monotherapy or adjunctive therapy for patients with initial presentation or milder forms of depression; however, it has not shown to be as effective as ECT. (C, D, E) TMS and pharmacotherapy are both optional treatment modalities with varying rates of remission.

6. **(D)** Cardinal features of parkinsonism include bradykinesia, tremor, rigidity, and postural instability. (A, B, C, E) These findings are commonly seen as Parkinson's disease progresses, however are not considered cardinal features.

7. **(C)** Optic neuritis in a young adult should raise suspicion for multiple sclerosis. Common presenting symptoms may also include weakness, paresthesias, unsteadiness in a limb, diplopia, and urinary urgency or hesitancy. (A, B, D, E) These conditions often have complex presentations as well but are not specifically associated with development of optic neuritis on initial evaluation.

8. **(B)** Guillain-Barré syndrome is an acute (or subacute) progressive diesease with neuopathy of multiple areas. Acute dysautonomia may be severe and life-threatening. The presenting complaint is proximal weakness of the legs. The weakness often progresses to involve the arms and one side of the face. Muscles of respiration may be affected, requiring mechanical ventilation. (A, C, D. E) Presentation of these conditions does not include symmetrical, proximal limb weakness as initial features.

9. **(B)** Bell's palsy is characterized by the sudden onset of facial palsy caused by lower motor neuron conduction blockade. The disorder is idiopathic in nature and most patients recover completely, often without treatment. When treatment is indicated, prednisone 60 mg orally for 5 days followed by a 5 day taper is administered. (A, C, D, E) These treatment options are not indicated in management of Bell's palsy.

10. **(B)** Syringomelia is often associated with Arnold-Chiari malformation, which includes displacement of cerebellar, medullar, and fourth ventricle brain tissue into the spinal canal. Meningomyelocele may also be seen. (B, C, D, E) These conditions are not associated with syringomyelia.

12

Pulmonary Review

Learning Objectives

In this chapter, you will review:

→ Pulmonary embolism
→ Virchow's triad
→ Sleep apnea
→ Types of asthma and treatment
→ Pulmonary tests

Pulmonary Embolism

A pulmonary embolism (PE) is defined as an obstruction in the pulmonary artery due to a thrombus, fat, air, and/or tumor, the most common of which is due to a thrombus. This topic focuses only on PE due to a thrombus. Most commonly, PEs originate from a deep vein thrombus in the lower extremities. It is the third most common cause of death amongst hospitalized patients and accounts for 100,000 deaths per year in the United States.

Pathophysiology

The pathogenesis of PE is defined by Virchow's triad, which consists of alterations in blood flow states (stasis), vascular endothelial injury, and altered blood constituents, such as loss of a protein leading to a hypercoagulable state.

Risk Factors for PE include:

- Smoking
- Fracture of lower limbs, hip, or knee replacement
- Active malignancy
- Major trauma
- Prior PE or deep vein thrombosis
- Prolonged immobility
- Spinal cord injury
- Older age
- Estrogen-containing contraceptives and hypercoagulable disorders, such as factor V Leiden and prothrombin gene mutation

Clinical Presentation

The most common symptoms include:

- Dyspnea at rest or exertion (73%)
- Pleurtic pain (66%)
- Cough (37%)
- Calf or thigh pain and/or swelling (44%)
- Orthopnea (28%)
- Hemoptyis (13%)14
- Dyspnea occurs rapidly, ranging from a few seconds to 15 minutes.

Common physical examination findings include:

- Tachypnea (54%)
- Calf or thigh swelling and/or erythema (47%)
- Tachycardia (24%)

Diagnostic and Lab Studies

The most useful diagnostic study is computed tomography pulmonary angiography (CTPA). It is relatively easy to obtain and has a high sensitivity (90%) and specificity (96%)

- In patients who are allergic to contrast, lower extremity duplex ultrasound is the diagnostic tool of choice.
- In pregnant patients, lower extremity duplex is the first test of choice to avoid radiation exposure to the fetus.

Laboratory tests by themselves are not diagnostic but may be useful. Due to strain on the right ventricle, brain natriuretic peptide (BNP) and troponin may be elevated. Elevated levels of BNP and troponin are associated with worse outcomes in PE. Another serum marker that may be useful in the management of PE is D-dimer.

D-dimers are breakdown proteins of cross-linked fibrin found in thrombus. While not sensitive or specific for PE, normal levels of D-dimer may be used to rule out PE in patients with low suspicion for PE.

Differential Diagnoses

Other conditions that presents with respiratory distress and chest pain include:

- Myocardial infarction (MI)
- Pneumothorax
- Pneumonia
- Aortic dissection
- Pericarditis

It is important to determine whether the symptoms began acutely or gradually. Acute onset of symptoms is more common in PE, MI, and aortic dissection, whereas pneumonia and pericarditis are more gradual in onset.

Treatment (Pharmaceutical and Clinical Intervention)

Prior to initiation of treatment, patients must be assessed for hemodynamic instability. In patients who are hypotensive or requiring vasopressors, tissue plasminogen activator (TPA) to break down the clot is the first step.

- TPA is then followed by anticoagulation.
- In patients who are normotensive, anticoagulation is the first step of choice.

Anticoagulation is divided into initial anticoagulation for 10 days and long-term anticoagulation for 3–6 months thereafter.

Common medications used during the initial period of anticoagulation include:

- Enoxaparin
- Rivaroxaban
- Apixaban
- Edoxaban
- Dabigatran

Long-term medications include:

- Warfarin
- Rivaroxaban
- Edoxaban
- Apixaban
- Dabigatran

Warfarin should not be started without bridging therapy. In general, anticoagulation is continued for 3–6 months. At the end of 3–6 months, patients must be assessed for the risk of recurrence. If patients have active cancer, hypercoagulable disorders, or recurrent DVT or PE, lifelong anticoagulation is necessary. Inferior vena cava (IVC) filters are an option in those who are not candidates for anticoagulation due to risk of bleeding. An IVC filter should not be routinely placed. While they decrease the risk of PE, they increase the risk of lower extremity DVT.

Other interventions during the acute phase of the PE include catheter-directed thrombolysis and surgical embolectomy. These interventions are limited to expert centers and performed on an individual case basis.

Health Maintenance and Patient Education

Patients should be followed up every 3–6 months to assess whether they need further anticoagulation for 2 years after the PE. Approximately 4% of patients develop chronic thromboembolic pulmonary hypertension (CTEPH), a complication of PE.

CTEPH should be suspected in patients who report persistent dyspnea despite being on anticoagulation for at least 3 months.

Professional Considerations

The choice of anticoagulation may be influenced by costs associated with the medication and also patient adherence. Unlike warfarin, which needs close monitoring and has multiple drug interactions, direct oral anticoagulants (DOACs) such as rivaroxaban, apixaban, edoxaban, and dabigatran do not need routine blood, making them convenient for patients. However, the costs associated with DOACs may prohibit their use in patients from lower socioeconomic statuses. In addition, the role of DOACs in the setting of renal failure or obesity has not been well studied.

Sleep Apnea

Sleep apnea refers to a condition in which patients suffer from a pathological number of breathing reductions (hypopneas) and/or complete breathing pauses (apneas) during their sleep. This results in short repetitive hypoxic episodes overnight, which cause arousal in the brain that in turn leads to sleep fragmentation, symptoms of daytime sleepiness, and adverse health outcomes.

It is estimated that about 15% of the US population has sleep apnea. There are two types of sleep apnea: obstructive sleep apnea (OSA) and central sleep apnea (CSA). If undiagnosed or left untreated, patients with sleep apnea are predisposed to developing hypertension, diabetes, myocardial infarction, and stroke. It has also been correlated with development of systolic and diastolic heart failure.

Pathophysiology

OSA is the most common type of sleep apnea. It is characterized by recurrent collapse of the upper airway during sleep that leads to hypopneas and/or apneas. These events occur due to relaxation of the tongue and upper airway muscles that occurs in sleep, which subsequently narrows or obstructs the airway. The resultant changes in oxygen and carbon dioxide, as well as sympathetic nervous system activation, trigger an arousal in the brain that interrupts sleep to open the airway and restore breathing. Although the strongest risk factor for OSA is obesity, other important risk factors include age older than 40 years old, male gender, smoking, and craniofacial and upper airway abnormalities.

CSA is also characterized by sleep-disordered breathing that is associated with decreased or absent respiratory effort. Therefore, rather than an obstruction impeding airflow, the airway is patent but breathing is shallow or absent due to a reduced or absent signal to breathe. CSA can be further classified into two categories: Hypocapnic and normocapnic-hypercapnic.

In hypocapnic CSA, apnea occurs due to the $PaCO_2$ transiently falling below the patient's apneic threshold (AT). The AT is the level of $PaCO_2$ below which respiration is not triggered during sleep. Patients with hypocapnic CSA have a smaller difference between their awake $PaCO_2$ and the AT. This narrow gap, along with a high ventilatory drive that blows off CO_2, causes CO_2 levels to drop below the AT and cause an apnea.

Nearly half of these patients experience a crescendo-decrescendo breathing pattern known as Cheyne-Stokes. Patients with CSA often have a history of heart failure with reduced ejection fraction (HFrEF), heart failure with preserved ejection fraction (HFpEF), or previous stroke. Normocapnic-hypercapnic CSA results from abnormal ventilatory control. This can result from respiratory centers that are immature (e.g., apnea of prematurity), damaged (e.g., brain tumor or infarct), or suppressed by drug or substance use (e.g., opioids or benzodiazepines).

Clinical Presentation

Symptoms

- A majority of patients with sleep apnea may report difficulty staying awake or alert throughout the day.
- This sleepiness is characterized by an increased propensity to doze off if not engaged in an activity and/or difficulty concentrating.

- This daytime sleepiness can be depicted with an Epworth Sleepiness Scale (ESS) score of more than 10.
- Additionally, patients often endorse trouble with sleep maintenance and episodes of waking up gasping for air.
- Bed partners frequently report loud snoring or witnessed apneas. Snoring alone, however, has a specificity below 50%; thus, patients who snore do not necessarily have sleep apnea.

Other symptoms can include:
- Morning headaches
- Nocturia
- Erectile dysfunction
- Resistant hypertension

Signs

- In addition to routine vital signs, note the BMI and neck circumference. Studies have demonstrated that a neck circumference of greater than 17 inches in males and greater than 16 inches in females is an increased risk factor for OSA.
- Physical exam should include a close examination of the mouth and upper airway, noting any retrognathia (retro-positioned jaw), micrognathia (small jaw), tongue enlargement, tonsillar hypertrophy, or other reason for a crowded airway.
- The Mallampati score conveys how crowded the upper airway is and higher Mallampati scores have been shown to have a positive correlation with the diagnosis of sleep apnea.

Differential Diagnosis/Formulating the Most Likely Diagnosis

Snoring, witnessed apneas, or gasping awake, includes primary snoring (snoring without symptoms or evidence of sleep disordered breathing), sleep apnea (obstructive or central), pulmonary (e.g., nocturnal asthma or COPD), or cardiac (e.g., arrhythmias).

Central sleep apnea moves up on the differential if the patient has known systolic or diastolic heart dysfunction, prior stroke, or is taking potent medications that cause respiratory suppression.

In patients presenting with a chief complaint of daytime sleepiness, the differential is broader and should include, but not be limited to, insufficient sleep, other sleep disorders, atypical depression, hypothyroidism, and vitamin D deficiency.

Diagnostic and Lab Studies

Sleep apnea is diagnosed with a sleep study, which can be done in the sleep lab (full channel polysomnography) or at home. Polysomnography (PSG) monitors brain activity, eye movements, muscle tone, airflow through the nose and mouth, respiratory effort, limb movements, oxygen levels, and heart rhythm.

- A home sleep test (HST) usually monitors airflow through the nose and mouth, respiratory effort, and oxygen levels.
- Use of respiratory effort on both PSG and HST helps differentiate obstructive vs. central sleep apnea.
- An apnea with preserved respiratory effort implies an obstructed airway. An apnea with absent respiratory effort suggests a central process.

Hypopneas and apneas are divided by total sleep time on PSG or total recording time on HST to yield the apnea-hypopnea index (AHI).

- In children, an AHI of > 1 is diagnostic of sleep apnea.
- In adults, an AHI of < 5 is considered normal, whereas an AHI > 5 confirms the diagnosis of sleep apnea.
- The higher the AHI depicts the severity as mild (AHI of 5 to < 15), moderate (AHI of 15 to < 30), or severe (AHI > 30).

Treatment (Pharmaceutical and Clinical Intervention)

Treatment is dependent on the etiology of the sleep apnea.

Treatments for OSA include
- Oral appliance (OA), positive airway pressure (PAP), and upper airway surgeries.
- Oral appliances are indicated for treatment of snoring, mild OSA, and moderate OSA. A dental practitioner with training in sleep medicine should manage the fitting of and treatment with this device.
- PAP is the treatment of choice for symptomatic mild OSA, as well as moderate and severe OSA.

PAP utilizes pressure to maintain airway patency, thus avoiding apneas. PAP devices are capable of varying pressures and pressure modalities to effectively treat OSA, and these devices can track adherence along with residual AHI. In patients who are not able to tolerate OA or PAP and have severe OSA, an evaluation by ENT or oral maxillofacial surgery is recommended for upper airway surgery. For pediatric OSA, the removal of the tonsils and adenoids can be very effective. Unfortunately, tonsillectomy and adenoidectomy in adults with OSA does not yield similar results because the level of obstruction is typically lower at the level of the tongue.

For central sleep apnea, always involve proper management of the underlying etiology (e.g., treating underlying heart failure, decreasing or removing respiratory suppressing medications). PAP is also useful to stabilize ventilation in CSA; however, advanced PAP modalities are often necessary.

Other Pulmonary Disorders

Asthma

Pathophysiology

Asthma is a common but heterogeneous disease characterized by chronic inflammation, airway hyper-responsiveness, bronchoconstriction, and mucus secretion. These changes are generally considered reversible but if left un- (or under-) treated, irreversible airway remodeling and airway smooth muscle hypertrophy can occur over time. Several inflammatory cell types are implicated in the host response in asthma, including airway epithelial cells, B and T lymphocytes, mast cells, neutrophils, and eosinophils. The pathogenesis is complex and varies both over time and between patients due to interactions between multiple genetic and environmental factors.

Clinical Presentation

Asthma can present at nearly any age and, not uncommonly, becomes asymptomatic in adolescence, returning later in adulthood. Males are twice as likely to have the disease as children, but the ratio is equal in adults. The symptoms are not specific and common to many conditions, but when due to asthma they will characteristically vary over time and in intensity and are often worse at night or early in the morning. A history of allergies or atopic diseases is often present, especially in younger patients.

Patients with asthma may be asymptomatic for weeks or even months at a time but commonly worsen in response to "triggers" such as:

- Allergens, respiratory irritants (smoke, strong odors)
- Respiratory viruses
- Exercise, among others

This can progress rapidly and result in episodic flare-ups that may be life-threatening. Commonly known as "exacerbations," they represent an acute or subacute worsening of both symptoms and more objective measures of lung function. While not as common, they can occur even in patients who have mild or previously well controlled disease. It may also be the initial presentation of asthma. Preventing exacerbations is one of the primary goals of asthma treatment, as they can result in irreversible loss of lung function and even death.

Symptoms
The most common symptoms of asthma are:

- Episodic shortness of breath
- Cough
- Wheezing
- Chest tightness

In the majority of cases, more than one symptom will be present.

Signs
The physical exam will often be normal in asthmatic patients.

The most common abnormal finding is expiratory wheezing, but this is nonspecific and can also be present with other conditions such as COPD, laryngospasm, infections, and inhaled foreign bodies. Other potential findings include manifestations of atopic diseases such as post nasal drip or eczema.

Diagnostic and Lab Studies

Since there are no reliable exam findings or pathognomonic symptoms, the diagnosis of asthma can only be made by documenting variable airflow limitation. The most common and widely available method is performing spirometry with post-bronchodilator testing, which will show an obstructive pattern that improves after an inhaled bronchodilator (typically a beta-agonist such as albuterol).

- Additional pulmonary function testing may be necessary if COPD is in the differential.
- Serial peak expiratory flow (PEF) measurements can also be used but are less reliable.
- Other diagnostic tests that may be employed in certain situations include bronchoprovocation or "challenge" testing using either exercise or inhaled agents, such as mannitol or methacholine.
- Chest radiography is only indicated when necessary to evaluate for other conditions (e.g., pneumonia).
- Routine laboratory testing is also not helpful for making the initial diagnosis.

Differential Diagnosis/Formulating the Correct Diagnosis

"All that wheezes is not asthma," and this finding can be the result of multiple other conditions, as noted above. Inspiratory wheezing in particular is an important diagnostic consideration as it is not a feature of asthma and suggests a vocal cord or other upper airway disorder. Patients with asthma also generally experience multiple symptoms; isolated dry cough with no other respiratory symptoms is rarely due to asthma, for example.

As such, asthma cannot be diagnosed clinically, and failure to get confirmatory testing is the most common source of diagnostic error. Spirometry pre/post-bronchodilator is the first-line test but may be normal when patients are asymptomatic. Bronchoprovocation tests do not have this limitation but are less widely available and require specialized equipment and trained staff. Note that in both cases using inhaled medications prior to testing may result in a falsely negative result. If suspected, chest radiography may reveal evidence of pneumonia or radio-opaque foreign body. Laryngoscopy and bronchoscopy are the modalities of choice to rule out vocal cord or other upper airway disorders.

Once the presence of obstruction has been established, the primary consideration is COPD vs. asthma. Unlike asthma, which can be asymptomatic for a significant length of time, COPD is characterized by chronic dyspnea and/or productive cough in an older patient with a history of smoking. A diffusion limitation seen on pulmonary function testing will also help differentiate between the two conditions. Classifying the severity of asthma is important for both treatment and prognostic considerations. For patients with chronic stable asthma, this is measured by the intensity of therapy required to keep their asthma under control.

Table 12.1 Criteria for Mild, Moderate, or Severe Asthma

Severity classification	Level of treatment
Intermittent	Step 1 therapy
Mild	Step 2 therapy
Moderate	Step 3 therapy
Severe	Step 4 or above

Note: Some classification schemes do not include an "intermittent" category and classify mild asthma as requiring step 1 or 2.

Health Maintenance and Patient Education

Patient education is crucial, particularly given the unique challenges inherent to treatment with inhaled medications. Up to 80% of asthma patients cannot use their inhalers correctly, and checking/correcting poor technique has been proven to improve asthma control.

- Guided skills training should be given to all patients with direct observation of their technique when possible.
- Similarly, poor adherence to inhaled medications is common, and the factors contributing to it (cost, side effects, etc.) should be identified and corrected.

Guided self-management is proven to reduce asthma-related morbidity. Patients should be educated on the rationale for use and differences between long-term "controller" medications and the fast-acting "relievers" in order to avoid overreliance on the latter. Self-monitoring of symptoms (which can include serial PEF measurement) should be emphasized so that any worsening can be detected and addressed early.

IMPORTANT

An important component of self-management is a written "action plan," which explains what patients should do in the case of worsening symptoms, including when to call their physician or present for emergency treatment for an exacerbation using "green," "yellow," and "red" zones. The recommended format and a number of printable and electronic action plans can be accessed at www.cdc.gov/asthma/actionplan.html.

Treatment (Pharmaceutical and Clinical Intervention)

Since asthma is characterized by airway inflammation, the mainstay in treatment is inhaled corticosteroids (ICS), either alone or in combination with a long-acting beta agonist (LABA). These agents reduce inflammation and the risk of exacerbations and are known as "controllers."

- Medications such as short-acting beta agonists (SABA) are classified as "relievers" as they have a more rapid onset of action for as-needed relief of breakthrough symptoms (they are also commonly known as "rescue inhalers").
- A standard treatment regimen will consist of one or more controllers every day paired with an as-needed reliever such as albuterol. Low risk patients with very mild asthma may be successfully treated with intermittent SABA alone, but that is a minority.

Chronic Therapy

- The primary goals of treatment are to prevent exacerbations and achieve good asthma "control," commonly defined as experiencing symptoms requiring reliever medication use two or fewer times a week with no or minimal impact on sleep or usual daily activities, such as work or school.
- The recommended controller medication regimens are divided into "steps" of increasing therapeutic intensity. (The ICS component is listed as "low," "medium," and "high" doses to account for the variation across age groups and individual formulations.)

An example of this "stepwise approach," listing the most commonly cited first-line recommendations, is seen below in Table 12.2.

Table 12.2 Simplified Stepwise Approach to Asthma Treatment ("Preferred" Regimens Only)

Step 1	Step 2	Step 3	Step 4	Step 5
As needed SABA alone	Daily low-dose ICS	Daily low-dose ICS + LABA	Medium dose ICS + LABA	High dose ICS + LABA

The initial step can be chosen based on the frequency of symptoms as seen in **Table 12.3**.

Table 12.3

Frequency of Symptoms	Initial Treatment Step
Less than twice a month	Step 1
More than twice a month but not daily	Step 2
Symptoms most days or waking up once a week or more	Step 3
Daily symptoms or high risk features*	Step 4

*Consider adding a short course of oral corticosteroids at this step if symptoms are very frequent or severe. High-risk features include reduced pulmonary function on spirometry and a history of life-threatening or frequent exacerbations.

Patients newly initiated on treatment should be reassessed after a short interval (no more than 3 months), and those who are not well-controlled on their current regimen should be moved up one step until control is achieved. For example, if a patient initiated on a step 2 regimen of daily low-dose ICS still reports persistent asthma symptoms requiring use of SABA 3 days a week, treatment should be stepped up to low-dose ICS + LABA (step 3).

Adding a LABA is considered more effective than increasing the dose of ICS but should only be used in this combination, as LABA monotherapy has been associated with an increased risk of asthma-related death. Oral medications such as leukotriene antagonists are listed as alternative or "add-on" options but are generally inferior to ICS (or the addition of a LABA) and are not recommended as a first-line treatment. A leukotriene antagonist or long-acting muscarinic antagonist can also be substituted for a LABA in those who are unable to tolerate one due to side effects such as tachycardia (or added as a third agent at higher steps).

Once a patient has been well controlled for a minimum of 3 months, therapy can be brought down one step on a trial basis in order to find the lowest effective regimen needed to maintain it. Periodic control assessments should continue when following patients already on long-term treatment.

Patients with severe asthma who remain uncontrolled despite high-dose inhaled therapy may be candidates for more advanced treatments such as monoclonal antibodies. Referral to a specialist is usually recommended for those who are not well controlled or continue to have exacerbations despite step 4 care or higher and can be considered at step 3. Other commonly suggested indications for specialist referral include a history of frequent or near-fatal exacerbations, need for more advanced diagnostic testing and/or treatment, or suspected subtypes of asthma (e.g., occupational or aspirin-sensitive).

In addition to asthma-specific treatment, all patients should be evaluated/treated for comorbid chronic rhinosinusitis, GERD, obesity, OSA, and depression/anxiety, as these conditions are known to worsen asthma symptoms and quality of life.

Recommended nonpharmacologic therapies include (when applicable) smoking cessation, weight loss, and avoidance of known triggers. Specific efforts to mitigate mold and rodents/insects known to be in the home have some evidence to support a clinical benefit, but more broad allergen avoidance measures such as HEPA filters and carpet removal are not recommended as a general treatment strategy.

- Exacerbations: Initial outpatient treatment of an exacerbation starts with an early increase in inhaled medications followed by a short course of oral corticosteroids (OCS), if needed.
- The recommended dose of OCS is 1–2 mg/kg/day up to a maximum of 50 mg (40 mg in children) for 5–7 days.
- Antibiotics are not recommended unless there is clear evidence of a bacterial infection.

Professional Considerations

Inhaler use is subject to issues with technique on top of general medication adherence, so it is important to review both components as often as possible, especially when a patient is not well controlled. These factors are a very common cause of poor control and should be evaluated before stepping up therapy. This also helps to differentiate between uncontrolled asthma (which may be due to noncompliance or other external factors) and severe asthma. Other considerations when a patient has persistent poor control are environmental or occupational exposures, including:

- Smoking
- Medications

Comorbid conditions such as:

- Obesity
- Sinus disease
- GERD

Aspirin and other NSAIDs are well tolerated by the majority of patients and are not generally contraindicated unless there is a documented adverse reaction. Beta-blockers (including ophthalmic formulations) should only be considered after a careful risk/benefit assessment and under the care of a specialist.

Pregnant patients with severe or uncontrolled asthma may warrant specialist referral, but most can be managed in primary care if closely monitored. One-third of these patients will have their disease worsen, One-third will see no change, and One-third will improve. The risk of uncontrolled asthma greatly outweighs any risk from usual asthma medications such as ICS and LABA, and they should not be discontinued during pregnancy. Pregnant women experiencing an exacerbation should be treated in an identical fashion to any other patient.

Practice Questions for Pulmonary Review

1. Asthma is characterized by episodic wheezing, shortness of breath, chest tightness, and cough along with

    (A) reversibility of airflow obstruction.
    (B) alveolar hyperextensibility.
    (C) intermittent pneumothorax.
    (D) cardiomyopathy.
    (E) intermittent fever.

2. Essential medications for long-term control of asthma symptoms include

    (A) inhaled albuterol.
    (B) inhaled ipratropium.
    (C) inhaled corticosteroids.
    (D) oral prednisone.
    (E) oral anti-allergy medications.

3. Bronchiectasis is associated with a chronic productive cough along with dyspnea and wheezing. There is radiographic evidence of dilated, thickened airways with scattered opacities. The disease, in non-cystic fibrosis patients, is most often associated with

    (A) *Staphylococcus aureus.*
    (B) pneumoniae.
    (C) *Pseudomonas aeruginosa.*
    (D) *Haemophilus influenzae.*
    (E) streptococcus.

4. Your patient is a 28-year-old female with a diagnosis of community-acquired pneumonia. She has no comorbid medical conditions, no medication allergies, and no increased risk factors for MRSA or pseudomonas. Recommended outpatient management of CAP in this patient includes

    (A) levofloxacin 500 mg po daily.
    (B) ceftriaxone 1–2 g every 12–24 hours.
    (C) cefpodoxime 200 mg BID.
    (D) amxicillin 1 g po TID.
    (E) azithromycin po × 7 days.

5. A person with no known risk factors for tuberculosis requires a skin test reaction of

    (A) > 5 mm.
    (B) > 10 mm.
    (C) > 15 mm.
    (D) > 25 mm.
    (E) none of the above.

6. Treatment of latent TB infection is critical in controlling disease spread and reducing progression to active disease. Isoniazid as monotherapy is recommended for

   (A) 3 months.
   (B) 6 months.
   (C) 24 months.
   (D) 8 months.
   (E) 9 months.

7. You are evaluating a 24-year-old male who presents to the ED complaining of unilteral chest pain and dsypnea. He is alert and oriented and has no ongoing medical problems. He is tall and thin and is seen "splinting" his right rib area with his arm. He denies a history of injury or trauma. On exam, there is limited chest expansion with inhalation on the right side only. Breath sounds are diminished on the right. The remainder of the exam is normal. He is afrebrile and oxygen saturation is 98%. The patient is uncomfortable but not in acute distress. Based on this presentation you suspect

   (A) tension pneumothorax.
   (B) iatrogenic pneumothorax.
   (C) spontaneous pneumothorax.
   (D) secondary pneumothorax.
   (E) pleurisy.

8. Patients with pleural effusion may present with chest pain and dyspnea, depending on the size of the effusion. Patients presenting with a new pleural effusion should initially undergo

   (A) CT of the thorax.
   (B) diagnostic thoracentesis.
   (C) radiographs of the chest.
   (D) MRI of the chest.
   (E) pulmonary function testing.

9. Symptoms of asthma may be exacerbated by all of the following classes of medications except

   (A) beta-blockers.
   (B) acetylcystine.
   (C) NSAIDs.
   (D) tricyclic antidepressants.
   (E) aspirin.

10. All of the following occupations have been associated with development of asbestosis except

   (A) welding.
   (B) mining.
   (C) insulation.
   (D) shipbuilding.
   (E) pipe fitting.

Answers Explained

1. **(A)** Reversibility of airflow obstruction, either sponteneously or with bronchodilator therapy, is a characteristic of asthma. (B) Air trapping may occur with severe disease; however, alveolar hyperextensibility is not a characteristic finding. (C, D) These conditions are not characteristic of asthma. (E) Fever is not associated with asthma unless an underlying infection is present.

2. **(C)** Inhaled corticosteroids are the mainstay for long-term control of asthma symptoms. (A, B, D, E) These agents are used to relieve acute symptoms of asthma.

3. **(D)** Bronchiectasis may be congenital or acquired, and the most common pathogen found in patients who do not have cystic fibrosis is *Haemophilus influenzae*. All other pathogens may be present but are less commonly seen than *H. influenzae*. (A, B, C, E) These pathogens may be present, but are less commonly seen than *H. influenzae*.

4. **(D)** First-line management of CAP in patients with no comorbidities and no increased risk for MRSA or pseudomonas includes amoxicillin 1 g TID. Other treatment options are doxycycline 100 mg po BID or a Z-pack. (A, B, C, E) These agents are used for patients with coexisting illnesses, increased risk for MRSA or pseudomonas, or who are severely ill, requiring inpatient care.

5. **(C)** An individual with no known risk factors for TB requires a skin reaction of > 15 mm to be considered positive. (A) A reaction of > 5mm is considered positive in patients who are HIV positive, recent contacts of someone with active TB, persons with radiographic indications of TB, organ transplant recipients, or those who are otherwise immunocompromised. (B) A reaction of > 10 mm is considered positive for recent immigrants from countries with high endemic rates of TB; injection drug users (who are HIV negative); residents and employees of high-risk congregate settings, such as prisons, hospitals, and long-term care facilities. Persons with medical conditions that pose a risk for severe, progressive TB and children younger than age 4; adolescents exposed to adults at high risk are also considered positive with a reaction of this size.

6. **(E)** A 9 month regimen of oral isoniazid is recommended for latent tuberculosis.

7. **(C)** Primary spontaneous pneumothorax occurs in the absence of injury, trauma, or underlying pathology. The condition occurs most often in young persons who are tall and thin. It occurs more commonly in males. (A) Tension pneumothorax usually occurs with penetrating trauma, positive-pressure mechanical ventilation, and CPR. (B) Iatrogenic pneumothorax occurs secondary to medical procedures, such as subclavian catheter placement, mechanical ventilation, or thoracentesis. (D) Secondary pneumothorax occurs as a complication of a pre-existing lung disease. (E) Pleurisy causes pain with respirations and a "rub" may or may not be auscultated on the affected side; however, breath sounds are not diminished, as this condition affects the pleural lining around the lung.

8. **(B)** Patients presenting with a new pleural effusion should undergo diagnostic thoracentesis, which will provide evidence of the type of effusion that is occurring. (A, C, D) Other imaging modalities may be indicated based on patient presentation following diagnostic thoracentesis. (E) PFTs are not indicated in the initial management of pleural effusion.

9. **(D)** Tricyclic antidepressants may cause central nervous system depression, decreasing pulmonary function. (A, B, C, E) These medications are associated with exacerbating symptoms of asthma.

10. **(A)** Welding has been associated with siderosis; however, not with asbestosis. (B, C, D, E) These occupations have all been implicated in asbestosis.

13

Renal Review

Learning Objectives

In this chapter, you will review:

→ Acute and chronic disorders

→ Congenital or structural kidney disorders

→ Fluid and electrolyte disorders

→ Neoplasms

Acute Disorders

Glomerulonephritis

Pathophysiology

Glomerulonephritis is an inflammation or scaring of the glomeruli inside the kidney resulting in disruptions to the filtration of the blood over days or weeks. This results in retention of waste products.

Clinical Presentation

Symptoms

- 50% of the patients are asymptomatic
- Decreased urinary output
- Reported dark urine output
- Nausea/vomiting
- Fatigue

Signs

- Swelling
- Shortness of breath
- Hypertension
- Tachycardia

Diagnostic and Lab Studies

Urinalysis

- Pyuria, proteinuria (24-hour collection), RBC casts on urine, white blood cell cast

Serum

Order CBC, electrolytes, blood urea nitrogen, check for anemia, antistreptolysin O titer, antinuclear antibody (ANA), hepatitis B surface antigen and antibody, hepatitis C antibody, rheumatoid factor, and HIV testing.

Biopsy

Kidney biopsy will help to confirm the diagnosis, determine the cause of the infection and amount of scaring, and estimate the potential for reversibility of the disease.

Differential Diagnosis/Formulating the Most Likely Diagnosis

Differential diagnosis may include:

- Underlying infections (untreated strep throat, hepatitis B, C, HIV)
- Vasculitis
- Immune disorders (Goodpasture syndrome, systemic lupus erythematous)

Health Maintenance and Patient Education

Low protein and sodium diet, routine blood pressure monitoring.

Treatment (Pharmaceutical and Clinical Intervention)

Treatment focusing on the underlying disease. Early intervention could preserve kidney function, and dialysis may not be warranted.

Professional Considerations

Major causes of acute glomerulonephritis include:

- Recent throat or skin infection with streptococcus infection
- Bacteria infection (staphylococcus and pneumococcus)
- Viral infection (chicken pox, hepatitis B, C, or HIV)
- Parasite infection (malaria)
- Vasculitis (blood vessel inflammation)
- Hereditary nephritis
- Drugs (quinine, gemcitabine, mitomycin C)

Nephrotic Syndrome

Pathophysiology

Nephrotic syndrome is the impairment of the podocytes (central to the filtration mechanism of the glomerular filtration barrier) resulting an increased glomerular permeability to protein in the blood especially albumin.

Clinical Presentation

Symptoms
- Anorexia
- Malaise
- Frothy urine (due to high concentrations of protein)

Signs
- Shortness of breath
- Arthralgia
- Abdominal pain (ascites)
- Edema

Diagnostic and Lab Studies

Urinalysis: urine random (spot) protein/creatinine ratio ≥ 3 or proteinuria ≥ 3 g/24 hours.

Differential Diagnosis/Formulating the Most Likely Diagnosis

Differential diagnosis includes nephrotic syndrome, which is more prevalent in children.

Primary causes: minimal changes disease, focal segmental glomerulosclerosis, and membranous nephropathy.
Secondary causes: ($> 50\%$ adult): diabetic nephropathy, preeclampsia, amyloidosis, and HIV-associated nephropathy.

Health Maintenance and Patient Education

Patients should receive pneumococcal vaccinations.

Treatment (Pharmaceutical and Clinical Intervention)

Treatment of the underlying disorder, angiotensin inhibition, statins, diuretics for fluids overload.

Professional Considerations

Sodium restriction (< 2 g per day) is recommended for patients with edema.

Pyelonephritis
Pathophysiology

Pyelonephritis occurs when there is an infection along the ascending urinary tract that could spread from the bladder to the kidney. Not all patients will show symptoms. The most common etiology pathogen for pyelonephritis is *E. coli* ($> 80\%$).

Clinical Presentation

Symptoms
- Fever
- Nausea/vomiting
- Flank pain
- Increased urinary frequency/urgency
- Dysuria

Signs
- Sudden onset of chills, fever
- Unilateral or bilateral flank pain with/without costovertebral tenderness

Diagnostic and Lab Studies

Urinalysis: pyuria, leukocytes cast, hematuria, nitrites, and mild proteinuria.

Differential Diagnosis/Formulating the Most Likely Diagnosis

Differential diagnosis may include:

- Obstructive uropathy
- Cholecystitis
- Acute pancreatitis
- Pelvic inflammatory disease
- Renal calculi
- Diverticulitis

Health Maintenance and Patient Education

Encourage patients' fluid intake and have them complete an entire course of antibiotic treatment. Patients with a history of frequent UTI may need additional urinalysis/urine culture to confirm the eradication of the infection upon completion of the treatment.

Treatment (Pharmaceutical and Clinical Intervention)

- Empiric treatment or treatment based on the urine culture with multidrug-resistant report
- Nitrofuran, fluoroquinolone, trimethoprim-sulfamethoxazole (TMP-SMX), or broad-spectrum β-lactam
- Analgesics
- Antipyretics

Professional Considerations

There is a high prevalence of asymptomatic bacteriuria among the elderly population, and urine culture is more reliable than in-house urine dipstick for the diagnosis of urinary tract infection. Other commonly associated conditions include indwelling catheters, renal calculi, and benign prostatic hyperplasia.

Congenital or Structural Renal Disorders

Hydronephrosis

Pathophysiology

Hydronephrosis could occur when there is a buildup of pressure in the urinary collecting system. If left untreated, the pressure can cause calyceal fornix rupture and resulting urinary extravasation.

Clinical Presentation

Symptoms
- Decreased urinary output
- Nausea/vomiting
- Fatigue
- Flank pain
- Abdominal pain
- Fever/chill (with coexisting infection)
- Anuria

Signs
- Abdominal mass
- Edema
- Shortness of breath
- Mental stage changes
- Tremors (from long-standing obstruction)
- Hypertension
- Diaphoresis

Diagnostic and Lab Studies

Urinalysis with Microscopy

- Hematuria, proteinuria, crystalluria, pyuria
- Urine culture and sensitivity
- Exclude UTI

Serum

- Ureamia, creatinine, hyperkalemia, hyperphosphatemia, and hypocalcemia
- US and non-contrast CT effective in diagnosing the presence or cause of obstruction

Differential Diagnosis/Formulating the Most Likely Diagnosis

Differential diagnosis may include:

- UTI, benign prostate hypertrophy, CKD, bladder outlet obstruction, and diabetes insipidus
- Cystosopy, retrograde pyelogram, uretoscopy, and biopsy could be used to determine the cause of obstruction or establish a pathologic diagnosis (mass lesion).

Health Maintenance and Patient Education

Patient will need to be monitored closely for kidney function and self-monitor blood pressure at home until renal function stabilizes.

Treatment (Pharmaceutical and Clinical Intervention)

Primary treatment is relief of obstruction and reducing the pressure in the urinary collecting system.

Professional Considerations

Major causes of hydronephrosis include:

- High urine output (diabetes insipidus, psychogenic polydipsia)
- Bacterial infections (UTI)
- Vesicoureteral reflux (VUR)
- Transplanted kidney (posttransplant period)
- Physiologic changes (pregnancy)

Polycystic Kidney Disease

Pathophysiology

Polycystis kidney disease is composed of a group of monogenic disorders that commonly result in renal cyst development. There are two genetically distinct conditions: autosomal dominant polycystic kidney disease (ADPKD) and autosomal recessive polycystic kidney disease (ARPKD). ADPKD: The most common inherited disorders, where the PKD1 and PKD2 mutations disrupt the function of polycystins on the primary cilium with clinical manifestation beginning at the third to fourth decade of life. ARPKD: More common in infants and children, where PKHD1 mutations cause the cystic dilation and liver enlargement.

Clinical Presentation

Symptoms and Signs

- Flank masses
- Hypertension

Diagnostic and Lab Studies

Urinalysis: Including urinary citrate
Serum: Evaluate electrolytes, BUN/creatinine
US, non-contrast CT, and MRI: Effective in diagnosing the presence of cyst or organ enlargement
Genetic testing: ADPKD: PKD1 and PKD2; ARPKD: PKHD1

Differential Diagnosis/Formulating the Most Likely Diagnosis

Differential diagnosis may include:

- Hypertension is one of the most common early manifestation of ADPKD.
- Tuberous sclerosis
- Nephronophthisis
- Renal cystic dysplasia
- Simple cysts
- Renal cystic neoplasms

Health Maintenance and Patient Education

- Blood pressure monitoring
- Encourage fluids
- Limit on caffeine intake
- Low protein diet
- Treat UTI and stone aggressively

Treatment (Pharmaceutical and Clinical Intervention)

No specific drug treatment.

- Symptomatic treatment (maintaining appropriate blood pressure, lipids level with statins a preferred choice)
- Referral to nephrologist, urologist, and genetic counseling

Professional Considerations

Patient presented with severe flank pain, gross hematuria with clots, will need to refer to emergency department.

A majority of the patients diagnosed with polycystic kidney disease will eventually develop end-stage kidney disease.

Hydration and BP management should be the main goals.

Renal Vascular Disease

Pathophysiology

Renal vascular disease compromises the blood flow into and out of the kidneys. A reduction of blood into the kidney will result in an increase of renin production, which is the strong hormone that raises blood pressure. If left untreated, this will result in kidney damage (short term), kidney failure (long term), and disrupt the body's homeostasis (high blood pressure). There are several vascular conditions: renal artery stenosis, renal artery thrombosis, renal vein thrombosis, renal artery aneurysm, and atheroembolic renal disease.

Renal artery stenosis: narrowing or blockage of an artery that functions as a passage to the kidney. This will result in kidney failure and high blood pressure.

Renal artery thrombosis: formation of blood clot(s) in an artery that replenishes blood flow to the kidney. It may reduce blood flow and cause kidney failure.

Renal vein thrombosis: formation of blood clot(s) in the vein to the kidney

Renal artery aneurysm: a weak surface area of an artery resulting in a formation of bulging, usually are small and does not cause symptoms

Atheroembolic renal disease: common cause of kidney problems in the elderly population when a piece of plaque detaches from an artery and blocks off small renal arteries

Renal Artery Stenosis

Clinical Presentation

Symptoms and Signs
- High blood pressure
- Uremia
- Unexplained kidney failure
- Sudden onset of kidney failure when first taking an angiotensin-converting enzyme (ACE) inhibitor

Renal Artery Thrombosis

Clinical Presentation

Symptoms and Signs
- High blood pressure
- Nausea/vomiting
- Hematuria
- Fever
- Flank pain
- Sudden decrease in kidney function

Renal Artery Aneurysm

Clinical Presentation

Symptoms and Signs
- No symptoms
- High blood pressure
- Flank pain
- Hematuria

Atheroembolic Renal Disease

Clinical Presentation

Symptoms and Signs

- Skin lesions
- Abdominal pain
- Weight loss
- Fatigue
- Myalgia
- Kidney failure
- Decreased skin perfusion on lower extremities
- Fever
- Confusion

Renal Vein Thrombosis

Clinical Presentation

Symptoms and Signs

- Most often causes no symptoms
- Decreased kidney function
- Severe flank pain with episodes of spasms at times
- Hematuria

Diagnostic and Lab Studies

- Renography

Imaging

Arteriogram, angiogram, magnetic resonance angiography (MRA)

US

Duplex ultrasound

Differential Diagnoses/Formulating the Most Likely Diagnosis

Differential diagnoses may include:

- Renal artery stenosis, renal artery thrombosis, renal vein thrombosis, renal artery aneurysm, atheroembolic renal disease, hypertensive, diabetes, chronic kidney disease
- The distinction between the narrowing or blockage of the artery or vein is important for proper diagnosis and treatment.

Health Maintenance and Patient Education

Lifestyle modification, low fat and sodium diet, routine blood pressure monitoring.

Treatment (Pharmaceutical and Clinical Intervention)

Blood pressure treatment, lipids lowering agents, diabetes management, thrombolytic medications, surgical procedure is based on the types of renal vascular disease that are present.

Professional Considerations

Untreated renal vascular disease can lead to kidney failure. Patients may require lifelong dialysis or a kidney transplant.

Neoplasms

Renal Cell Carcinoma

Pathophysiology

Renal cell carcinoma is a hereditary autosomal dominant arising from parenchyma of the kidney. It accounts for almost 85% of all primary kidney cancer. The two most common genes involved in the pathogenesis of this disease are Von Hippel–Lindau (VHL) and the protein polybromo-1 (PBRM-1) genes.

Clinical Presentation

Symptoms

- Decreased urinary output
- Nausea/vomiting
- Abdominal pain
- Flank pain
- Hematuria

Signs

- Swelling
- Hypertension
- Tachycardia

Diagnostic and Lab Studies

Urinalysis

Urine cytology

Serum

CBC, Chem-7, LDH, liver function tests

US

Differentiate between solid or cystic

Imaging

X-ray, CT, MRI

Differential Diagnosis/Formulating the Most Likely Diagnosis

Differential diagnosis may include diabetes, hypertension, benign renal masses, simple/simple renal cysts, pyelonephritis, hydronephrosis, renal abscess, Wilms tumor, melanoma metastatic disease, lymphoma, and liposarcomas. Incorporating the Bosniak classification (I, II, IIF, III, IV) and TNM classification of malignant tumors as part of the diagnosis formulation is important.

Health Maintenance and Patient Education

Lifestyle modification: smoking cessation, low fat, low meat, weight management, moderation in analgesic use.

Treatment (Pharmaceutical and Clinical Intervention)

Active monitoring is recommended for small renal masses (less than < 4 cm).

Medications
- Immunotherapy
- Antiangiogenic

Surgery
- For removal of masses on the affected sites
- For nonsurgical candidates: cryoablation, radiofrequency ablation
- Supportive care

Professional Considerations

Renal cell carcinoma metastasis through lymphatic spreading. The most common site of the metastatic is the lung.

Practice Questions for Renal Review

1. Red cell casts found in urinalysis is indicative of

   (A) insterstitial nephritis.
   (B) chronic kidney disease.
   (C) acute tubular necrosis.
   (D) glomerulonephritis.
   (E) acute kidney injury.

2. Acute kidney injury is defined and identified by

   (A) rapid increase in serum creatinine.
   (B) widespread peripheral edema.
   (C) decrease in blood urea nitrogen (BUN) level.
   (D) hypokalemia.
   (E) decreased glomerular filtration rate (GFR).

3. Obstruction within the urinary tract is a common cause of

   (A) prerenal azotemia.
   (B) intrinsic renal disease.
   (C) postrenal azotemia.
   (D) acute tubular necrosis.
   (E) renal artery stenosis.

4. Acute tubular necrosis occurs in up to 25% of hospitalized patients treated with

   (A) cephalosporins.
   (B) aminoglycosides.
   (C) acyclovir.
   (D) all chemotherapeutic agents.
   (E) salicylates.

5. Chronic kidney disease is a progressive disorder that may go undetected for years as compensatory mechanisms work to maintain homeostasis. Medication classes used to help reduce injury and slow progression of CKD include angiotensin receptor blockers (ARBs) and

   (A) ACE inhibitors.
   (B) corticosteroids.
   (C) calcium channel blockers (CCBs).
   (D) beta-blockers (BBs).
   (E) metformin.

6. A patient starting ACE inhibitor therapy who develops acute kidney injury should be evaluated for

   (A) glomerulonephritis.
   (B) chronic kidney disease.
   (C) renal artery stenosis.
   (D) end-stage renal disease.
   (E) acute tubular necrosis.

7. Diabetic nephropathy develops after approximately 10 years in many patients with poor glycemic control. One of the first indications is

   (A) hematuria.
   (B) a decrease in GFR.
   (C) overt proteinuria.
   (D) hypokalemia.
   (E) an increase in GFR.

8. The most common cause of renal disease associated with proteinuria in children is minimal change disease. Electron microscopy of kidney tissue reveals which characteristic finding?

   (A) Foot-process effacement
   (B) Necrosis of renal bed
   (C) Diffuse polycysitic disease
   (D) Neoplastic tissue changes
   (E) Gross hematuria

9. Postinfectious glomerulonephritis is most often due to prior infection with

   (A) *Staphylococcus aureus*.
   (B) *Pseudomonas aeruginosa*.
   (C) group B beta-hemolytic strep.
   (D) cytomegalovirus.
   (E) adenovirus.

10. Patients with diabetes mellitus should be screened annually for nephropathy. Screening should be done through

   (A) microalbuminuria testing.
   (B) renal ultrasound.
   (C) GFR.
   (D) CT of the kidneys.
   (E) urine culture.

Answers Explained

1. **(D)** Red cell casts in microscopic urine sample indicates glomerulonephritis. (A) White blood cell casts is indicative of interstitial nephritis. (B) Chronic kidney disease often presents with broad waxy casts in the urine. (C) Renal tubular cell casts is characteristic of acute tubular necrosis. (E) AKI is not specifically associated with the presence of red cell casts in urine.

2. **(A)** Acute kidney injury produces a rapid increase in serum creatinine. Usually an increase by 0.3 mg/dL or more within 48 hours. (B) As waste products of metablism accumulate, patients experience uremia, which is nausea, vomiting, malaise, and altered level of consciousness. Widespread edema is not characteristic of initial AKI. (C) The BUN may rise with AKI; it should not decrease. (D) Hyperkalemia is seen with AKI, not hypokalemia. (E) GFR decrease develops progressively over time and with ongoing renal disease. A decreased GFR on presentation of AKI should lead to a suspicion of underlying chronic disease.

3. **(C)** Postrenal azotemia is most often a result of obstruction in the urinary tract. (A) Causes of prerenal azotemia include poor renal perfusion, from a number of causes. (B) Intrinsic renal disease includes acute tubular necrosis, acute glomerulonephritis, and acute interstitial nephritis. (D) Acute tubular necrosis is an intrinsic cause of azotemia. (E) Renal artery stenosis is an area of blockage or narrowing of the renal artery and is not associated with intrarenal obstruction.

4. **(B)** ATN is seen in approximately 25% of patients receiving aminoglycoside therapy. Kidney injury usually occurs after 5–10 days of therapy and is nonoliguric in most cases. Risk factors include preexisting kidney disease, advanced age, and volume depletion. (A, C, D, E) These agents may be nephrotoxic for individuals with or without preexisting renal disease; however, the incidence of injury is not as high as with aminoglycosides.

5. **(A)** ARBs and ACE inhibitors reduce hyperfiltration renal injury and help to slow the progression of CKD. (B, C, D) These medications are not associated with slowing the progression of CKD. (E) Metformin is an oral agent used in the treatment of type 2 diabetes mellitus. Strict control of serum glucose levels reduces long-term damage to the kidneys; however, the indication for administration is diabetes mellitus, not to prevent or slow progression of CKD.

6. **(C)** Stenosis of the renal artery is caused by atheroscleoritc disease in most cases. Patients present with new onset hypertension, usually after age 45 years. The hypertension is often refractory to treatment. A patient in this setting who develops AKI after starting ACE inhibitor therapy should be evaluated for renal artery stensosis, which is often bilateral. (A, B, D, E) These conditions are not associated with ACEI-induced AKI.

7. **(E)** One of the first indications of diabetic nephropathy is an increase in the GFR caused by hyperfiltration. This increase is then followed by a decrease in GFR along with overt proteinuria and electrolyte imbalances (A, B, C, D).

8. **(A)** The characteristic finding on tissue biopsy with minimal change disease is "foot-process" effacement on electron microscopy. (B, C, D, E) These findings are not characteristic of minimal change disease.

9. **(C)** Previous infection with group B beta-hemolytic strep is the most common cause of postinfectious glomerulonephritis. (A, B, D, E) These pathogens are occasionally implicated; however, they are not the most common cause.

10. **(A)** All patients with diabetes mellitus should be screened annually for microalbuminuria. (B, C, D) These studies may be used to evaluate known or progressive renal function decline or to rule out structural abnormalities of the kidney. (E) Urine culture is useful in the setting of a urinary tract infection to determine the offending pathogen and direct treatment.

14

Reproductive Review

Cervical Disorders

Cervicitis

Cervicitis is an inflammation of the uterine cervix. It can have infectious and noninfectious causes. Most often, the bacterial and viral infections that cause cervicitis are transmitted by sexually transmitted infections (STIs), including gonorrhea, chlamydia, trichomoniasis, and genital herpes.

Pathophysiology

Mycoplasma gonorrhea spares the vaginal epithelium and primarily infects the columnar, transitional, and epithelial cervical cells. This is a gram-negative organism.

- *Chlamydia trachomatis* is a gram-negative, obligate parasite that infects the columnar epithelial cells.
- *Mycoplasma genitalium* cannot be detected by Gram stain and infects endocervical columnar cells. This agent was previously thought to be a biologic XY organism; however, more studies have pointed to this agent as a biologic XX infectious factor.

A patient may also have a cervical irritant from a retained foreign body; however, this is readily seen on exam and removed.

Clinical Presentation

Patients with cervicitis will generally present with persistent and substantial discharge. This is white to yellow in color, and odor is minimal. It is not irritating. Patients may also experience intermenstrual bleeding, particularly after intercourse. Patients with chlamydia report urinary frequency and urgency. In *Mycoplasma gonorrhea* and *genitalium*, the patient may be asymptomatic. Skin lesions and bleeding are apparent. On physical exam, discharge may be noted from an edematous, erythematous cervix (*Chlamydia trachomatis*), or the patient may have minimal to no discharge noted with a normal appearing cervix. A significant differentiator in cervicitis versus pelvic inflammatory disease is the absence of pelvic or abdominal pain. There should also be no cervical motion tenderness.

Diagnostic and Lab Studies

For all three forms of cervicitis, nucleic acid amplification testing (NAAT) is the preferred method of diagnosing the specific organism causing symptomatology.

- Pelvic and bimanual exam
- A specimen can be collected from the endocervix, the urethra, or the initial stream void of urine.

> **Of note, urine is least preferred if the endocervix or urethra is available.**
>
> In patients with known exposure to *Mycoplasma genitalium* or cervicitis that is persistent despite negative NAAT, *Mycoplasma genitalium* should be strongly considered as agent, as the United States does not have an FDA approved NAAT for this organism. In all patients, consider screening in other areas of sexual entry (anus and oropharynx).

Differential Diagnosis

The differential diagnosis of cervicitis includes vaginitis (particularly atrophic vaginitis), desquamative inflammatory vaginitis, contact dermatitis, allergy, and lichen planus.

Health Maintenance and Patient Education

Patients should be screened for GC/CT if they are less than 24 years of age, have another sexually transmitted infection, are sexually active with a partner with a known sexually transmitted infection, have multiple or new partners, are engaging in sexual activity (oral, anal, or rectal) without a barrier method, or are employed as a sex worker.

- If at any time their sexual behavior changes, they should be offered repeat screening. Patients with symptoms should also be screened.
- Education regarding transmission of GC/CT and decreased rates of transmission via barrier methods should be discussed at patient encounters.
- Patients should also be made aware to abstain from intercourse until both or all partners have been able to complete pharmaceutical therapy and become asymptomatic.

Treatment (Pharmaceutical and Clinical Intervention)

Mycoplasma gonorrhea has had recent updates to treatment guidelines in the United States. The 2021 Centers for Disease Control STI recommendations for uncomplicated gonorrhea no longer recommend a standard two drug regimen due to increasing antibiotic resistance. Patients found to be gonorrhea positive should be treated with a single 500 mg intramuscular dose of ceftriaxone and, if a chlamydia culture was not performed or has not been returned negative at time of treatment, should also receive an additional prescription for 100 mg oral doxycycline to be taken twice daily for a total of 7 days.

- If the patient is allergic to cephalosporins, or the penicillin class, they may be given 240 mg gentamicin IM for one dose followed by an oral dosage of azithromycin 2 grams to be taken at one time.
- Expedited partner treatment, the prescribing of medication to a patient's sexual partner(s) without the physical evaluation of the partner in the practice, can be performed via 800 mg oral cefixime for one dose and a follow-up of doxycycline 100 mg oral twice daily for 7 days.

Chlamydia has less resistance in the United States and requires a one-drug treatment regimen. The preferred therapeutic for this infection is azithromycin 500 mg, taken two tablets at the same time.

- Alternatively, a patient can be given doxycycline 100 mg twice daily for 7 days or erythromycin 500 mg taken four times daily for 7 days.
- Expediated partner treatment can be performed here as well, with the same treatment used, and a test of cure is recommended at 3 months due to reinfection rates.

Mycoplasma genitalium follows a similar treatment regimen with exception of increasing resistance to doxycycline. Additionally, since there is no FDA approved NAAT confirmation test for this infection in the United States, patients are treated for this following a known exposure in a male partner or through clinical suspicion following continued symptoms in absence of negative NAAT for other infections. Treatment consists of azithromycin 500 mg taken two tablets at one time or moxifloxacin 400 mg taken once daily × 7–14 days.

Cervical Dysplasia

Pathophysiology

Most dysplastic lesions of the cervix are due to human papillomavirus (HPV) infections. Of these, a subset of high-risk (HPV-HR) strains have been particularly shown to enact changes in the squamous epithelium of the cervix. HPV types 16 and 18 are two such HR types with a high progression to invasive neoplasia. Other risk factors include cigarette smoking, poor access to cervical cancer screening, high-risk sexual behavior, combined oral contraceptive use, and low socioeconomic status. Involvement of dysplastic lesions can be broken into three categories. Cervical intraepithelial neoplasia I (CIN I), or mild dysplasia, involves the lower one-third of the intraepithelium. CIN II, moderate, extends into the middle half, and CIN III, or severe dysplasia, extends into the upper one-third. Carcinoma in situ involves the full thickness of the squamous intraepithelium. This terminology refers to the histologic result received on a colposcopic biopsy. Persistent CIN II or CIN III is concerning for the development of invasive carcinoma and necessitates more thorough workup and treatment than CIN I or self-limiting CIN II.

> **NOTE**
>
> **It should be noted that expedited partner treatment is not legal in every state. Test of cure should be definitively performed on patients with oropharyngeal gonorrhea at 7–14 days and due to high reinfection rates, should be performed at 3 months for rectal and cervical infections.**

Clinical Presentation

The vast majority of patients with early dysplasia will not have any noticeable symptoms.
Patients with persistent dysplasia may go on to develop:

- A noticeable foul-smelling vaginal discharge with necrotic material
- Abnormal vaginal bleeding
- Pelvic pain
- Weight loss.

Physical exam is generally without abnormality in early to middle stages. Advanced dysplasia may have visible neovascularity on the cervix.

- CIN II can present with flat, bright white lesions visible in the transformation zone, while CIN III lesions have a duller, grey border.
- Tumors generally do not visibly erode through the endocervix until much later in the diagnostic period.

Diagnostic and Lab Studies

The liquid-based pap smear is the current standard for cervical pathology abnormalities, in addition to HPV testing. Current guidelines are to begin screening at age 21 and continue until age 65, with HPV testing routinely at age 30. Newer guidelines were recommended by the American Cancer Society in 2021 to begin routine testing at age 25 every 5 years, with primary HPV testing as the cornerstone. Any abnormal pap smear is evaluated according to the patient's age, prior pap smears, and HPV status. Patients will either enter surveillance or further evaluation protocols. Further evaluation is performed via colposcopy and possible cervical biopsy for histologic evaluation. Surveillance will change the period of time between pap smear screenings.

Differential Diagnosis

The differential diagnosis of cervical dysplasia includes neoplasia of other origin, cervical polyp, cervical leiomyoma, cervical ectopic pregnancy, vaginal cancer, and cervical lymphoma.

Health Maintenance and Patient Education

- Patients should be educated on the appropriate screening for their age group and any co-existing medical conditions.
- Referrals for low cost pap smears should be performed.
- Cultural/language barriers must be evaluated, especially given the high rates of Black and Hispanic women with invasive cervical cancer.

Treatment (Pharmaceutical and Clinical Intervention)

Treatment of cervical dysplasia is based on the degree of abnormality. Recent significant changes to both abnormal pap smear and colposcopic biopsy management in October 2020 have focused on persistent CIN II and the prevention of CIN III development. Preinvasive lesions can be treated with cold knife conization or loop electricoexcision of the cervix. This functions to remove these lesions from the transitional zone. Lesions that have progressed into invasive may require hysterectomy and/or adjunctive therapies. Preventative vaccines are available against HPV. These include two bivalent and one quadrivalent vaccines that are aimed at adolescents ages 9–14.

Contraceptive Methods

Non-hormonal methods include:

- Timed ovulation
- Breastfeeding (lactational amenorrhea)
- Barrier contraception
- Spermicides
- Diaphragms
- Cervical caps
- Periodic abstinence
- Body temperature monitoring

Failure rates are highest with these methods.

- These methods require the most involvement on the part of the patient. Timed fertility methods include basal body temperature monitoring, cervical mucous monitoring, and timed intercourse.
- These methods are dependent on a consistent menstrual cycle and adequate instruction of the patient.
- Barrier methods including male and female condoms require correct usage with each sexual act.
- Diaphragms and cervical caps require an appointment with a provider for correct fit and placement, as well as a limited time for their usage

Progesterone based oral contraceptive pills:

- For use in a limited population, including lactating mothers
- Effectiveness of these agents as single-use items is decreased (up to 50%).
- These "mini-pills" are most effective as a backup to lactational amenorrhea or for use with a barrier method.
- Benefits include decreased risk of estrogen-based adverse events, including thromboembolic activity, hypertension, cholelithiasis, and liver tumors.
- Adverse effects include increased rates of intermenstrual bleeding and unintentional pregnancy. Progestin sensitive tumors will also be responsive to these agents.

Progesterone based injection:

- This is a depot formulation of synthetic progestin that inhibits anterior pituitary function.
- It is commonly given as a dose of 150 mg every 3 months via intramuscular route.
- Unpredictable bleeding is the most common adverse reaction with this formulation, followed by headache, mood changes, and weight gain.
- There is a black box warning against using this agent for more than 5 years, as bone loss may be irreversible.
- This method has a 97% success rate when given within correct parameters.
- Patients have a 2-week window in which to receive an injection if a dose is missed.

Combined Oral Contraceptives (COCs)

These agents are comprised of synthetic estrogens and progestins to act on the hypothalamus to suppress pulsatile GnRH and thus prevent pituitary secretion of FSH and LH (inhibiting ovulation). They are generally considered highly effective due to having multiple effects on contraception. COCs come in monophasic form (all pills have the same amount of synthetic hormone until the last days of placebo pills designed to induce a withdrawal bleed), biphasic form (a higher level of synthetic hormone for the first 2 weeks before the second lower level leads into the placebo week), or triphasic, which most closely mimics the hormone phasing of the menstrual cycle. COC form should be chosen based on all aspects desired to control for the patient.

COCs can be used for more than contraception. They have indication for dysmenorrhea, heavy menstrual bleeding, premenstrual dysphoric disorder, acne, ovarian cyst formation, hirsutism, and treatment in other diseases (endometriosis and leiomyomata when used continuously).

Due to the estrogen influence, COCs have many potential adverse effects and interactions. Increased rates of thromboembolic events, including deep venous thrombosis, pulmonary embolus, and cerebrovascular accident have been reported; and, thus, patients should be screened for outside risk factors. Those with increased risk for VTE or smokers over age 35 should have an alternative form of contraception issued. Other common adverse effects include changes in the menstrual cycle, breast tenderness, headache, and cholelithiasis. Patients must be cautioned that COCs alone only prevent conception and not STIs.

Transdermal/Mucosal Combined Agents
These include both the transdermal patch and the vaginal ring. Both contain estrogen/progestin agents. The transdermal patch has the highest levels of estrogen/progestin, while the vaginal ring has the lowest levels of hormone. These varying rates in hormone are due to the methods of delivery system.

Progesterone Implant
There is currently a one-rod implant system using levonorgestrel. This thin, flexible rod is implanted just under the skin of the upper arm and remains in place for up to 3 years or until the patient desires fertility. Adverse effects include the highest rates of menstrual cycle changes of any of the hormonal methods, headache, and weight changes. Efficacy is significantly high as the patient does not have to follow up with any other method following placement.

Long Acting Reversible Contraceptives (LARCs)
Intrauterine devices (IUDs) are available in both a hormonal (progesterone) and a non-hormonal (copper) form. The mechanism of action is variable depending on which LARC is being used. Efficacy is quite high, with little follow-up needed after insertion for either form. A 1-month string check is common. Failure rates remain at 1–1.5% with correct insertion. Adverse effects for both forms include uterine perforation, ectopic pregnancy, higher rates of spontaneous abortion if pregnancy occurs, and pelvic infection. Changes in menstrual cycle are common to both forms but for differing reasons. The copper LARC does not have a hormonal effect on the patient's menses; thus, they return to a baseline function. If the patient has not experienced baseline menses in some time, the patient may experience a heavier flow than usual. The progesterone LARC does exert hormonal influence on the patient; and, particularly in the first 6 months, menstrual flow may be irregular with development of oligo or amenorrhea following the seventh month. There are currently four progesterone-based LARCs available for use, with one having an additional indication for the treatment of heavy menstrual bleeding (Mirena). The other three are only indicated for the use of contraception. The copper LARC (ParaGard) is only indicated for contraception and can be used for emergency contraception if inserted within 5 days of unprotected intercourse.

Sterilization
A patient who is certain of the desire against future fertility can be offered permanent sterilization. This is done via a bilateral tubal ligation. The fallopian tubes are interrupted in a multitude of ways, and scar tissue forms, preventing the transfer of an ovum into the uterus.

Emergency Contraception

Patients who have unprotected or unplanned intercourse and are not already on another form of hormonal contraception can be given emergency contraception. As above, if a patient does not desire fertility in the next 5 years, a copper LARC can be placed for long-term contraception and can act as emergency contraception at the same time. Alternatively, oral synthetic estrogen/progestin combination pills or progestin only pills can be given. There are multiple regimens of these agents available as stand-alone forms, or many prescription COCs or POPs can be given individually in higher doses. Patients should be cautioned against the common adverse reaction of nausea and vomiting. Additionally, a pregnancy that is already in place will not be disrupted by the use of COCs or POPs, but the placement of the LARC would be detrimental. As such, a pregnancy test must be performed prior to placement.

Uterine Disorders

Endometriosis

Pathophysiology

The primary cause of endometriosis is poorly differentiated. It is characterized by the presence of normal endometrial tissue outside of the endometrial cavity that still responds to cyclic hormonal changes.

Five theories have been generally accepted including:

- Retrograde menstruation
- Coelomic metaplasia
- Hematogenous spread
- Stem cell derivation
- Mullerian remnant differentiation

Retrograde menstruation is the most accepted theory, with a vast majority of women who experience some form of lower outflow tract obstruction having at least a minimal degree of endometriosis.

Coelomic metaplasia is the second most accepted theory, allowing for patients who have not yet entered menarche, as well as those who have never had a uterus but have been treated with estrogen, to develop endometriosis. This theory is based in the thought that the parietal peritoneum contains pluripotent cells that can undergo transformation to be matched to endometrial tissue.

Endometriosis develops when implants of endometrial tissue grow outside of the endometrium, including, but not limited to, the cul-de-sac, peritoneum, ovaries, ligaments, rectum, ureters, bladder, and other structures as high as lung pleura. These implants can be superficial or deep. They can also form endometriomas, or cysts of chocolate brown fluid on the ovaries.

Clinical Presentation

Symptoms

- A small number of patients with endometriosis will be asymptomatic; the majority of patients presenting with endometriosis will complain of pain.
- Will range from dysmenorrhea, dyspareunia, dyschezia, dysuria (both particularly associated with menses), and anterior abdominal wall pain
- Pain will generally precede menses and steadily worsen throughout. This pain also progressively becomes longer in duration as adhesions and scar tissue develops, becoming chronic in nature.

- The majority of women with chronic pelvic pain will have endometriosis (70%).

Signs
- Infertility will be a primary sign for a majority of the asymptomatic patients.
- Physical exam is unreliable for signs to be consistent with the degree of endometriosis present.
- Patients may have red or blue powder burn lesions on the cervix or posterior vaginal fornix.
- Bimanual exam may reveal uterosacral ligament nodularities and tenderness.
- Adhesions may have redirected uterine position to axial or retroverted positioning and decreased mobility.
- The adnexa may be enlarged and tender, particularly if an endometrioma is present.

Diagnostic and Lab Studies

There are no specific laboratory markers for endometriosis. Studies should be performed to rule out infections and pregnancy. Upcoming studies are evaluating the use of microRNAs for the diagnosis of endometriosis via serum. The transvaginal ultrasound is useful for the diagnosis of endometriomas but not endometriosis.

An endometrioma will have a classic appearance of a cyst with homogeneous, low-level echoes, or the "ground glass" presence. Laparoscopy is the gold standard for diagnosing endometriosis. This is the only definitive diagnosis for visualizing endometriosis of all types. Lesions can be clear, red, black, or white. Laparoscopy can also be therapeutic and allow for removal of adhesions and cautery of lesions.

Differential Diagnosis/Formulating the Most Likely Diagnosis

Differential diagnosis of endometriosis may include:

- Chronic pelvic pain of unknown etiology
- Dysmenorrhea
- Pelvic adhesions
- Serositis
- Uterine malformation
- Adenomyosis
- Pelvic malignancies

Health Maintenance and Patient Education

Patients with endometriosis should be counseled on goals for treatment and desire for future fertility. Treatment is based on both of these items. Discussion around chronic pelvic pain and recurrence of symptoms, even following most aggressive therapy, must be held with patient. Risks of recurrent symptoms following hysterectomy/bilateral salpingoophorectomy is high, and patients must be counseled against possible resurgence of symptoms if using estrogen add-back therapy.

Treatment (Pharmaceutical and Clinical Intervention)

The primary consideration when beginning treatment is the desire of the patient for fertility. Patients must take into consideration desire for current or future childbearing. Patients who desire fertility may need referral to reproductive endocrinology or laparoscopy with excision/ablation of lesions or intrauterine insemination. Patients who do not desire fertility must be evaluated on pain status. Patients with mild pain can be managed expectantly with NSAIDS.

This is a small category of patients. Patients with moderate pain should be started on GnRH agonists; and, if this fails, they will move on to the severe pain workup. Patients with severe pain are treated with laparoscopy excision and then moved into postoperative treatment with either continuous cycling oral contraceptives, GnRH agonists, or aromatase inhibitors. Patients who are unable to tolerate symptoms after the above should be offered definitive therapy such as a hysterectomy/BSO, after childbearing is complete.

Leiomyomas

Pathophysiology

These commonly-occurring benign smooth muscle neoplasms arise from the myometrium in as high as 80% of women. They have poor blood supply and are easily separated from the uterine tissue by their own thin outer connective layer. They can be easily seen from normal myometrium due to the difference in cellularity. Leiomyomas have spindled, smooth muscle cells with long, blunt nuclei that intersect at right angles. They have higher cell levels than surrounding tissue. These tumors are highly sensitive to both estrogen and progesterone, with progesterone being the hormone responsible for leiomyoma growth and estrogen helping upregulate the progesterone receptor. Thus, conditions increasing exposure to estrogen will encourage tumor growth (obesity, early menarche, nulliparity). Leiomyomas are classified based on location in and around the uterus. These classifications include sub serosal, intramural, submucous, pedunculated, and parasitic.

Clinical Presentation

While a large number of patients are asymptomatic, many women will present with changes in the menstrual cycle with a tendency toward heavy menstrual bleeding.

Additionally, patients will complain of these:

Symptoms
- Pelvic pain
- Pressure
- Urinary frequency
- Incomplete emptying
- Incontinence
- Constipation
- Pelvic pain that is generally chronic in nature

Patients who present with sudden and severe pelvic pain in the setting of leiomyoma will also have fever and leukocytosis due to a degenerating and prolapsing fibroid.

Signs
- Patients with leiomyomas will generally have an irregularly hard uterus that is not freely mobile.
- If the leiomyoma is degenerating, there may also be significant tenderness to palpation and a necrotic mass protruding from the cervix.

Diagnostic and Lab Studies

In the setting of uterine enlargement and irregular contour, a pregnancy test should be performed in the office to exclude pregnancy. There are no serologic evaluations to diagnosis leiomyomas.

Patients with suspected degenerating leiomyomas should have a complete blood count performed to monitor leukocytosis. Imaging via transvaginal ultrasound is the initial modality for uterine enlargement. If the entire uterus is unable to be visualized, it may become necessary to utilize a transabdominal viewing screen as well. A leiomyoma can be hypo-or hyperechoic and may contain calcifications.

Further imaging resolution may be obtained using magnetic resonance imaging, particularly when mapping out treatment strategies in patients with enlarged body habitus, patients who desire fertility and need uterine-sparing options, or patients who have unclear transvaginal ultrasound images.

Differential Diagnosis

The differential diagnosis of leiomyoma is:

- Leiomyosarcoma
- Adenomyosis
- Endometrial carcinoma
- Uterine carcinosarcoma

Health Maintenance and Patient Education

Patients should be counseled regarding general slow growth of leiomyoma and overall benign nature. Expectant management is a viable option for patients without symptoms and who do not have issues with fertility. Patients who are symptomatic and who have not responded to conservative options should be offered surgical intervention.

Treatment (Pharmaceutical and Clinical Intervention)

Patients who are **asymptomatic** or who are approaching menopause may opt for expectant management with annual pelvic exam or ultrasound. **Symptomatic** patients must decide whether to pursue fertility-sparing measures or not. Patients who desire fertility can choose a myomectomy, the removal of the leiomyoma itself, depending on location and size. Medication can be used to help decrease the size of a leiomyoma prior to surgery. This may reduce the amount of uterus that is removed, improving the success of a pregnancy. Conversely, medications alone may be used to decrease the leiomyoma (typically GnRH agonists). Patients who do not desire fertility may also have pre-operative medication to reduce the size of the leiomyoma in order to have a less invasive surgical approach or to avoid surgery completely. Continuous cycling oral contraceptives followed by GnRH agonists are typical approaches to medication therapy. Surgical approaches include uterine artery embolization, myomectomy, and hysterectomy. These patients may maintain their ovaries and do not require add-back estrogen therapy for vasomotor instability due to surgery alone.

NOTE

Leiomyosarcoma, a malignant growth, is difficult to differentiate on imaging and should be suspected in patients who fail to respond to conservative treatment.

Practice Questions for Reproductive Review

1. A 24-year-old female presents to your clinic requesting emergency contraception. She reports unprotected sexual intercourse 2 days ago. She does not desire pregnancy at this time. She has no ongoing chronic medical conditions. She is gravida 0, para 0. Based on this presentation, you order levonorgestrel 1.5 mg orally as a single dose. Emergency contraceptives are used to decrease risk of pregnancy after intercourse but before establishment of pregnancy. These agents should be started as soon as possible and within

   (A) 120 hours after unprotected coitus.
   (B) 200 hours after unprotected coitus.
   (C) 2 weeks after unprotected coitus.
   (D) 30 days after unprotected coitus.
   (E) 48 hours after unprotected coitus.

2. First-line treatment for endometriosis includes

   (A) laproscopic ablation of endometrial implants.
   (B) hysterectomy with bilateral salpingo-oophrectomy.
   (C) danazol.
   (D) combined hormonal contraceptives.
   (E) dilatation and curettage (D&C).

3. A female patient presents with a complaint of heavy uterine bleeding, irregular periods, pelvic pain and pressure, and fatigue. On gynecologic exam, you note an irregular enlargement of the uterus. All other physical findings are unremarkable. CBC reveals a mild iron-deficiency anemia. Based on this information, your differential diagnoses include

   (A) cervical dysplasia.
   (B) sexually transmitted infection.
   (C) uterine leiomyoma.
   (D) ovarian cancer.
   (E) cervical polyps.

4. Which of the following conditions presents an absolute contraindication for use of combined oral contraceptive agents for birth control?

   (A) Diabetes mellitus
   (B) Gallbladder disease
   (C) Migraine without aura
   (D) Thrombophlebitis
   (E) Antiretroval administration

5. Cervical cancer is the third most common cancer in the world and, in developing nations, the leading cause of cancer death. Cervical cancer has demonstrated evidence of secondary to HPV infection, primarily HPV types 16 and

   (A) 12.
   (B) 14.
   (C) 36.
   (D) 31.
   (E) 18.

6. A female patient, aged 78 years, presents with a complaint of "something bulging" in the vaginal area. She also complains of urinary incontinence. The sensation of "bulging" gets worse when she coughs or sneezes. She is worried something is "falling out." On pelvic examination, you note a soft anterior fullness in the anterior vaginal wall. Based on history and your physical exam, you suspect

    (A) enterocele.
    (B) cystocele.
    (C) rectocele.
    (D) urethrocele.
    (E) uterine prolapse.

7. According to the National Institutes of Health, the Rotterdam criteria are endorsed in the diagnosis of polycystic ovarian syndrome (PCOS). Key diagnostic features, according to these criteria, include polycystic ovaries, hyperandrogenism, and

    (A) primary dysmenorrhea.
    (B) endometriosis.
    (C) pelvic inflammatory disease (PID).
    (D) ovulatory dysfunction.
    (E) hirsutism.

8. You are managing care for a 26-year-old female with a new diagnosis of pelvic inflammatory disease (PID). She reports lower abdominal pain and pressure, and your physical examination reveals uterine, adnexal, and cervical motion tenderness. Based on this diagnosis, recommended first-line outpatient treatment is

    (A) ceftriaxone 250 mg IM plus doxycycline 100 mg BID po for 14 days.
    (B) Augmentin 875 mg po BID for 21 days.
    (C) Levaquin 750 mg po QD for 14 days.
    (D) ciprofloxacin 750 mg po BID for 14 days.
    (E) azithromycin 500 mg po × 1 day, then 250 mg po QD × 4 days.

9. Your patient is a 65-year-old female who presents to your clinic with complaints of fairly new onset of intermittent constipation and occasional mild diarrhea. She reports increased abdominal bloating. Her physical exam is negative; however, the patient reports that her mother died of ovarian cancer in her late 40s. Based on patient history and your physical exam, you order which of the following to rule out ovarian cancer?

    (A) Abdominal radiographs
    (B) Complete metabolic panel
    (C) Transvaginal ultrasound
    (D) Complete blood count with differential
    (E) CT of the pelvis

10. You are seeing a 14-year-old female patient with a chief complaint of severe cramping pain in her lower abdomen that occurs when she having her period. She began menses 1 year ago and has noticed the cramping pain is getting worse. She describes the pain as occurring in "waves of cramping" in her lower abdomen. She sometimes also experiences a headache along with the cramping. She denies fever, weight loss, or other medical comorbidities. She reports that she is not sexually active. She states the pain usually gets better when she takes ibuprofen and, also, that the pain goes away by the fourth day of her menses, only to return the next month. She is worried she may have cancer or another serious illness. Your physical examination reveals mild generalized tenderness over the lower abdomen without guarding or rebound. Urinalysis is negative for infection. Based on this presentation, your most likely diagnosis is

   (A) polycystic ovarian syndrome (PCOS).
   (B) endometriosis.
   (C) primary dysmenorrhea.
   (D) sexually transmitted infection (STI).
   (E) urinary tract infection.

Answers Explained

1. **(A)** Emergency contraceptives should be administered as soon as possible after unprotected sexual intercourse and no later than 120 hours. These agents do not have evidence of persistent effectiveness after 120 hours.

2. **(D)** First-line treatment for endometriosis is combined hormonal contraceptives. These agents suppress ovulation and inhibit stimulation of endometrial tissue. (A, B, C) These options may be appropriate based on poor response to first-line agents. (E) D&C is not indicated in the management of endometriosis as first-line treatment.

3. **(C)** Uterine leiomyoma involves development of discrete, usually round, tumors of the uterine cavity. Tumors are composed of smooth muscle and connective tissue and are not cancerous. Patients may present with irregular menses or heavy bleeding with menses. They may report pelvic pressure, dysmenorrhea, or pain; however, often leiomyomas are asymptomatic. Ultrasound is the diagnostic imaging of choice and will confirm the presence of uterine myomas. (A) Cervical dysplasia is often diagnosed with PAP screening and confirmed through cervical biopsy. (B) STIs are identified by characteristic symptoms and physical exam findings such as vaginal discharge, cervical friability, and adnexal tenderness. (D) Ovarian cancer is often asymptomatic until advanced. Symptoms, when present, may include vague abdominal discomfort, bloating, and bowel changes. (E) Cervical polyps are associated with postcoital bleeding and are visible on the cervical os with speculum examination.

4. **(D)** Combined oral contraceptives are very effective in preventing pregnancy with consistent use. The "perfect use" failure rate is 0.3%; however, the failure rate with typical use is 8%. Many women have difficulty remembering to take the contraceptive every day at the same time, leading to this discrepancy in effectiveness. Absolute contraindications for use of oral combined hormonal contraceptives include the presence or history of thrombophlebitis. Other absolute contraindications include pregnancy, estrogen-dependent cancer (or history of), stroke or coronary artery disease, undiagnosed abnormal vaginal bleeding, migraine with aura (increased risk of stroke), and uncontrolled hypertension, among others. (A, B, C) All are relative contraindications for OCP use; however, they may be prescribed with appropriate warnings and ongoing monitoring of medical conditions. (E) Antiretroviral medications, among many others, may decrease the effectiveness of OCP in preventing pregnancy. Patients should be counseled accordingly.

5. **(E)** Cervical cancer is considered a sexually transmitted diesase because both adenocarcinoma and squamous cell carcinoma are associated with infection with HPV types 16 and 18. Women with HIV or other forms of immunosuppression are at increased risk. Smoking also increases risk for this type of cancer. Early cervical cancer is often asymptomatic and may be found on PAP screening. Vaccination with Gardasil-9 can prevent cervical cancer by targeting HPV types associated with this disease. (A, B, C, D) These HPV types are not implicated in the development of cervical cancer.

6. **(B)** Pelvic organ prolapse may include all of these conditions. They are often seen in multiparous women. Based on physical exam findings of anterior vaginal wall softness, cystocele is the most likely pathology, as the bladder wall herniates into the vaginal area. This creates a finding of "fullness or softness" on exam. (A) Enterocele is herniation of a portion of the small intestine into the vaginal vault. Findings include an abnormality of the posterior vaginal wall. (C) Rectocele involves herniation of the terminal rectum into the vaginal vault. On exam there is often a collapsible pouch-like fullness noted of the posterior vaginal wall.

(D) Urethrocele may occur along with a cystocele and is not an actual herniation but is seen following childbirth when the urethra is detached from the pubic symphysis. (E) Uterine prolapse is readily discovered on vaginal examination with findings of uterine tissue coming through the cervix to varying degrees.

7. **(D)** PCOS is a relatively common endocrine disorder characterized by polycystic ovaries, hyperandrogenism, and chronic anovulation. Patients may present with complaints of heavy menstrual bleeding or problems with fertility. Dermatologic conditions associated with PCOS include hirsutism and acne. Individuals with PCOS may show signs of insulin resistance or hyperinsulinemia. Patients with untreated PCOS have an increased risk for endometrial cancer because of long-term exposure to unopposed estrogen. The Rotterdam criteria are endorsed by the NIH for diagnosis of PCOS. (A, B, C, E) These are not included in the Rotterdam criteria profile.

8. **(A)** Recommended first-line treatment for PID includes ceftriaxone 250 mg IM plus doxycycline 100 mg po BID for 14 days. The other recommendation for first-line treatment is a single dose of cefoxitin 2g IM with probenecid 1 gram po plus doxycycline 100 mg po BID for 14 days. The other antibiotics listed are not indicated in the treatment of PID. It is important to remember that all sexual partners must also be treated appropriately. (B, C, D, E) These antibiotics are not indicated in the treatment of PID.

9. **(C)** Ovarian cancer is often asymptomatic in early stages; however, women sometimes report vague abdominal symptoms such as bloating, constipation, or pelvic pressure. Transvaginal sonography is useful in screening women who are at higher risk for ovarian cancer. Lab tests include CA 125, which is elevated in approximately 50% of women with early disease and 80% of those with epithelial ovarian cancer. (A, B, D, E) These studies may be useful in overall assessment; however, they do not add significant data to aide in the diagnosis of ovarian cancer.

10. **(C)** Primary dysmenorrhea is lower abdominal pain and cramping associated with menses and in the absence of pathologic findings. (A) PCOS is a disorder associated with hyperandrogenism. Patients with PCOS usually report oligomenorrhea or amenorrhea. On ultrasound, the ovaries are found to have numerous cysts. (B) Endometriosis results from aberrant growth of endometrial tissue outside the uterus. This tissue attaches to pelvic structures and causes cyclic pain with menses. (D) Sexually transmitted infections often (though not always) present with vaginal discharge and odor. There is usually a history of unprotected sexual intercourse. STIs produce symptoms that usually resolve with appropriate therapy. (E) UTIs present with urinary frequency and urgency along with burning with urination. Systemic symptoms may or may not be present.

Practice Tests

ANSWER SHEET
Practice Test 1

1. Ⓐ Ⓑ Ⓒ Ⓓ Ⓔ	26. Ⓐ Ⓑ Ⓒ Ⓓ Ⓔ	51. Ⓐ Ⓑ Ⓒ Ⓓ Ⓔ	76. Ⓐ Ⓑ Ⓒ Ⓓ Ⓔ
2. Ⓐ Ⓑ Ⓒ Ⓓ Ⓔ	27. Ⓐ Ⓑ Ⓒ Ⓓ Ⓔ	52. Ⓐ Ⓑ Ⓒ Ⓓ Ⓔ	77. Ⓐ Ⓑ Ⓒ Ⓓ Ⓔ
3. Ⓐ Ⓑ Ⓒ Ⓓ Ⓔ	28. Ⓐ Ⓑ Ⓒ Ⓓ Ⓔ	53. Ⓐ Ⓑ Ⓒ Ⓓ Ⓔ	78. Ⓐ Ⓑ Ⓒ Ⓓ Ⓔ
4. Ⓐ Ⓑ Ⓒ Ⓓ Ⓔ	29. Ⓐ Ⓑ Ⓒ Ⓓ Ⓔ	54. Ⓐ Ⓑ Ⓒ Ⓓ Ⓔ	79. Ⓐ Ⓑ Ⓒ Ⓓ Ⓔ
5. Ⓐ Ⓑ Ⓒ Ⓓ Ⓔ	30. Ⓐ Ⓑ Ⓒ Ⓓ Ⓔ	55. Ⓐ Ⓑ Ⓒ Ⓓ Ⓔ	80. Ⓐ Ⓑ Ⓒ Ⓓ Ⓔ
6. Ⓐ Ⓑ Ⓒ Ⓓ Ⓔ	31. Ⓐ Ⓑ Ⓒ Ⓓ Ⓔ	56. Ⓐ Ⓑ Ⓒ Ⓓ Ⓔ	81. Ⓐ Ⓑ Ⓒ Ⓓ Ⓔ
7. Ⓐ Ⓑ Ⓒ Ⓓ Ⓔ	32. Ⓐ Ⓑ Ⓒ Ⓓ Ⓔ	57. Ⓐ Ⓑ Ⓒ Ⓓ Ⓔ	82. Ⓐ Ⓑ Ⓒ Ⓓ Ⓔ
8. Ⓐ Ⓑ Ⓒ Ⓓ Ⓔ	33. Ⓐ Ⓑ Ⓒ Ⓓ Ⓔ	58. Ⓐ Ⓑ Ⓒ Ⓓ Ⓔ	83. Ⓐ Ⓑ Ⓒ Ⓓ Ⓔ
9. Ⓐ Ⓑ Ⓒ Ⓓ Ⓔ	34. Ⓐ Ⓑ Ⓒ Ⓓ Ⓔ	59. Ⓐ Ⓑ Ⓒ Ⓓ Ⓔ	84. Ⓐ Ⓑ Ⓒ Ⓓ Ⓔ
10. Ⓐ Ⓑ Ⓒ Ⓓ Ⓔ	35. Ⓐ Ⓑ Ⓒ Ⓓ Ⓔ	60. Ⓐ Ⓑ Ⓒ Ⓓ Ⓔ	85. Ⓐ Ⓑ Ⓒ Ⓓ Ⓔ
11. Ⓐ Ⓑ Ⓒ Ⓓ Ⓔ	36. Ⓐ Ⓑ Ⓒ Ⓓ Ⓔ	61. Ⓐ Ⓑ Ⓒ Ⓓ Ⓔ	86. Ⓐ Ⓑ Ⓒ Ⓓ Ⓔ
12. Ⓐ Ⓑ Ⓒ Ⓓ Ⓔ	37. Ⓐ Ⓑ Ⓒ Ⓓ Ⓔ	62. Ⓐ Ⓑ Ⓒ Ⓓ Ⓔ	87. Ⓐ Ⓑ Ⓒ Ⓓ Ⓔ
13. Ⓐ Ⓑ Ⓒ Ⓓ Ⓔ	38. Ⓐ Ⓑ Ⓒ Ⓓ Ⓔ	63. Ⓐ Ⓑ Ⓒ Ⓓ Ⓔ	88. Ⓐ Ⓑ Ⓒ Ⓓ Ⓔ
14. Ⓐ Ⓑ Ⓒ Ⓓ Ⓔ	39. Ⓐ Ⓑ Ⓒ Ⓓ Ⓔ	64. Ⓐ Ⓑ Ⓒ Ⓓ Ⓔ	89. Ⓐ Ⓑ Ⓒ Ⓓ Ⓔ
15. Ⓐ Ⓑ Ⓒ Ⓓ Ⓔ	40. Ⓐ Ⓑ Ⓒ Ⓓ Ⓔ	65. Ⓐ Ⓑ Ⓒ Ⓓ Ⓔ	90. Ⓐ Ⓑ Ⓒ Ⓓ Ⓔ
16. Ⓐ Ⓑ Ⓒ Ⓓ Ⓔ	41. Ⓐ Ⓑ Ⓒ Ⓓ Ⓔ	66. Ⓐ Ⓑ Ⓒ Ⓓ Ⓔ	91. Ⓐ Ⓑ Ⓒ Ⓓ Ⓔ
17. Ⓐ Ⓑ Ⓒ Ⓓ Ⓔ	42. Ⓐ Ⓑ Ⓒ Ⓓ Ⓔ	67. Ⓐ Ⓑ Ⓒ Ⓓ Ⓔ	92. Ⓐ Ⓑ Ⓒ Ⓓ Ⓔ
18. Ⓐ Ⓑ Ⓒ Ⓓ Ⓔ	43. Ⓐ Ⓑ Ⓒ Ⓓ Ⓔ	68. Ⓐ Ⓑ Ⓒ Ⓓ Ⓔ	93. Ⓐ Ⓑ Ⓒ Ⓓ Ⓔ
19. Ⓐ Ⓑ Ⓒ Ⓓ Ⓔ	44. Ⓐ Ⓑ Ⓒ Ⓓ Ⓔ	69. Ⓐ Ⓑ Ⓒ Ⓓ Ⓔ	94. Ⓐ Ⓑ Ⓒ Ⓓ Ⓔ
20. Ⓐ Ⓑ Ⓒ Ⓓ Ⓔ	45. Ⓐ Ⓑ Ⓒ Ⓓ Ⓔ	70. Ⓐ Ⓑ Ⓒ Ⓓ Ⓔ	95. Ⓐ Ⓑ Ⓒ Ⓓ Ⓔ
21. Ⓐ Ⓑ Ⓒ Ⓓ Ⓔ	46. Ⓐ Ⓑ Ⓒ Ⓓ Ⓔ	71. Ⓐ Ⓑ Ⓒ Ⓓ Ⓔ	96. Ⓐ Ⓑ Ⓒ Ⓓ Ⓔ
22. Ⓐ Ⓑ Ⓒ Ⓓ Ⓔ	47. Ⓐ Ⓑ Ⓒ Ⓓ Ⓔ	72. Ⓐ Ⓑ Ⓒ Ⓓ Ⓔ	97. Ⓐ Ⓑ Ⓒ Ⓓ Ⓔ
23. Ⓐ Ⓑ Ⓒ Ⓓ Ⓔ	48. Ⓐ Ⓑ Ⓒ Ⓓ Ⓔ	73. Ⓐ Ⓑ Ⓒ Ⓓ Ⓔ	98. Ⓐ Ⓑ Ⓒ Ⓓ Ⓔ
24. Ⓐ Ⓑ Ⓒ Ⓓ Ⓔ	49. Ⓐ Ⓑ Ⓒ Ⓓ Ⓔ	74. Ⓐ Ⓑ Ⓒ Ⓓ Ⓔ	99. Ⓐ Ⓑ Ⓒ Ⓓ Ⓔ
25. Ⓐ Ⓑ Ⓒ Ⓓ Ⓔ	50. Ⓐ Ⓑ Ⓒ Ⓓ Ⓔ	75. Ⓐ Ⓑ Ⓒ Ⓓ Ⓔ	100. Ⓐ Ⓑ Ⓒ Ⓓ Ⓔ

ANSWER SHEET
Practice Test 1

101. Ⓐ Ⓑ Ⓒ Ⓓ Ⓔ   126. Ⓐ Ⓑ Ⓒ Ⓓ Ⓔ   151. Ⓐ Ⓑ Ⓒ Ⓓ Ⓔ   176. Ⓐ Ⓑ Ⓒ Ⓓ Ⓔ
102. Ⓐ Ⓑ Ⓒ Ⓓ Ⓔ   127. Ⓐ Ⓑ Ⓒ Ⓓ Ⓔ   152. Ⓐ Ⓑ Ⓒ Ⓓ Ⓔ   177. Ⓐ Ⓑ Ⓒ Ⓓ Ⓔ
103. Ⓐ Ⓑ Ⓒ Ⓓ Ⓔ   128. Ⓐ Ⓑ Ⓒ Ⓓ Ⓔ   153. Ⓐ Ⓑ Ⓒ Ⓓ Ⓔ   178. Ⓐ Ⓑ Ⓒ Ⓓ Ⓔ
104. Ⓐ Ⓑ Ⓒ Ⓓ Ⓔ   129. Ⓐ Ⓑ Ⓒ Ⓓ Ⓔ   154. Ⓐ Ⓑ Ⓒ Ⓓ Ⓔ   179. Ⓐ Ⓑ Ⓒ Ⓓ Ⓔ
105. Ⓐ Ⓑ Ⓒ Ⓓ Ⓔ   130. Ⓐ Ⓑ Ⓒ Ⓓ Ⓔ   155. Ⓐ Ⓑ Ⓒ Ⓓ Ⓔ   180. Ⓐ Ⓑ Ⓒ Ⓓ Ⓔ
106. Ⓐ Ⓑ Ⓒ Ⓓ Ⓔ   131. Ⓐ Ⓑ Ⓒ Ⓓ Ⓔ   156. Ⓐ Ⓑ Ⓒ Ⓓ Ⓔ   181. Ⓐ Ⓑ Ⓒ Ⓓ Ⓔ
107. Ⓐ Ⓑ Ⓒ Ⓓ Ⓔ   132. Ⓐ Ⓑ Ⓒ Ⓓ Ⓔ   157. Ⓐ Ⓑ Ⓒ Ⓓ Ⓔ   182. Ⓐ Ⓑ Ⓒ Ⓓ Ⓔ
108. Ⓐ Ⓑ Ⓒ Ⓓ Ⓔ   133. Ⓐ Ⓑ Ⓒ Ⓓ Ⓔ   158. Ⓐ Ⓑ Ⓒ Ⓓ Ⓔ   183. Ⓐ Ⓑ Ⓒ Ⓓ Ⓔ
109. Ⓐ Ⓑ Ⓒ Ⓓ Ⓔ   134. Ⓐ Ⓑ Ⓒ Ⓓ Ⓔ   159. Ⓐ Ⓑ Ⓒ Ⓓ Ⓔ   184. Ⓐ Ⓑ Ⓒ Ⓓ Ⓔ
110. Ⓐ Ⓑ Ⓒ Ⓓ Ⓔ   135. Ⓐ Ⓑ Ⓒ Ⓓ Ⓔ   160. Ⓐ Ⓑ Ⓒ Ⓓ Ⓔ   185. Ⓐ Ⓑ Ⓒ Ⓓ Ⓔ
111. Ⓐ Ⓑ Ⓒ Ⓓ Ⓔ   136. Ⓐ Ⓑ Ⓒ Ⓓ Ⓔ   161. Ⓐ Ⓑ Ⓒ Ⓓ Ⓔ   186. Ⓐ Ⓑ Ⓒ Ⓓ Ⓔ
112. Ⓐ Ⓑ Ⓒ Ⓓ Ⓔ   137. Ⓐ Ⓑ Ⓒ Ⓓ Ⓔ   162. Ⓐ Ⓑ Ⓒ Ⓓ Ⓔ   187. Ⓐ Ⓑ Ⓒ Ⓓ Ⓔ
113. Ⓐ Ⓑ Ⓒ Ⓓ Ⓔ   138. Ⓐ Ⓑ Ⓒ Ⓓ Ⓔ   163. Ⓐ Ⓑ Ⓒ Ⓓ Ⓔ   188. Ⓐ Ⓑ Ⓒ Ⓓ Ⓔ
114. Ⓐ Ⓑ Ⓒ Ⓓ Ⓔ   139. Ⓐ Ⓑ Ⓒ Ⓓ Ⓔ   164. Ⓐ Ⓑ Ⓒ Ⓓ Ⓔ   189. Ⓐ Ⓑ Ⓒ Ⓓ Ⓔ
115. Ⓐ Ⓑ Ⓒ Ⓓ Ⓔ   140. Ⓐ Ⓑ Ⓒ Ⓓ Ⓔ   165. Ⓐ Ⓑ Ⓒ Ⓓ Ⓔ   190. Ⓐ Ⓑ Ⓒ Ⓓ Ⓔ
116. Ⓐ Ⓑ Ⓒ Ⓓ Ⓔ   141. Ⓐ Ⓑ Ⓒ Ⓓ Ⓔ   166. Ⓐ Ⓑ Ⓒ Ⓓ Ⓔ   191. Ⓐ Ⓑ Ⓒ Ⓓ Ⓔ
117. Ⓐ Ⓑ Ⓒ Ⓓ Ⓔ   142. Ⓐ Ⓑ Ⓒ Ⓓ Ⓔ   167. Ⓐ Ⓑ Ⓒ Ⓓ Ⓔ   192. Ⓐ Ⓑ Ⓒ Ⓓ Ⓔ
118. Ⓐ Ⓑ Ⓒ Ⓓ Ⓔ   143. Ⓐ Ⓑ Ⓒ Ⓓ Ⓔ   168. Ⓐ Ⓑ Ⓒ Ⓓ Ⓔ   193. Ⓐ Ⓑ Ⓒ Ⓓ Ⓔ
119. Ⓐ Ⓑ Ⓒ Ⓓ Ⓔ   144. Ⓐ Ⓑ Ⓒ Ⓓ Ⓔ   169. Ⓐ Ⓑ Ⓒ Ⓓ Ⓔ   194. Ⓐ Ⓑ Ⓒ Ⓓ Ⓔ
120. Ⓐ Ⓑ Ⓒ Ⓓ Ⓔ   145. Ⓐ Ⓑ Ⓒ Ⓓ Ⓔ   170. Ⓐ Ⓑ Ⓒ Ⓓ Ⓔ   195. Ⓐ Ⓑ Ⓒ Ⓓ Ⓔ
121. Ⓐ Ⓑ Ⓒ Ⓓ Ⓔ   146. Ⓐ Ⓑ Ⓒ Ⓓ Ⓔ   171. Ⓐ Ⓑ Ⓒ Ⓓ Ⓔ   196. Ⓐ Ⓑ Ⓒ Ⓓ Ⓔ
122. Ⓐ Ⓑ Ⓒ Ⓓ Ⓔ   147. Ⓐ Ⓑ Ⓒ Ⓓ Ⓔ   172. Ⓐ Ⓑ Ⓒ Ⓓ Ⓔ   197. Ⓐ Ⓑ Ⓒ Ⓓ Ⓔ
123. Ⓐ Ⓑ Ⓒ Ⓓ Ⓔ   148. Ⓐ Ⓑ Ⓒ Ⓓ Ⓔ   173. Ⓐ Ⓑ Ⓒ Ⓓ Ⓔ   198. Ⓐ Ⓑ Ⓒ Ⓓ Ⓔ
124. Ⓐ Ⓑ Ⓒ Ⓓ Ⓔ   149. Ⓐ Ⓑ Ⓒ Ⓓ Ⓔ   174. Ⓐ Ⓑ Ⓒ Ⓓ Ⓔ   199. Ⓐ Ⓑ Ⓒ Ⓓ Ⓔ
125. Ⓐ Ⓑ Ⓒ Ⓓ Ⓔ   150. Ⓐ Ⓑ Ⓒ Ⓓ Ⓔ   175. Ⓐ Ⓑ Ⓒ Ⓓ Ⓔ   200. Ⓐ Ⓑ Ⓒ Ⓓ Ⓔ

ANSWER SHEET
Practice Test 1

201. Ⓐ Ⓑ Ⓒ Ⓓ Ⓔ
202. Ⓐ Ⓑ Ⓒ Ⓓ Ⓔ
203. Ⓐ Ⓑ Ⓒ Ⓓ Ⓔ
204. Ⓐ Ⓑ Ⓒ Ⓓ Ⓔ
205. Ⓐ Ⓑ Ⓒ Ⓓ Ⓔ
206. Ⓐ Ⓑ Ⓒ Ⓓ Ⓔ
207. Ⓐ Ⓑ Ⓒ Ⓓ Ⓔ
208. Ⓐ Ⓑ Ⓒ Ⓓ Ⓔ
209. Ⓐ Ⓑ Ⓒ Ⓓ Ⓔ
210. Ⓐ Ⓑ Ⓒ Ⓓ Ⓔ
211. Ⓐ Ⓑ Ⓒ Ⓓ Ⓔ
212. Ⓐ Ⓑ Ⓒ Ⓓ Ⓔ
213. Ⓐ Ⓑ Ⓒ Ⓓ Ⓔ
214. Ⓐ Ⓑ Ⓒ Ⓓ Ⓔ
215. Ⓐ Ⓑ Ⓒ Ⓓ Ⓔ
216. Ⓐ Ⓑ Ⓒ Ⓓ Ⓔ
217. Ⓐ Ⓑ Ⓒ Ⓓ Ⓔ
218. Ⓐ Ⓑ Ⓒ Ⓓ Ⓔ
219. Ⓐ Ⓑ Ⓒ Ⓓ Ⓔ
220. Ⓐ Ⓑ Ⓒ Ⓓ Ⓔ
221. Ⓐ Ⓑ Ⓒ Ⓓ Ⓔ
222. Ⓐ Ⓑ Ⓒ Ⓓ Ⓔ
223. Ⓐ Ⓑ Ⓒ Ⓓ Ⓔ
224. Ⓐ Ⓑ Ⓒ Ⓓ Ⓔ
225. Ⓐ Ⓑ Ⓒ Ⓓ Ⓔ

226. Ⓐ Ⓑ Ⓒ Ⓓ Ⓔ
227. Ⓐ Ⓑ Ⓒ Ⓓ Ⓔ
228. Ⓐ Ⓑ Ⓒ Ⓓ Ⓔ
229. Ⓐ Ⓑ Ⓒ Ⓓ Ⓔ
230. Ⓐ Ⓑ Ⓒ Ⓓ Ⓔ
231. Ⓐ Ⓑ Ⓒ Ⓓ Ⓔ
232. Ⓐ Ⓑ Ⓒ Ⓓ Ⓔ
233. Ⓐ Ⓑ Ⓒ Ⓓ Ⓔ
234. Ⓐ Ⓑ Ⓒ Ⓓ Ⓔ
235. Ⓐ Ⓑ Ⓒ Ⓓ Ⓔ
236. Ⓐ Ⓑ Ⓒ Ⓓ Ⓔ
237. Ⓐ Ⓑ Ⓒ Ⓓ Ⓔ
238. Ⓐ Ⓑ Ⓒ Ⓓ Ⓔ
239. Ⓐ Ⓑ Ⓒ Ⓓ Ⓔ
240. Ⓐ Ⓑ Ⓒ Ⓓ Ⓔ
241. Ⓐ Ⓑ Ⓒ Ⓓ Ⓔ
242. Ⓐ Ⓑ Ⓒ Ⓓ Ⓔ
243. Ⓐ Ⓑ Ⓒ Ⓓ Ⓔ
244. Ⓐ Ⓑ Ⓒ Ⓓ Ⓔ
245. Ⓐ Ⓑ Ⓒ Ⓓ Ⓔ
246. Ⓐ Ⓑ Ⓒ Ⓓ Ⓔ
247. Ⓐ Ⓑ Ⓒ Ⓓ Ⓔ
248. Ⓐ Ⓑ Ⓒ Ⓓ Ⓔ
249. Ⓐ Ⓑ Ⓒ Ⓓ Ⓔ
250. Ⓐ Ⓑ Ⓒ Ⓓ Ⓔ

251. Ⓐ Ⓑ Ⓒ Ⓓ Ⓔ
252. Ⓐ Ⓑ Ⓒ Ⓓ Ⓔ
253. Ⓐ Ⓑ Ⓒ Ⓓ Ⓔ
254. Ⓐ Ⓑ Ⓒ Ⓓ Ⓔ
255. Ⓐ Ⓑ Ⓒ Ⓓ Ⓔ
256. Ⓐ Ⓑ Ⓒ Ⓓ Ⓔ
257. Ⓐ Ⓑ Ⓒ Ⓓ Ⓔ
258. Ⓐ Ⓑ Ⓒ Ⓓ Ⓔ
259. Ⓐ Ⓑ Ⓒ Ⓓ Ⓔ
260. Ⓐ Ⓑ Ⓒ Ⓓ Ⓔ
261. Ⓐ Ⓑ Ⓒ Ⓓ Ⓔ
262. Ⓐ Ⓑ Ⓒ Ⓓ Ⓔ
263. Ⓐ Ⓑ Ⓒ Ⓓ Ⓔ
264. Ⓐ Ⓑ Ⓒ Ⓓ Ⓔ
265. Ⓐ Ⓑ Ⓒ Ⓓ Ⓔ
266. Ⓐ Ⓑ Ⓒ Ⓓ Ⓔ
267. Ⓐ Ⓑ Ⓒ Ⓓ Ⓔ
268. Ⓐ Ⓑ Ⓒ Ⓓ Ⓔ
269. Ⓐ Ⓑ Ⓒ Ⓓ Ⓔ
270. Ⓐ Ⓑ Ⓒ Ⓓ Ⓔ
271. Ⓐ Ⓑ Ⓒ Ⓓ Ⓔ
272. Ⓐ Ⓑ Ⓒ Ⓓ Ⓔ
273. Ⓐ Ⓑ Ⓒ Ⓓ Ⓔ
274. Ⓐ Ⓑ Ⓒ Ⓓ Ⓔ
275. Ⓐ Ⓑ Ⓒ Ⓓ Ⓔ

276. Ⓐ Ⓑ Ⓒ Ⓓ Ⓔ
277. Ⓐ Ⓑ Ⓒ Ⓓ Ⓔ
278. Ⓐ Ⓑ Ⓒ Ⓓ Ⓔ
279. Ⓐ Ⓑ Ⓒ Ⓓ Ⓔ
280. Ⓐ Ⓑ Ⓒ Ⓓ Ⓔ
281. Ⓐ Ⓑ Ⓒ Ⓓ Ⓔ
282. Ⓐ Ⓑ Ⓒ Ⓓ Ⓔ
283. Ⓐ Ⓑ Ⓒ Ⓓ Ⓔ
284. Ⓐ Ⓑ Ⓒ Ⓓ Ⓔ
285. Ⓐ Ⓑ Ⓒ Ⓓ Ⓔ
286. Ⓐ Ⓑ Ⓒ Ⓓ Ⓔ
287. Ⓐ Ⓑ Ⓒ Ⓓ Ⓔ
288. Ⓐ Ⓑ Ⓒ Ⓓ Ⓔ
289. Ⓐ Ⓑ Ⓒ Ⓓ Ⓔ
290. Ⓐ Ⓑ Ⓒ Ⓓ Ⓔ
291. Ⓐ Ⓑ Ⓒ Ⓓ Ⓔ
292. Ⓐ Ⓑ Ⓒ Ⓓ Ⓔ
293. Ⓐ Ⓑ Ⓒ Ⓓ Ⓔ
294. Ⓐ Ⓑ Ⓒ Ⓓ Ⓔ
295. Ⓐ Ⓑ Ⓒ Ⓓ Ⓔ
296. Ⓐ Ⓑ Ⓒ Ⓓ Ⓔ
297. Ⓐ Ⓑ Ⓒ Ⓓ Ⓔ
298. Ⓐ Ⓑ Ⓒ Ⓓ Ⓔ
299. Ⓐ Ⓑ Ⓒ Ⓓ Ⓔ
300. Ⓐ Ⓑ Ⓒ Ⓓ Ⓔ

Practice Test 1

> **DIRECTIONS:** Find a quiet place to take this practice test. For each question, select the choice that best answers the question and mark that answer on the sheet provided. There are 300 questions and a review of the correct answers suggested upon test completion. You have a total of 5 hours to complete this test. Allow 1 minute per question and take breaks. Good luck!

1. A 25 year-old man has dyspnea and chest pain of 2 days duration. Pain is sharp and not worsened by activity. He feels better laying down. There is no associated nausea or diaphoresis. He has a past medical history of eczema, and he had influenza 3 weeks ago.

   Exam:

   Blood pressure: 100/75 mmHg, heart rate 110 bpm, respiratory rate 24 rpm

   Lungs: crackles at bases

   Cardiac: tachycardia, no murmurs, + S3 gallop, normal pulses, + pitting edema in the shins

   Lab data: Complete blood count (CBC) and basic metabolic profile (BMP) are normal.

   Brain natriuretic peptide (BNP) is elevated.

   High sensitivity (HS) troponin is elevated at time 0, 1, and 3 hr – (22, 18, 23) (Normal HS troponin is less than 14.)

   Chest X-ray shows bilateral pulmonary congestion.

   EKG shows sinus tachycardia, with normal ST segments.

   What is the most likely diagnosis?

   (A) Myocarditis
   (B) Non ST elevation myocardial infarct (NSTEMI)
   (C) Pericarditis
   (D) ST elevation MI
   (E) Pulmonary embolism

2. You are seeing a patient with leg symptoms. There is discoloration and pitting edema that is equal in both legs up to shin level, the condition is an annoyance but non-painful and has been present for 2 years. There are normal dorsalis pedis pulses bilaterally. The appearance of the legs are shown below.

What is the most likely cause of this condition?

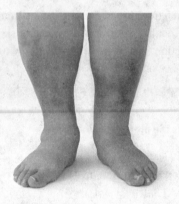

(A) Peripheral arterial occlusive disease
(B) Venous stasis dermatitis
(C) Deep venous thrombosis
(D) Cellulitis
(E) Vitiligo

3. Mr. Jones is a 45-year-old Caucasian man recently diagnosed with hypertension. He has tried 2 months of lifestyle changes without benefit, so his PA is considering drug therapy. He has no past medical history and no known drug allergies. Which antihypertensive medication should be avoided as a first-line therapy for him?

(A) Benazepril (ACE inhibitor)
(B) Amlodipine (Ca++ channel blocker)
(C) Chlorthalidone (thiazide diuretic)
(D) Metoprolol (beta-blocker)
(E) Clonidine (alpha-1 blocker)

4. Which of the following explains why hydralazine is a poor choice for reducing the symptoms of stable angina?

(A) It has been shown to counteract the vasodilation effects of nitroglycerine.
(B) Its peripheral arterial vasodilation may result in tachycardia increasing myocardial demand.
(C) It decreases the HR, BP, and contractility, which decreases myocardial oxygen demand.
(D) It reduces afterload by vasodilation, decreases the preload, and vasodilates the coronary tree, which reduces the oxygen consumption of the myocardium.
(E) It increases peripheral vascular resistance.

5. Mr. U is a 60-year-old man who successfully underwent maxillary sinus surgery today. In the recovery room, the nurse notes an arrhythmia, but the patient feels no symptoms and is behaving normally. On exam, HR 135 bpm, BP 120/75 mmHg, RR 14 rpm, and 02 saturation of 98% on room air. An EKG shows atrial flutter. Which of the following is the best immediate intervention?

(A) Synchronized cardioversion
(B) Calcium channel blocker (CCB)
(C) Heparin (anticoagulant)
(D) Alpha antagonist
(E) Angiotensin converting enzyme inhibitor (ACE inhibitor)

6. A 65 year-old woman with confusion, headache, and vomiting is in the emergency department. Her vital signs:

   Blood pressure 190/112 mmHg

   Heart rate 54 bpm

   Resp rate 14 rpm and unlabored

   Oxygen saturation 96% on room air

   What would be the most appropriate drug to initiate for this patient?

   (A) Chlorthalidone (thiazide diuretic)
   (B) Metoprolol succinate (long-acting beta-blocker)
   (C) Eplerenone (aldosterone receptor blocker)
   (D) Sodium nitroprusside (vasodilator)
   (E) Amlodipine (calcium channel blocker)

7. Who should be screened for an abdominal aortic aneurysm with an ultrasound of the abdomen?

   (A) A child with a much higher blood pressure in the right arm than the left arm
   (B) An adult patient with cardiac tamponade
   (C) A 70-year-old man who quit smoking 4 years ago
   (D) A 60-year-old woman with a family history of abdominal aortic aneurysm
   (E) An 88-year-old woman with BP 125/85 who smoked for 6 months in high school and none since

8. Which of the following patients, with known hypertension, needs an evaluation for secondary causes of hypertension?

   (A) 45-year-old man with anxiety who has a BP of 140/80 and takes no medication
   (B) 28-year-old woman with an abdominal bruit and renal failure
   (C) 55-year-old woman with obesity whose BP is 140/85 despite taking one medication
   (D) 70-year-old man who has controlled HTN using three drugs for 20 years
   (E) 57-year-old woman who is obese and has a thyroid dysfunction

9. A 50-year-old man with no history of heart disease has a greater than 15% risk of developing a myocardial infarction in the next 10 years as predicted by the ASCVD risk calculator. He currently takes no medication. Which plan is the best primary prevention strategy for this patient?

   (A) Aspirin 81 mg oral daily, exercise 30 min 5 days a week, high intensity statin therapy
   (B) Aspirin 325 mg oral daily, high protein diet, low dose statin therapy
   (C) Assure smoking cessation, cardiac rehabilitation, no medication at this time
   (D) Metoprolol (beta-blocker), exercise 90 minutes daily, red yeast rice for cholesterol lowering
   (E) Lower high density lipoproteins and control blood glucose.

10. Mrs. Ferrari is 62. She has substernal pressure radiating to the jaw intermittently for 8 hours. She also reports dyspnea and nausea. She has had angina in the past relieved by nitroglycerin and rest. These treatments did not work today. Her BP now is 160/85 mmHg, HR 50 bpm. Her EKG strip shows sinus bradycardia with T-wave inversion and 1 mm of ST segment depression. Three high sensitivity troponin tests over 3 hours are 10, 12, and 10 (normal less than 14). At this time, what is the best diagnosis?

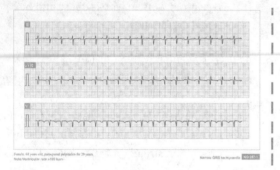

(A) Stable angina

(B) Normal ECG tracing

(C) Non ST elevation MI

(D) ST elevation MI

(E) Unstable angina

11. Which is the best initial treatment for acute pericarditis?

(A) Beta-blocker

(B) Ibuprofen (nonsteroidal anti-inflammatory)

(C) Surgical pericardiectomy

(D) Prednisone (glucocorticoid)

(E) Chest tube placement

12. A 26-year-old athlete wants counseling about risks associated with hypertrophic obstructive cardiomyopathy. Which of the following statements gives false information to the patient?

(A) A genetic problem with proteins can result in abnormal swelling of the wall between the ventricles.

(B) Stroke from an abnormal increase in blood pressure during exercise may occur.

(C) Heart failure from developing a thick, stiff heart as well as a murmur can occur.

(D) Beta-blockers are the main medical therapy but are likely to cause drowsiness and reduce endurance of young athletes.

(E) Palpitations may occur.

13. What is the most appropriate next step when seeing a patient who has the type of vascular condition depicted in the figure?

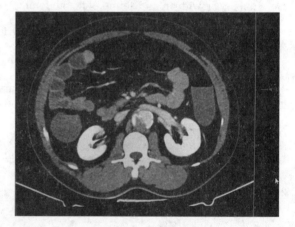

(A) Complete blood count (CBC)

(B) Order electrocardiogram

(C) Prescribe a calcium channel blocker

(D) Lipid panel and dietary consultation

(E) Surgical consultation

14. Which of the following would be expected to increase preload (venous return) to the right heart?

(A) Furosemide (diuretic)

(B) Intravenous saline

(C) High intrathoracic pressures

(D) Nitroglycerin (nitrate)

(E) Angiotensin receptor blockers

15. All of the patients below have a 10-year history of systolic heart failure with reduced ejection fraction. Which one do you predict to have the best prognosis?

    (A) A man has just been found to have syncope related to ventricular dilation and tachyarrhythmia.
    (B) A woman's brain natriuretic peptide (BNP) levels go from 202 to 467 over 6 months despite being on an ace inhibitor, beta-blocker, and diuretic (normal BNP less than 100).
    (C) A woman has just had her beta-blocker and ace inhibitor dose increased to reduce her blood pressure, which was 145/85 mmHg.
    (D) A man has developed nausea and malnutrition as a result of edema in his small intestine.
    (E) A man with aortic stenosis

16. A 58-year-old woman has been having stable angina for 2 years. Today she had an ST elevation acute myocardial infarction (STEMI). Which of the following best describes what happened today in her coronary artery?

    (A) A plaque rupture that recruited platelets to the area and eventually occluded a coronary artery
    (B) Foam cells clustered under the endothelial lining to cause a bulge called a fatty streak
    (C) A dissection of the descending aorta blocked blood flow to a coronary artery
    (D) Oxidized triglycerides in the subendothelial space are taken up by macrophages blocking the lumen of the coronary artery.
    (E) Endocardial necrosis

17. A patient with which of the following conditions is most likely to have a fourth heart sound (S4)?

    (A) Left ventricular hypertrophy from hypertension
    (B) Postpartum cardiomyopathy
    (C) Myocarditis from parvovirus
    (D) Patent foramen ovale in a patient with a deep vein thrombosis
    (E) Brugada syndrome

18. The physician assistant is called at 1:00 A.M. to a patient's room to evaluate dyspnea, hypotension, and confusion. The EKG shows bradycardia (HR 39) and no relationship between the P-waves and QRS complexes. What would be the best course of action?

    (A) Establish an airway.
    (B) Draw Basic Metabolic Panel (BMP) and Troponin. Observe for any worsening in condition.
    (C) Give adenosine IV to temporarily block the AV node.
    (D) Place a cardiac pacer on the patient's chest and call a cardiologist.
    (E) Give an angiotensin-converting enzyme inhibitor.

19. A 56-year-old patient is recovering from prostate surgery. He has left calf swelling and tenderness for the past 3 days. He denies fevers or trauma to the leg. On exam, you palpate normal pulses and note redness, warmth, and edema in the left leg up to the mid-calf. His right leg is normal. He has labs showing an elevated d-dimer. Based on these findings what would be the most appropriate test to confirm the diagnosis?

    (A) CT angiogram
    (B) Duplex ultrasonography
    (C) Bacterial culture of the skin
    (D) Ankle Brachial Index
    (E) Blood pressure reading of left lower extremity

20. You are seeing a 38-year-old patient in the ED who is unresponsive to your voice. Vitals are: BP 88/40, HR 135, oxygen saturation 92%, and RR-26. On exam, you note muffled heart sounds and jugular venous distention. You note that his systolic BP drops to 65 mmHg during inspiration. Chest X-ray is below. His complete blood count (CBC), chemistries, and cardiac enzymes (troponin) are normal. What is the most likely diagnosis?

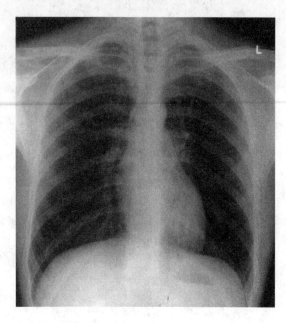

(A) Pulmonary embolism
(B) Pericarditis
(C) Asthma
(D) Pericardial tamponade
(E) Bronchiectasis

21. A 66-year-old woman is seen in a clinic for dyspnea and leg pain after walking 50 feet. She has a 20-year history of coronary artery disease. She has severe COPD and osteoarthritis. An EKG from today shows ST segment depression and inverted T-waves both now and present 1 year ago. She has a stable angina pattern. Troponin blood tests are normal when checked at hours 0, 1, and 3.

What test to determine the presence of myocardial ischemia would be best for this patient?

(A) Transesophageal echocardiogram
(B) Pharmacologic nuclear stress test
(C) Exercise treadmill stress test
(D) Cardiac MRI
(E) Repeat ECG

22. A patient with which of the following conditions is most likely to have a third heart sound (S3)?

(A) Hypertension with hyperkalemia
(B) Pericarditis resulting from an acute respiratory virus
(C) Aortic stenosis
(D) Hypertrophic cardiomyopathy caused by abnormal protein deposits
(E) Chronic heart failure with low ejection fraction from an myocardial infarct

23. Blood pressure differences of greater than 10–15 mmHg between the right and left arm suggests which of the following?

(A) Systolic hypertension
(B) Aortic dissection
(C) Coarctation of the aorta
(D) Auscultatory gap
(E) White coat syndrome

24. A 57-year-old woman, with a past medical history significant for bicuspid aortic valve, presents to the office with complaints of low-grade fever for 2 weeks accompanied by malaise and increasing dyspnea. Physical examination is remarkable for a temperature of 101°F and an IV/VI systolic murmur which represents a change from an II/VI murmur on her last visit 4 months ago. Funduscopic examination reveals Roth spots. The ECG shows no acute changes.

    Which of the following is the most likely diagnosis?

    (A) Acute MI
    (B) Infectious endocarditis
    (C) Chagas disease
    (D) Congestive heart failure
    (E) Pulmonary stenosis

25. A patient with a 27% chance of having a coronary event in the next 10 years is taking a high intensity statin (HMGcoA inhibitor). She begins to have muscle aching after walking that her provider says is due to the drug. Her lab testing shows the statin has been effective, and there is no liver or muscle inflammation. What is the best recommendation for this patient?

    (A) Keep the statin dose the same, no change in therapy.
    (B) Lower the statin dose to a moderate intensity, monitor closely.
    (C) Stop taking statin; no other interventions warranted.
    (D) Stop taking statin; maintain her reduced LDL with diet and exercise no medication.
    (E) Change statin and add grapefruits to diet.

26. Which patient most likely has a nonischemic cardiomyopathy caused by infiltration of the heart muscle?

    (A) A young man with granulomas in his heart has shortness of breath and edema; today he has ventricular tachycardia.
    (B) A woman treated for breast cancer has left ventricle ejection fraction of 35% 1 year after treatment.
    (C) An elderly man has ST elevation in leads II and III on EKG, and his high sensitivity troponin is 63 and rising 3 hours after the onset of pain.
    (D) A college student, dependent on alcohol, has orthopnea and JVD that started about 4 months ago.
    (E) A male patient with diabetes and hypothyroidism

27. Your patient had a viral-like illness, and you suspect there is now pericarditis. You want a test that will detect a pericardial effusion and, if present, determine its impact on the heart. Which is the preferred test for this workup?

    (A) Transthoracic echocardiogram
    (B) Fluid sampling of the pericardium
    (C) Cardiac MRI
    (D) Electrocardiogram
    (E) Cardiac CT scan

28. Which patient with a systolic murmur most likely has tricuspid regurgitation?

    (A) A 60-year-old woman with a dilated right ventricle has JVD and a new murmur that gets louder with inspiration.
    (B) A child with a history of a "heart defect" has a systolic crescendo-decrescendo murmur at the left upper sternal border.
    (C) An 80-year-old man has dyspnea on exertion attributed to calcifications that significantly narrowed one of his heart valves.
    (D) A teenager learns their murmur represents a condition that lowers blood pressure when exercising and can cause syncope or death.
    (E) A 50-year-old male patient who gets lightheaded when leaning forward and exhaling

29. A 45-year-old man comes to the clinic for reevaluation of his hypertension. He reports his home BP readings have been 145/90, 160/95, and 150/90 and he has occasional headaches. He is currently taking lisinopril 10 mg (ACE inhibitor). Today, temperature is 36.6°C (98°F), pulse rate is 88/min and regular, respirations are 18/min and unlabored, and blood pressure is 138/88 mmHg.

Which of the following should be monitored when increasing the medication dosage?

(A) Sodium
(B) Magnesium
(C) Calcium
(D) Potassium
(E) Glucose

30. An infarction in the inferior wall of left ventricle should correlate to a blockage of which coronary artery? (All other sections of the heart appear to be contracting normally on echo.)

(A) Left main
(B) Left anterior descending
(C) Right
(D) Left circumflex
(E) Right anterior descending

31. A 57-year-old male presents to the emergency department with acute onset of palpitations and dyspnea lasting 3 hours. PMH is significant for atrial flutter and atrial fibrillation with an unsuccessful ablation procedure 5 years ago. Medications include diltiazem 180 mg daily and Eliquis 5 mg twice a day. Patient notes that he forgot to take diltiazem twice this week while on vacation. He has no known allergies. On physical examination, VS: HR 150, irregularly irreg, BP 90/40 mm/Hg, and O_2 sat is 94%. Patient is in mild distress and dyspneic. Cardiac exam reveals +S1/S2, without murmurs, rubs, or gallops. The remainder of the PE is unremarkable. Cardiac monitor shows a saw-tooth appearance to the cardiac rhythm. Which of the following is appropriate management for this patient?

(A) Administer 180 mg oral diltiazem.
(B) Administer IV diltiazem bolus followed by diltiazem drip.
(C) Perform electrical cardioversion.
(D) Initiate pharmacologic cardioversion with IV sotalol (Betapace).
(E) Instruct patient to perform valsalva maneuver.

32. A 45-year-old patient, without diabetes or heart disease, was started on an Ace inhibitor and calcium channel blocker at the same time. What initial blood pressure should the patient have had in order to justify this two-drug therapy for hypertension?

(A) 165/95
(B) 140/85
(C) 130/80
(D) 120/80
(E) 110/60

33. All of these patients have been determined to need further cardiac testing. In which patient would a treadmill stress test (exercise EKG) be the best next test?

(A) A 22-year-old has syncope. He has an abnormal EKG with an elevated rate of 120 bpm. His dad has a defibrillator.

(B) A 68-year-old female patient has an elevated high-sensitivity troponin and ST elevation on electrocardiogram today. She had angina at rest yesterday and has a history of coronary bypass surgery.

(C) A 43-year-old female patient has chest pain immediately after eating. Her electrocardiogram is normal sinus rhythm. She has a left knee replacement and uses a scooter to ambulate.

(D) A 50-year-old male patient has many CAD risk factors. He recently had a normal electrocardiogram and three normal troponin levels when he visited an urgent care center after having angina during weight lifting.

(E) A 75-year-old male patient with diabetes, prolonged QRS intervals on electrocardiogram

34. Which drug class improves symptoms and reduces hospital visits for heart failure but does not improve survival (mortality)?

(A) Beta-blockers

(B) Thiazide type diuretic

(C) Aldosterone (mineralocorticoid) blocker

(D) Angiotensin receptor blocker

(E) Alpha-blockers

35. A 63-year-old woman presents to the office complaining of increasing dyspnea and fatigue on exertion for 1 month. She had a syncopal episode yesterday, which prompted the office visit. Her prior medical history is significant for COPD. Physical examination of the heart shows narrow splitting of the second heart sound, accentuation of the pulmonary component, and a systolic ejection click. Jugular venous distension is present. ECG reveals right ventricular hypertrophy. Which of the following is the most likely diagnosis?

(A) Pulmonary hypertension

(B) Pulmonary embolism

(C) Bronchiectasis

(D) Pulmonary vasculitis

(E) Aortic dissection

36. A patient has a blood pressure that is consistently 35/20 mmHg above her goal BP. Which medication regimen is best at reducing her risk of death from a cardiovascular cause?

(A) Chlorthalidone (diuretic) + benazepril (ACE inhibitor)

(B) Benazepril (ACE inhibitor) + valsartan (angiotensin receptor blocker)

(C) Chlorthalidone (diuretic) + amlodipine (Ca channel blocker)

(D) Amlodipine (Ca channel blocker) + benazepril (ACE inhibitor)

(E) Amlodipine (Ca channel blocker) + chlorthalidone (diuretic)

37. Which of the following patients most likely has had a type 2 myocardial infarction? High sensitivity troponin I—normal range (less than 14).

(A) 72-year-old woman has angina. EKG shows sinus tachycardia and acute ischemia. Troponin levels are elevated and rising rapidly over 3 hours.

(B) A 58-year-old man had ventricular tachycardia, rate 140 bpm, as a result of hyperkalemia. His heart rate is controlled now at 90 bpm. Troponin levels (21, 21, 17) at 0, 1 and 3 hr.

(C) A man in the cardiac cath lab has chest pain while having a stent placed. After opening the artery, pain is resolved. The first troponin after the procedure is 88.

(D) A woman has ST elevations on an EKG done in an ambulance. She smokes. She reports symptoms of classic angina. The medic draws blood, but troponin results are not back yet.

(E) A man with diabetes who is asymptomatic and has abnormal Q-waves on EKG

38. All patients below are currently having a non-ST elevation myocardial infarction (NSTEMI). Which should go to the cath lab as soon as possible for a coronary revascularization?

(A) Woman has ST segment depression persisting after starting six drugs appropriate for NSTEMI.

(B) Man has troponin levels that peak then begin to decline after 8 hours of medical therapy.

(C) Woman has a TIMI risk score of 2 (1 point for risk factors and 1 for EKG changes).

(D) Man has a history of heart failure with preserved ejection fraction (HFpEF). EF right now is 55%.

(E) Woman with two anginal episodes in prior 24 hours and presence of ST segment deviation on admission electrocardiogram.

39. Which blockage of a coronary artery is most likely to result in an ST elevation myocardial infarction (STEMI) while the person is walking up two flights of stairs?

(A) A lipid-rich plaque in the wall of the right coronary is covered by a firm fibrous cap after months of therapy with a statin.

(B) A circumflex artery narrowing is only seen when a woman is given a provoking medication during cardiac catheterization.

(C) An atheroma is soft with no fibrous cap and blocks 75% of the circumflex artery.

(D) A lesion in the right coronary artery is described as a calcified callus that blocks 40% of the artery.

(E) A vasospasm of the right anterior descending artery

40. When counseling a patient with heart disease, which advice is most accurate based on current nutritional guidelines?

(A) Western (standard American) diet reduces arterial inflammation.

(B) All vegetarian diets are equivalent in reduction of cardiovascular disease risk.

(C) Replace as many meat and dairy servings as possible with whole grains, legumes, fruit, and vegetables.

(D) Refined sugars are consistently found in studies to be healthier than lean meat.

(E) Avoid nutritional supplements.

41. When adding an HMG CoA reductase inhibitor (statin) as a preventative medication for coronary artery disease, what major side effects should the patient be warned about and observed for?

(A) Muscle pain and liver failure

(B) Arrhythmia and angina

(C) Hypotension and hyperkalemia

(D) Heart failure resulting in renal failure

(E) Alterations in blood glucose

42. After several weeks of tetracycline treatment for acne, an obese 20-year-old man develops a bright red scaling groin rash involving the scrotum with satellite pustules. He has been applying a non-prescription ointment without relief. A KOH prep shows budding yeast and pseudohyphae. What is the most likely diagnosis?

    (A) Contact dermatitis
    (B) Tinea cruris
    (C) Psoriasis
    (D) *Candidiasis*
    (E) Eczema

43. An 86-year-old female presents to her primary care clinic complaining of an annoying, dull pain over the left side of her face for the past 2 days with fever and a painful rash that started yesterday. Your exam shows a vesicular rash on an erythematous base in a characteristic distribution on the left side of her face extending to the nasal tip. What is the most important next course of action?

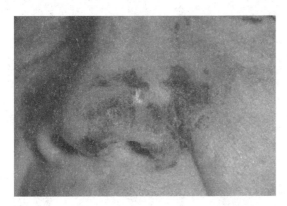

    (A) Initiate oral antiviral therapy and refer emergently to dermatology.
    (B) Initiate oral antibiotics and send the patient home to rest.
    (C) Initiate oral antiviral and refer emergently to ophthalmology.
    (D) Initiate antibiotics and return to clinic in 1 week to reevaluate.
    (E) Initiate ophthalmic drops and provide eye patch.

44. A superficial form of cellulitis that occurs classically on cheek caused by beta hemolytic streptococci, which may appear first as firm red spots then enlarges and coalesces to form a circumscribed, red lesion with a raised border.

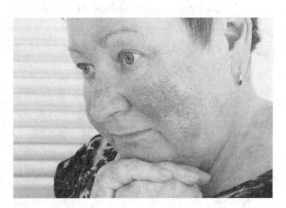

    (A) Erythrasma
    (B) Erysipelas
    (C) Acne rosacea
    (D) Impetigo
    (E) Eczema

45. A 25-year-old male presents to the clinic with a very itchy rash on his hands and abdomen for 2 weeks. You perform a physical exam and see numerous erythematous scaling patches with excoriations on the hands, web spaces of the fingers, and around the waistline of his abdomen. You perform a scrape test and microscopy reveals this pictured below. Which of the following drugs would you use to treat this patient?

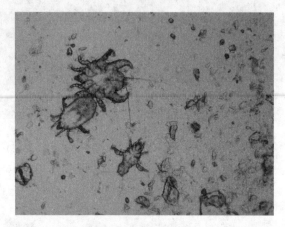

(A) Cephalexin (antibiotic)
(B) Ketoconazole (antifungal)
(C) Permethrin cream (antiparasitic)
(D) Selenium sulfide (antiseborrheic)
(E) Prednisone (corticosteroid)

46. This type of psoriasis is most commonly seen in children and may be associated with streptococcal pharyngitis. Usually appears as shown in the picture below: coalescing erythematous scaling papules and plaques of the trunk and extremities.

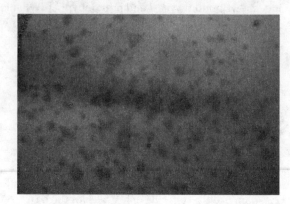

(A) Pustular psoriasis
(B) Guttate psoriasis
(C) Exfoliative psoriasis
(D) Inverse psoriasis
(E) Nummular psoriasis

47. You are seeing an 8-year-old child in clinic. The patient's mother describes a rash of 6 months duration on the arms and backs of the legs. It is very itchy at times, and the child is visibly scratching during the exam. The child has allergic rhinitis, but no other pertinent medical history. Mom reports she has asthma also. On exam, you note erythematous scaling patches with excoriations on the antecubital spaces of the upper extremities and popliteal fossae. What is the most likely diagnosis?

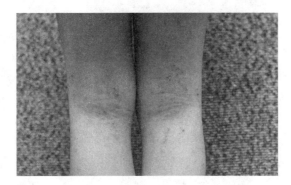

(A) Contact dermatitis

(B) Psoriasis

(C) Lichen simplex chronicus

(D) Tinea corporis

(E) Atopic dermatitis

48. Which of the following dermatophyte infections should always be treated using systemic antifungals?

(A) Tinea capitis

(B) Tinea corporis

(C) Tinea cruris

(D) Tinea pedis

(E) Mycosis fungoides

49. Which of the following is an indication for the use of Mohs micrographic surgery to treat cutaneous malignancies?

(A) Clearly defined clinical margins

(B) High-risk locations

(C) Low risk for recurrence

(D) Small lesion size

(E) Multiple freckles

50. A carbuncle is best described as which of the following?

(A) A collection of infected hair follicles that form a draining abscess

(B) A fungal or dermatophyte infection of the nail plate

(C) A pigmented scaly lesion that develops on sun-exposed skin

(D) Scaly, yellowish, inflammatory plaques of the scalp

(E) Dark lesion with undefined borders

51. A 30-year-old male presents to the clinic with complaints of discoloration on back and chest. He states these areas are not tanning as usual and itch. On exam, you note scaly, hypopigmented macules on the trunk and proximal extremities. You perform a KOH and note the rounded yeast and pseudohyphae "spaghetti and meatballs." What treatment would you recommend for this patient?

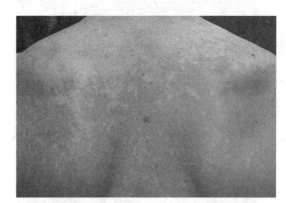

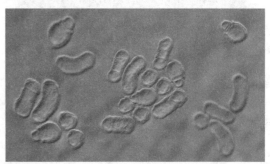

(A) Topical hydrocortisone cream

(B) Phototherapy

(C) Topical mupirocin (antibiotic) cream

(D) Selenium sulfide shampoo/lotion

(E) Oral cephalosporin

52. This condition may be caused by HSV or adverse drug reactions that present with epidermal "target lesions" primarily on the extremities. Refer to the photos below.

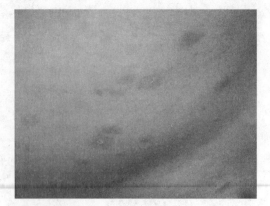

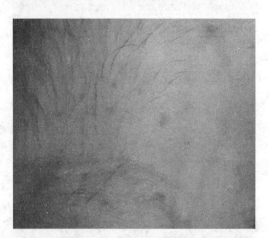

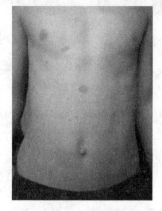

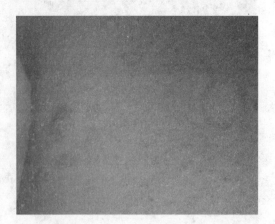

(A) Pityriasis rosea
(B) Lupus erythematosus
(C) Erythema multiforme
(D) Exfoliative erythroderma
(E) Vitiligo

53. You were at a friend's house and were bitten by this animal (cat). What is the likely pathogen associated with this cat?

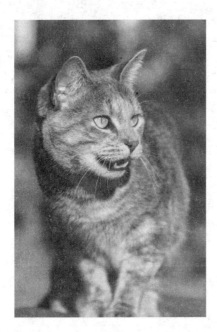

(A) Vibrio vulnificus
(B) Aeromonas hydrophila
(C) *Staphylococcus aureus*
(D) Vibrio multiforme
(E) *Pasteurella multocida*

54. These lesions commonly occur in infants and immunocompromised adults as discrete white patches on the buccal mucosa that can be scraped off, leaving a bright red surface.

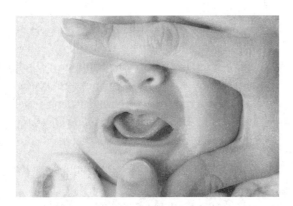

(A) Oropharyngeal tinea
(B) Oropharyngeal cytomegalovirus
(C) Oropharyngeal herpes
(D) Oropharyngeal candidiasis
(E) Oropharyngeal cancer

55. A sexually transmitted disease with an eroded, crusted papule that may appear 18–21 days after infection. If left untreated, this disease can have other skin manifestations as well as potentially serious, systemic manifestations. It is often referred to as the "great imitator."

(A) Herpes simplex
(B) Herpes whitlow
(C) Syphilis
(D) Herpes gladitorium
(E) Candidiasis

56. A 27-year-old white male presents to your clinic today with a 2 month history of itchy, dry skin on the top of his feet. He is a construction worker and wears heavy boots daily. He reports that the itching is becoming extreme and is affecting his work. He has tried OTC foot creams to include triple antibiotic, antifungal, and hydrocortisone but they have not helped. A photo of his feet is shown below. What is the most appropriate first step in treating this patient?

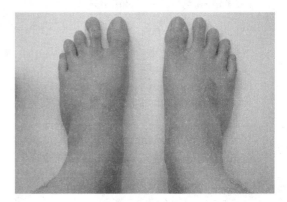

(A) Treat with Lotrisone (antifungal + corticosteroid) for 2 weeks, then return to clinic for recheck.
(B) Scrape scale, perform KOH, then treat for contact dermatitis (–) vs fungus if (+).
(C) Scrape scale for culture and treat for contact dermatitis with mid-high potency corticosteroid.
(D) Refer to podiatrist.
(E) Check blood glucose.

57. A 72-year-old female is noted to have elevated calcium on routine laboratories during a routine annual examination. Additional labs demonstrate an elevated PTH. Which of the following clinical findings is most likely related?

    (A) Anxiety
    (B) Diarrhea
    (C) Kidney stones
    (D) Weight gain
    (E) Hyperthyroidism

58. A 22-year-old female graduate student presents for evaluation of hirsutism. She has noted the gradual development of facial hair over the past 5–6 years. She had menarche at age 13, and her menses have been irregular ever since. Her most recent menstrual period was 3 months ago. On a physical exam, she is 5'4" tall and weighs 150 lb. She has a few acne cysts on her chin. She also has terminal hair on her upper lip and around the areola. The remainder of the exam is normal. Given these clinical findings which of the following is the most likely diagnosis?

    (A) Addison's disease
    (B) Conn syndrome
    (C) Graves' disease
    (D) Polycystic ovary syndrome (PCOS)
    (E) Fragile X syndrome

59. Which of the following physical exam findings would be consistent with hypocalcemia?

    (A) Carpopedal spasm
    (B) Brisk deep tendon reflexes
    (C) Hypertension
    (D) Tachycardia
    (E) Wrist pain

60. Which of the following test results is diagnostic for primary chronic adrenal insufficiency?

    (A) Low 8:00 A.M. plasma cortisol level accompanied by elevated ACTH levels
    (B) Elevated morning plasma cortisol levels accompanied by elevated ACTH levels
    (C) Elevated 8:00 A.M. plasma cortisol level accompanied by low ACTH levels
    (D) Low 8:00 A.M. plasma cortisol level accompanied by low ACTH levels
    (E) Low plasma cortisol level accompanied by elevated calcium levels

61. A 25-year-old male presents to your clinic complaining of extreme weakness, 20 pound weight loss, light-headedness and dizziness for the past 8–9 months. On physical examination, his BP is 90/68 mmHg. He has dark skin and there is hyperpigmentation of the creases of his palms. Laboratory studies reveal low serum sodium and elevated potassium. Which of the following is the most likely diagnosis?

    (A) Addison's disease
    (B) Cushing's syndrome
    (C) Hyperaldosteronism
    (D) Pheochromocytoma
    (E) Kallmann syndrome

62. A 21-year-old female presents complaining of amenorrhea over the past year and a milky discharge from her left nipple. She is not taking any medications. She is sexually active but does not want to become pregnant. Other than a milky discharge from her left breast, the physical examination is normal. A urine pregnancy test is negative. Labs reveal her prolactin level is 300 mg/dL (normal: 525 ng/dL). Which of the following tests is the best way to confirm the suspected diagnosis?

    (A) Overnight dexamethasone suppression test
    (B) PET scan
    (C) Transsphenoidal resection
    (D) MRI
    (E) Mammogram

63. What is the most appropriate test to monitor adequate dosing of levothyroxine (Synthroid)?

    (A) TBG
    (B) FT4
    (C) TRH
    (D) TSH
    (E) Free T4

64. According to the ADA guidelines, what is the target A1C value for most patients with diabetes mellitus?

    (A) < 6.5%
    (B) < 7.0%
    (C) < 7.5%
    (D) < 8.0%
    (E) > 10.0%

65. Which of the following hormones is secreted from the anterior pituitary gland?

    (A) ACTH
    (B) Vasopressin
    (C) Aldosterone
    (D) PTH
    (E) ADH

66. Which of the following is a least likely characteristic of Turner syndrome?

    (A) Small stature
    (B) Gynecomastia
    (C) Webbed neck
    (D) Bicuspid aortic valve
    (E) Cataracts

67. A 45-year-old female presents with a very painful neck. She also reports difficulty swallowing. Upon questioning, you find that she recently had an upper respiratory infection but otherwise she is healthy. What is the most likely diagnosis?

    (A) Postpartum thyroiditis
    (B) Sporadic thyroiditis
    (C) Sick euthyroid syndrome
    (D) Subacute thyroiditis
    (E) Thyroid nodules

68. A 16-year-old boy presents to the clinic for a sports physical. On the physical exam, you document Tanner stage 3 gonad development with firm testes. Labs reveal low testosterone, high LH and FSH. Which of the following etiologies most likely explains the lab results and exam findings?

    (A) Klinefelter syndrome
    (B) Prader-Willi syndrome
    (C) Kallmann syndrome
    (D) Anabolic steroid abuse
    (E) Hypercholesterolemia

69. Patients with endocrine abnormalities are at greater risk for which of the following?

    (A) Psychiatric problems
    (B) Autoimmune disorders
    (C) Cancer
    (D) Genetic anomalies
    (E) Cystic fibrosis

70. Which of the following physical findings is most suggestive of thyroid carcinoma in a patient with a thyroid nodule?

    (A) Painless, diffuse swelling of the thyroid
    (B) Lymphedema
    (C) Symmetrical thyroid enlargement
    (D) Surrounding erythema
    (E) Ecchymosis of neck

71. A 35-year-old female presents with increased intense thirst, craving ice water and polyuria of several months duration. Urine dipstick shows specific gravity < 1.005 and is negative for glucose. What is the most likely diagnosis?

    (A) Diabetes mellitus type 2
    (B) Iron deficiency anemia
    (C) Hyperthyroidism
    (D) Diabetes insipidus
    (E) Addison's disease

72. A 34-year-old woman presents to the office with complaints of fatigue, constipation, dry skin, and weight gain. Physical examination shows delayed deep tendon reflexes. Which of the following is the most likely diagnosis?

    (A) Adrenal insufficiency
    (B) Cushing's syndrome
    (C) Hypoparathyroidism
    (D) Hyperaldosteronism
    (E) Hypothyroidism

73. A 57-year-old man presents with occipital headache, muscle weakness, lower leg cramping, and elevated blood pressure of 184/112 that has not been responsive to diuretic or ACE inhibitor treatment. Serum electrolytes show low potassium. Which of the following is the most likely diagnosis?

    (A) Addison's disease
    (B) Pheochromocytoma
    (C) Hyperparathyroidism
    (D) Hyperthyroidism
    (E) Hyperaldosteronism

74. Which of the following is the most common cause of Cushing's syndrome?

    (A) Pheochromocytoma
    (B) Adrenocortical tumor
    (C) Pituitary tumor
    (D) Corticosteroid use
    (E) Renal tumor

75. The positive finding of TPO antibodies is most specific confirming the diagnosis of

    (A) Graves' disease.
    (B) Addison's disease.
    (C) cystic fibrosis.
    (D) Hashimoto's thyroiditis.
    (E) thyroid cancer.

76. A 28-year-old female is being evaluated for infrequent menstrual periods. Additionally, she complains of headaches, fatigue, and breast discharge. She does not take any medications regularly. Which lab is most likely to be evaluated?

    (A) LH and FSH
    (B) Oxytocin
    (C) Prolactin
    (D) TSH
    (E) Hemoglobin A1C

77. An asymptomatic 30-year-old female, who is 6 weeks pregnant, is found to have the following lab results:

    Free T4: 3.3ng/dL (normal 0.9–2)

    TSH: < 0.01 IU/mL (normal 0.5–4.5)

    What is the most appropriate treatment for this patient?

    (A) Levothyroxine
    (B) Propranolol
    (C) Propylthiouracil (PTU)
    (D) Radioactive iodine
    (E) Prenatal vitamins

78. What is the test for checking mean plasma glucose concentration over the last 8–10 weeks?

    (A) Fasting plasma glucose
    (B) Fructosamine test
    (C) Hemoglobin A1C
    (D) Oral glucose tolerance test
    (E) Finger stick

79. A patient presents to your clinic with a chief complaint of left eye pain, blurred vision, tearing, redness, foreign body sensation, and photophobia for the past 4 days. The image depicts the fluorescein stain. What is the most likely diagnosis?

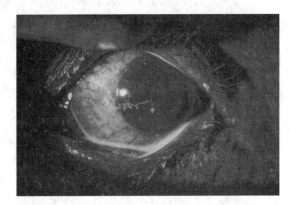

(A) Acanthamoeba keratitis
(B) Bacterial keratitis
(C) Herpes simplex keratitis
(D) Fungal keratitis
(E) Conjunctival hemorrhage

80. Which of the following types of burns causes worse corneal injury and why?

(A) Alkali burns, liquefaction
(B) Acidic burns, coagulation
(C) Acidic burns, liquefaction
(D) Alkali burns, coagulation
(E) Alkali burns, lens disruption

81. An ocular condition associated with blunt trauma that is characterized by blood in the anterior chamber and a possible increase in intraocular pressure is called

(A) chalazion.
(B) hyphema.
(C) ectropion.
(D) hypopyon.
(E) retinal detachment.

82. The most common area to be affected by dental caries is which of the following?

(A) Mandibular anterior incisors
(B) Canines
(C) Permanent third molars
(D) Permanent first molars
(E) Central incisors

83. Primary medical management of open angle glaucoma consists of which of the following?

(A) Topical beta-blockers
(B) Topical steroids
(C) Topical antibiotics
(D) Topical antivirals
(E) Diuretic

84. The Dix-Hallpike maneuver is useful for assessing which one of the following conditions?

(A) Acute otitis media
(B) Benign paroxysmal positional vertigo
(C) Otitis externa
(D) Tinnitus
(E) Hip pain

85. An 18-month-old girl is brought to your clinic by her mother who reports that she has been irritable, tugging on her left ear, and has had fever for the last 3 days. Otoscopic examination reveals a red, bulging tympanic membrane with decreased mobility (see image). Which of the following would be your first choice of therapy?

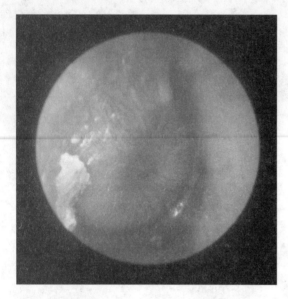

(A) Amoxicillin
(B) Ciprofloxacin
(C) Doxycycline
(D) Sulfonamide
(E) Erythromycin

86. A 24-year-old male presents to your office with a chief complaint of ear pain. What is your impression of the following otoscopic examination?

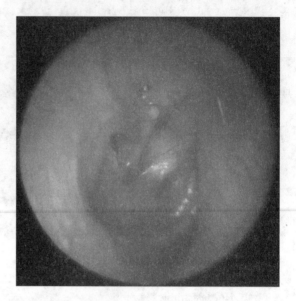

(A) Bulging of the tympanic membrane with loss of landmarks
(B) Fluid collection behind the tympanic membrane
(C) Normal tympanic membrane
(D) Scar tissue on the tympanic membrane
(E) Perforation of the tympanic membrane

87. Which of the following would be the most likely location for squamous cell carcinoma to develop intra-orally?

(A) Buccal mucosa
(B) Gingiva
(C) Hard palate
(D) Tongue
(E) Torus mandibularis

88. A patient presents to your clinic with white plaques on the tongue, palate, and buccal mucosa for 3 days. The patient can wipe the plaques off, but they keep coming back. The patient is currently undergoing chemotherapy for colon cancer. What is the most likely diagnosis?

(A) Herpes stomatitis
(B) Oral candidiasis
(C) Oral lichen planus
(D) Oral leukoplakia
(E) Erythema migrans

89. A 32-year-old man presents to your ER 45 minutes after being struck in the nose by a softball. He had a nose bleed, which has since stopped. On inspection of the nasal cavity you note the lesion depicted in this image. Given this clinical picture, which of the following is the most appropriate to avoid damage of the nasal septum?

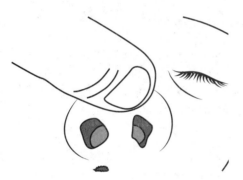

(A) Broad-spectrum intravenous antibiotics
(B) Ice compress and head elevation
(C) Incision and drainage
(D) Radiograph to rule out a fracture
(E) Cryotherapy treatment

90. During the physical exam of a 15-year-old male, you notice clear rhinorrhea, pale blue discoloration, and moderate edema of the mucosa covering the nasal turbinates. He also has mild redness and swelling to the lower eyelid area. Given these physical findings, which of the following is considered the first line of treatment?

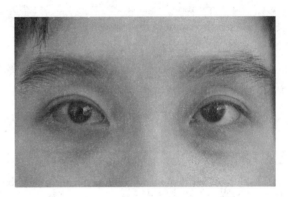

(A) Antibiotics (azithromycin)
(B) Topical steroids (Flonase)
(C) Allergy shots
(D) Oral steroids (prednisone)
(E) Will resolve spontaneously

91. A patient presents with a 3-day history of sores in the mouth, located along the inner, gingival aspect of the lower lip. On the exam, you notice 3–4 ulcers with a yellow pseudomembranous covering and surrounding erythematous halo. What is the most likely diagnosis?

(A) Aphthous stomatitis
(B) Erythema migrans
(C) Herpes labialis
(D) Oral candidiasis
(E) Pseudomembranous enterocolitis

92. A patient presents to the emergency department with complaints of left-sided earache and headache. The patient has an associated fever of 101.9°F and was diagnosed with an ear infection a few weeks prior but only took a few days of the antibiotics. On exam, you note that the left ear is protruding forward and there is significant mastoid tenderness to palpation. The most appropriate management of this patient is

(A) oral antibiotics.
(B) referral to ENT.
(C) steroids.
(D) supportive care.
(E) intubation.

93. Primary medical management of open angle glaucoma consists of intraocular application of which of the following?

(A) Alpha 2 agonists
(B) Beta-blockers
(C) Prostaglandin analogs
(D) Steroids
(E) Diuretics

94. The most common pathogen associated with malignant otitis externa is

(A) Klebsiella.
(B) Pseudomonas.
(C) *Staphylococcus aureus.*
(D) *Streptococcus pneumoniae.*
(E) *Haemophilus influenza.*

95. Periodontitis differs from gingivitis by evidence of

(A) alveolar involvement.
(B) bone loss.
(C) necrotic gum tissue.
(D) nerve damage.
(E) tooth decay.

96. A 67-year-old man presents to the ED with sudden painless loss of vision in the left eye. He has a past medical history of hyperlipidemia and carotid stenosis. Visual acuity is 20/20 in the right eye and light perception only in the left eye. Fundoscopic exam of the right eye is normal. The left eye shows a pallid retinal swelling with a cherry red spot in the area of the fovea. What is the most likely diagnosis?

(A) Amaurosis fugax
(B) Central retinal vein occlusion
(C) Retinal detachment
(D) Angle closure glaucoma
(E) Central retinal artery occlusion

97. A patient presents with episodic vertigo that lasts anywhere from 20 minutes to several hours. They also complain of hearing loss, tinnitus, and a sensation of fullness in the right ear. Which of the following is the most likely diagnosis?

(A) Acoustic neuroma
(B) Benign positional vertigo
(C) Labyrinthitis
(D) Ménière's disease
(E) Migraine headache

98. Management of auricular hematoma includes

(A) incision and drainage.
(B) ice.
(C) warm compress.
(D) watchful waiting.
(E) topical antibiotic.

99. A toddler is brought to the emergency department, accompanied by their parents; the family recently emigrated and vaccine status is unknown. The patient has had a decreased appetite and a sore throat since last night.

Vital signs: pulse 112, respirations 35, BP 100/60, O2 saturation 98% on room air.

On the exam, you find the child sitting on the exam table leaning forward and breathing rapidly. While talking to the parents, you notice the mother wiping drool from the child's mouth. Neck films show a "thumb print" sign. What is the most likely diagnosis?

(A) Acute epiglottitis
(B) Asthma exacerbation
(C) Croup
(D) Viral pharyngitis
(E) Foreign body

100. An 18-year-old male patient presents to the office complaining of mildly tender swelling at the base of his spine, which seems to be getting bigger over the past month. On examination, you note a sinus tract opening in the midline over the coccyx, which has a "halo" of erythema surrounding the sinus opening. A small amount of purulent drainage is easily expressed. Which of the following is the most likely diagnosis?

(A) Coccygeal carcinoma
(B) Pilonidal cyst
(C) Syphilitic chancre
(D) Herpes simplex
(E) Anorectal fissure

101. A patient presents to the office with right upper quadrant pain, nausea, and mild diarrhea. History of present illness is significant for moderate fatigue, myalgia, and anorexia. No one else at home is sick. Diet is usually healthy with fresh fruits and vegetables as a staple. Physical exam demonstrates some cervical lymph node enlargement, mild hepatomegaly, and slight tenderness to palpation over the liver. Lab workup is significant for elevations in ALT (alanine aminotransferase) and AST (aspartate aminotransferase). Which of the following is most likely responsible for these findings?

(A) Hepatitis A
(B) Hepatitis B
(C) Hepatitis C
(D) Hepatitis D
(E) Hepatitis E

102. A patient with worsening nighttime cough for the last 6 months also notes that they have not been able to eat or drink anything, including water, for the last 3 months without having prolonged belching and an epigastric burning sensation. The symptoms worsen when lying down. There have not been any associated bowel changes. Which of the following most likely represents the diagnosis?

(A) Cholelithiasis
(B) Gastroesophageal reflux disease
(C) Irritable bowel syndrome
(D) Peptic ulcer disease
(E) Kidney cyst

103. A 46-year-old female presents with intermittent abdominal pain for 8 months. She has not noted precipitating factors. She has associated fatigue and malaise. She denies blood or mucus in her "runny stools." She usually feels better after a bowel movement. Physical exam is unremarkable. Which of the following is the next best step in the evaluation of this patient?

(A) Abdominal X-ray
(B) Colonoscopy
(C) Blood work
(D) Ultrasound of abdomen
(E) None of the above

104. A 50-year-old male is brought to the emergency department following a seizure this morning. He does not have a history of seizures. His wife reports he has been complaining about joint pain for several weeks in addition to intermittent abdominal pain and diarrhea. This morning he had a temperature of 99.8°F. On exam, you find nystagmus, cervical lymphadenopathy, clear lungs, and a systolic murmur 2/6. He has some muscle wasting and bilateral knee effusions. Which of the following tests will confirm your diagnosis?

    (A) Biopsy of the duodenum
    (B) Biopsy of the jejunum
    (C) Hydrogen breath test
    (D) Serology for IgA tTG (tissue transglutaminase)
    (E) Rheumatoid factor test

105. A 20-year-old male presents with a 6-week history of colicky abdominal pain, hematochezia, fecal urgency, and two episodes of fecal incontinence. He has had three to four stool episodes daily. On exam, he is found to have mild abdominal tenderness without focal mass. He is afebrile, HR 90, BP 110/78, RR 17. Colonoscopy is scheduled and findings are consistent with diffuse ulcerations that begin at the anal verge and continue through the sigmoid colon. What is the most likely diagnosis?

    (A) Crohn's disease
    (B) Celiac sprue
    (C) Microscopic colitis
    (D) Ulcerative colitis
    (E) Cholecystitis

106. Which of the following is considered the drug of choice for first-line therapy in a patient with mild-to-moderate ulcerative colitis above the sigmoid colon?

    (A) Oral 5-ASA (e.g., pentasa) and rectal 5-ASA
    (B) Oral corticosteroids (e.g., prednisone) only
    (C) Anti-TNF (e.g., infliximab) plus rectal corticosteroids
    (D) Anti-integrins (e.g., vendoluzimab) plus rectal 5-ASA
    (E) Adulimabab (Humira) only

107. A patient presents with persistent dysphagia and regurgitation. The following image is obtained on esophagram. Which of the following best describes the condition?

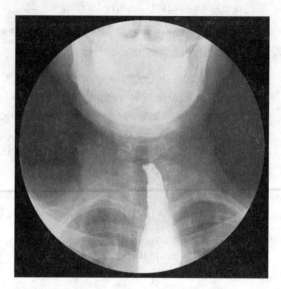

    (A) Achalasia
    (B) Eosinophilic esophagitis
    (C) Scleroderma
    (D) Zenker's diverticulum
    (E) Celiac disease

108. A patient comes to your office with complaints of feeling full after eating just a little bit of his meals. This is accompanied by frequent nausea and occasional emesis. There are rare episodes of abdominal pain with meals. Past medical history is significant for a diagnosis of diabetes with your office about 6 years ago with suboptimal control. Which of the following is this patient most likely suffering from?

    (A) Pancreatitis
    (B) Cholecystitis
    (C) Diverticulosis
    (D) Gastroparesis
    (E) Intestinal obstruction

109. A patient with prior medical history of eczema and asthma has developed dysphagia to solid foods and reflux. What is the first-line treatment for this condition?

    (A) Endoscopic myotomy
    (B) Topical steroids puffed and swallowed two times daily
    (C) A lactose free diet
    (D) Proton pump inhibitor daily for 8 weeks
    (E) Feeding tube placement

110. What is the best imaging technique for a middle-aged mother of three children who has postprandial right upper quadrant pain?

    (A) Abdominal CT scan
    (B) Abdominal ultrasound
    (C) Endoscopic retrograde cholangiopancreatography (ERCP)
    (D) Upright and supine abdominal X-ray
    (E) Abdominal MRI

111. The patient is a 26-year-old with an 8-day history of crampy abdominal discomfort, flatulence, and diarrhea. She has not noticed any blood in her stool but she has lost 3 pounds. She has recently returned from a camping trip in a national park. She is a vegetarian and all her meals were cooked over a campfire. She does not have a fever and her white blood cell count is normal. What is the most likely cause of diarrhea?

    (A) Rotavirus
    (B) *Giardia lamblia*
    (C) *Campylobacter jejuni*
    (D) *Salmonella* non-typhi species
    (E) *Entamoeba histolytica*

112. You are evaluating an 83-year-old patient with a 100.8°F temperature, abdominal cramps, and frequent, high-volume watery stools who is a resident of a nursing home. The roommate returned to the home 4 days ago after a hospital stay for pneumonia. What is the most likely pathogen causing your patient's symptoms?

    (A) *Vibrio cholera*
    (B) *Clostridium difficile*
    (C) *Staphylococcus aureus*
    (D) Enterotoxigenic *Escherichia coli*
    (E) *Giardia*

113. A patient was previously treated for gastritis caused by *H. pylori* with 2 antibiotics and a proton pump inhibitor for 14 days. After a 2-week waiting period since the completion of treatment, what is the simplest and most available method for determining if the infection has been eradicated?

    (A) An endoscopic examination of the upper GI tract (EGD)
    (B) *H. pylori* culture and sensitivities
    (C) D-xylose breath test
    (D) *H. pylori* stool antigen
    (E) Eradication completed with time

114. A 67-year-old woman has 8 pounds of unintentional weight loss over 4 months. She has a history of iron deficiency anemia, but has no changes in bowel habits, no epigastric pain, and no heartburn. She has blood detected in her stool by antigen testing. Her vital signs are normal, her abdomen is soft and without rebound or guarding. Which procedure/test would you order to confirm your suspected diagnosis?

    (A) Colonoscopy with biopsy suspecting adenocarcinoma
    (B) CT scan of the abdomen to confirm diverticulitis
    (C) Barium enema suspecting adenomatous polyps
    (D) CBC suspecting Plummer-Vinson syndrome
    (E) Echocardiogram suspecting endocarditis

115. All patients below have abdominal pain. Which patient is most likely to have a serum lipase level that is three times above the upper limit of normal?

    (A) A person with a CT scan showing walled off necrosis near the second part of the duodenum

    (B) A woman with loss of villi and presence of crypt abscesses on biopsy of the small intestine

    (C) A patient with pruritus has a bile duct with multifocal strictures and dilations on magnetic resonance cholangiopancreatography (MRCP)

    (D) A patient who had an esophagogastroduodenoscopy (EGD) that shows a nonhealing duodenal ulcer after 12 weeks of treatment

    (E) A patient with pancreatic cancer

116. Which cause of acute pancreatitis is not associated with the development of chronic pancreatitis?

    (A) An anatomic defect in drainage of the pancreatic duct (pancreas divisum)

    (B) Autoimmune-mediated pancreatic inflammation

    (C) Choledocholithiasis after cholecystectomy

    (D) Alcohol and nicotine dependence

    (E) Hypertrigyceridemia

117. Which of the following symptoms is considered the most concerning alarm symptom in the evaluation of irritable bowel syndrome?

    (A) Abdominal pain relieved by stooling

    (B) Abdominal pain with nighttime awakening

    (C) Change in stool frequency

    (D) Change in stool consistency

    (E) Continuous abdominal pain

118. Mom brings her 3-year-old to the clinic concerned about possible dehydration. The child has had vomiting and diarrhea for 2 days. She has missed day care. Mom notes the stool is bright green and profuse. She has lost count of the number of stools the child has had today. What is the likely pathogen present?

    (A) *Campylobacter*

    (B) *Salmonella*

    (C) Norovirus

    (D) Rotavirus

    (E) *Giardia*

119. A patient well known to your emergency room for multiple episodes of acute alcohol intoxication is now presenting for mid-epigastric pain that radiates to the back. This pain has been occurring intermittently for the last few weeks, but tonight it is severe. The patient engaged in significant alcohol intake in the last 24 hours. Which of the following therapies is most beneficial for this patient?

    (A) Aggressive fluid resuscitation

    (B) Administration of antibiotics

    (C) Emergent laparoscopy

    (D) Emergent lactulose administration

    (E) Activated charcoal

120. A 54-year-old patient with rectal bleeding, change in bowel habits, abdominal pain, and weight loss should undergo which of the following tests?

    (A) CT colonography

    (B) Flexible sigmoidoscopy

    (C) Flexible sigmoidoscopy with fecal immunochemical test of the stool

    (D) Abdominal ultrasound

    (E) Colonoscopy

121. A patient undergoes a colonoscopy. The following image displays the results. Which of the following complications is the patient at a higher risk of?

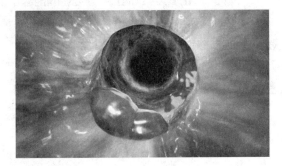

   (A) Gastroparesis
   (B) Diverticulitis
   (C) Toxic megacolon
   (D) Fistula formation
   (E) Crohn's disease

122. A patient undergoes a laparoscopic cholecystectomy and returns to the office with right upper quadrant pain 2 weeks later. Labs demonstrate an elevated bilirubin. What is the cause of this problem?

   (A) Gallstone ileus
   (B) Chole-enteric fistula
   (C) Gallstone within common bile duct
   (D) Biliary cyst
   (E) Dissolving suture

123. A 53-year-old patient presents to the emergency department with gross hematemesis. Which of the following is the most appropriate imaging test?

   (A) Esophagogastroduodenoscopy (EGD)
   (B) Barium swallow
   (C) Colonoscopy
   (D) Abdominal ultrasound
   (E) Abdominal CT

124. A patient with a history of well-controlled diabetes has become very difficult to manage over the past 2 months. They endorse a 10 lb weight loss in the same time period along with some persistent right upper quadrant pain. For the past week, stools have been difficult to flush ("floating") and the patient has noticed that the whites of his eyes have looked yellow. Which of the following conditions is most likely the cause of these symptoms?

   (A) Gallbladder neoplasm
   (B) Liver neoplasm
   (C) Splenic neoplasm
   (D) Pancreatic neoplasm
   (E) Abdominal neoplasm

125. High-pitched bowel sounds found on physical exam accompanied by abdominal distention should raise suspicion for which of the following?

   (A) Volvulus
   (B) Small bowel obstruction
   (C) Diverticular abscess
   (D) Large bowel obstruction
   (E) Intussusception

126. A patient with a rigid, distended abdomen is found to have the following image. What is the diagnosis?

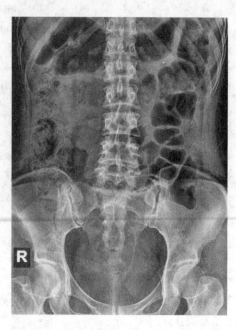

(A) Volvulus
(B) Large bowel obstruction
(C) Small bowel obstruction
(D) Toxic megacolon
(E) Foreign body

127. A 66-year-old male presents to the ED for evaluation of altered mental status and seizure. On physical exam, you find Trousseau sign. Which of the following is the most likely diagnosis?

(A) Hypercalcemia
(B) Hyperkalemia
(C) Hypocalcemia
(D) Hypokalemia
(E) Hypernatremia

128. A 21-year-old male presents to student health with severe flank pain and vomiting since the pain began 5 hours ago. He states that he had blood in his urine this morning. He has severe right-sided CVA tenderness on examination. What is the currently preferred diagnostic test to confirm your suspected diagnosis?

(A) Renal ultrasound
(B) Kidney, ureter, and bladder X-ray (KUB)
(C) Magnetic resonance imaging (MRI)
(D) Non-contrast computed tomography (CT)
(E) Intravenous urogram

129. A 22-year-old male is diagnosed with testicular cancer. Which of the following aspects of his history is a key risk factor for this condition?

(A) Multiple STDs
(B) Tobacco abuse
(C) Undescended testis
(D) Uncircumcised penis
(E) Vasectomy

130. A 26-year-old female presents to the ED with complaints of progressively worsening fever, intractable vomiting, left-sided flank pain, and dysuria x 3 days. Physical exam revealed a temperature of 101.4°F, heart rate of 140, and moderate CVA tenderness. The remainder of the physical exam is unremarkable. A urinalysis is obtained and shows +++ leukocytes and trace blood. The microscopy reveals 10–20 WBC per high power field, too numerous to count bacteria and a few white blood cell casts. The WBC count on CBC is elevated. What is the most appropriate treatment plan for this patient?

(A) Carbapenems and discharge
(B) Cephalosporin and admit
(C) Penicillins and discharge
(D) Quinolone and admit
(E) Glucocorticoid therapy

131. A 26-year-old female patient presents with a 24-hour history of dysuria, urinary hesitancy, and urgency. She has some associated suprapubic pressure as well. She denies fever, chills, nausea, and vaginal symptoms. A urinalysis reveals positive nitrites and large leukocyte esterase. The remainder of the urinalysis is unremarkable. What is the most likely infectious organism?

    (A) *Enterobacter*
    (B) *Escherichia coli*
    (C) *Staphylococcus*
    (D) Proteus
    (E) HIV

132. A 46-year-old mother of three children complains of small amounts of urine leaking when she coughs or laughs. Her physical examination reveals no remarkable findings of the genitourinary system. Urinalysis is normal. Which of the following is the most appropriate first step in management of her condition?

    (A) Recommend pelvic floor therapy
    (B) Recommend hormonal replacement therapy
    (C) Refer for cystoscopy
    (D) Pessary placement
    (E) Hormonal supplements

133. In a patient who has been vomiting, and now presents with metabolic alkalosis and BP of 82/40 mm HG, what is the most appropriate initial phase of treatment?

    (A) 3% saline
    (B) D5W
    (C) Furosemide
    (D) Abnormal saline
    (E) Normal saline

134. A 13-year-old male presents to the ED with acute pain in the right side of his "private parts." He denies any trauma. The symptoms have been present for approximately 1–2 hours and have gotten progressively worse. On exam, he has no cremasteric reflex and negative Prehn sign on the right side. Which of the following is the diagnostic study of choice to confirm your suspected diagnosis?

    (A) CT of the pelvis with contrast
    (B) Ultrasound with doppler
    (C) Urinalysis
    (D) Voiding cystourethrogram
    (E) CBC

135. A 24-year-old male presents with fever, dysuria, and perineal pain x 4 days. On exam, you note prostate tenderness on rectal examination, and a urinalysis reveals pyuria, bacteriuria, and 2+ hematuria. What is the most likely diagnosis?

    (A) Acute bacterial prostatitis
    (B) Benign prostatic hyperplasia
    (C) Prostate cancer
    (D) Pyelonephritis
    (E) UTI

136. Which of the following scrotal masses presents as a nontender mass?

    (A) Epididymitis
    (B) Hydrocele
    (C) Orchitis
    (D) Testicular torsion
    (E) Testicular cancer

137. A 75-year-old patient with PMH of constipation presents for evaluation of nausea. An ECG is obtained revealing a prolonged PR interval and tall T-waves. Physical exam shows absent deep tendon reflexes. Which of the following is the most likely underlying electrolyte disorder?

    (A) Hyperphosphatemia
    (B) Hypermagnesemia
    (C) Hypokalemia
    (D) Hypomagnesemia
    (E) Hypoglycemia

138. A 70-year-old male with PMH of dementia presents for increased lethargy and generalized weakness. At baseline, the patient does not communicate verbally or ambulate independently. On exam, he has notable orthostatic hypotension and dry mucous membranes. Labs show a high serum osmolality. Which of the following electrolyte disorders is most likely?

    (A) Hypocalcemia
    (B) Hypomagnesemia
    (C) Hyperkalemia
    (D) Hypernatremia
    (E) Hyponatremia

139. Which of the following would be considered a complicated UTI?

    (A) Pregnant patient
    (B) Male patient
    (C) Immunosuppressed patient
    (D) All of the above
    (E) None of the above

140. A 58-year-old male with a past medical history of diabetes complains of recent onset peripheral edema and abdominal bloating. Blood chemistries reveal serum albumin of 2.4 g/dL, total serum protein of 5 mg/dL, and a serum cholesterol of 290 mg/dL. Which of the following is the most likely diagnosis?

    (A) Nephrotic syndrome
    (B) Nil disease
    (C) Tubulointerstitial nephritis
    (D) Medullary sponge kidney
    (E) Acute glomerulonephritis

141. A 72-year-old poorly controlled diabetic presents to the emergency department for concerns of a wound for the last 4 days that has grown in size. On exam, you note a black, eschar-appearing wound with necrosis and foul-smelling purulent discharge. BP is 84/58 and HR is 138 bpm. What would be the most appropriate next course of action for this patient?

    (A) Initiate broad-spectrum antibiotics and admit to the floor.
    (B) Initiate broad-spectrum antibiotics and surgical debridement.
    (C) Perform a scrotal incision, and drainage.
    (D) Order an ultrasound.
    (E) Manage blood pressure and consult dermatology.

142. A 34-year-old woman is seen for evaluation of anemia. You suspect iron deficiency as the cause. Which one of the following laboratory results would support this diagnosis?

    (A) Decreased total iron binding capacity
    (B) Decreased percent iron saturation
    (C) Elevated MCV
    (D) Elevated reticulocyte count
    (E) MCV = 90 fL

143. Which of the following is true about disorders of primary homeostasis?

    (A) Can be caused by aspirin
    (B) Causes bleeding into large spaces (i.e., the joints)
    (C) Normal bleeding time
    (D) Prolonged PT or PTT
    (E) Von Willibrand factor decrease

144. A 68-year-old woman presents to the emergency department complaining of recurrent right-sided headaches for 3 weeks. She states that it hurts to touch her skin between the right eye and ear when the headache is present. She also notes jaw pain when chewing. Physical examination shows a temperature of 101 orally. Visual acuity diminished in the right eye, and there is tenderness to palpation lateral to the right eye. Which of the following should be administered pending diagnostic studies?

(A) Daily aspirin therapy
(B) Oral opioid analgesics
(C) IV antibiotics
(D) Oral glucocorticoids
(E) Oral NSAIDs

145. A 3-year-old African-American male is brought to the emergency room by his parents with an abrupt onset of severe pain in both of his legs, both arms, and low back. He has had episodes like this in the past. He is febrile, tachypneic, and vomits while you are in the exam room. Hemoglobin electrophoresis on this patient would most likely reveal which of the following genotypes?

(A) Hb AA
(B) Hb AS
(C) Hb DS
(D) Hb SS
(E) Hb ST

146. An established patient presents for her annual physical exam. She is a 32-year-old Asian female with no complaints. Routine labs reveal:

Test	Result	Reference Range
WBC	4.3×10^3	
Hgb	9.3	
HCT	29	
MCV	67	80–96 fL/cell
MCH	25	27–33 pg/cell
RDW	12	11.5–14.5%
Platelets	200	
Neutrophils	70	45–73%
Bands	3	3–5%
Monocytes	2	2–8%
Eosinophils	0	0–4%
Basophils	0	0–4%
Lymphocytes	25	20–40–4%
Serum Iron	75	50–150 mcg/dL
TIBC	300	250–410 mcg/dL
Transferrin Saturation	45	30–50%
Serum Ferritin	15	10–20 mcg/L

What test would you order to confirm your suspected diagnosis?

(A) Bone marrow biopsy
(B) Hemoglobin electrophoresis
(C) Methylmalonic acid level
(D) Serum protein electrophoresis
(E) Schilling test

147. A 23-year-old female presents to the clinic with complaints of fatigue and yellowing of her skin.

   Social History: She is in a dorm with her roommate who is not ill. She goes to college classes and has been doing well. She denies smoking or any illicit drug use. She states that she drinks approximately two drinks each weekend.

   Past Medical History: She is up to date on her immunizations and routine physical exams. She has no medical illnesses.

   Family History: HTN in her mother, DM in her father.

   Labs: Electrolytes: Mild hyperkalemia, otherwise normal

   Liver Profile: Elevated LDH, elevated indirect bilirubin, normal direct bilirubin

   Coombs test: Positive

   What is your diagnosis?

Test	Result	Reference Range
WBC	5.0	
Hgb	8.5	
HCT	25.6	
MCV	88	80–96 fL/cell
MCH	30	27–33 pg/cell
RDW	12	11.5–14.5%
Platelets	200	
Neutrophils	55	45–73%
Bands	3	3–5%
Monocytes	2	2–8%
Eosinophils	3	0–4%
Basophils	3	0–4%
Lymphocytes	34	20–40–4%
Peripheral Smear	Spherocytosis and nucleated RBC	
Reticulocyte Count	6%	0.5–2.5%
Reticulocyte Index	4.2	1

(A) Aplastic anemia
(B) Autoimmune hemolytic anemia
(C) Non-autoimmune hemolytic anemia
(D) Iron-deficiency anemia
(E) Megaloblastic anemia

148. What is your presumptive diagnosis after examining this slide under your microscope?

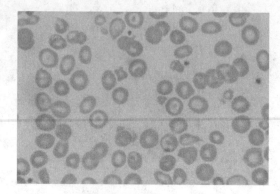

(A) Aplastic anemia
(B) Iron-deficiency anemia
(C) Sickle cell anemia
(D) Thalassemia
(E) Anemia of chronic illness

149. A 12-year-old boy comes into your office for evaluation of epistaxis. He states that he has had to come home from school on two separate occasions because they couldn't get the bleeding to stop. Upon further questioning, you discover that he also has gingival bleeding quite frequently when brushing his teeth. His ROS is otherwise negative. His 16-year-old sister has a history of heavy menstruation, and his father has frequent nosebleeds. His physical exam is unremarkable. What is your diagnosis?

(A) Hemophilia A
(B) Hemophilia B
(C) Idiopathic thrombocytopenia purpura
(D) Von Willebrand's disease
(E) Hemolytic anemia

150. You are rounding on a patient that is post-op day 3 following amputation of the right leg due to a traumatic crush injury. You notice that the patient's IV site is oozing blood as is the surgical site. In addition, you notice petechiae. You order labs and discover the following: PT – prolonged, PTT – prolonged, platelet count – low, D-dimer – elevated. Which of the following is the diagnosis?

(A) Acute DIC
(B) Hemophilia
(C) ITP
(D) Vitamin K deficiency
(E) Factor V deficiency

151. A 69-year-old Black male has been experiencing increased weakness, intermittent fevers, and weight loss in addition to progressive back pain over the course of the last several months. An X-ray of the back shows compression fractures in the thoracic spine as well as lytic lesions within the thoracic and lumbar spine. Labs show hypercalcemia and increased total serum protein. What is the best next step to confirm this patient's diagnosis?

(A) Hemoglobin electrophoresis
(B) PET scan
(C) Serum protein electrophoresis
(D) Urinalysis
(E) X-ray

152. Your patient is receiving a blood transfusion. The nurse comes to tell you that the patient has started running a fever of 102.6 with chills. You go to assess the patient and see dark colored urine in the Foley bag. Your patient is complaining of back pain and chest tightness. What is the first thing you should do?

(A) Get an EKG
(B) Stop the transfusion
(C) Start IV fluids
(D) Order a diuretic
(E) Start chest compressions

153. A 52-year-old female presents to your office with complaints of fatigue. Her vital signs are stable. You obtain a CBC, which is included here. What is the best next step for this patient?

Test	Result	Reference Range
WBC	5.2	
Hgb	8.4	
HCT	25	
MCV	77	80–96 fL/cell
MCH	22	27–33 pg/cell
RDW	15.2	11.5–14.5%
Platelets	158	
Neutrophils	72	45–73%
Bands	3	3–5%
Monocytes	5	2–8%
Eosinophils	0	0–4%
Basophils	0	0–4%
Lymphocytes	20	20–40%
Reticulocyte Count	6.5	0.5–2.5%
Reticulocyte Index	2.41	1
Serum Iron	44	50–150 mcg/dL
TIBC	451	250–410 mcg/dL
Transferrin Saturation	14	30–50%
Serum Ferritin	5.2	10–20 mcg/L

(A) Follow up in 3 weeks without treatment
(B) Give IV iron
(C) Search for the site of bleeding
(D) Transfuse packed red blood cells
(E) No action needed

154. A 30-year-old woman presents with frequent, easy bruising and menorrhagia for the last 6 months.

Medications: None

Allergies: No known drug allergies

Family Hx: No history of bleeding

Surgical History: No prior surgeries

Current labs:

Test	Result	Reference Range
WBC	4.3×10^3	
Hgb	15	
HCT	45	
Platelets	25×10^3	
PT	12	11–13.5 seconds
INR	1	0.8–1.1
PTT	65	60–70
TT	27	25–35 seconds
D-Dimer	27	<200 ng/mL

Her CBC 1 year ago was normal.

What is the most likely diagnosis?

(A) Disseminated intravascular coagulation (DIC)
(B) Immune-mediated thrombocytopenia (ITP)
(C) Liver disease
(D) Thrombotic thrombocytopenic purpura (TTP)
(E) Cancer

155. You are asked to provide hematology consultation to evaluate anemia in a 54-year-old hospitalized woman. She has a long history of renal failure and rheumatoid arthritis. She denies blood in her urine or stool or heavy menstrual periods.

Her CBC:

Test	Result	Reference Range
WBC	6.2×10^3	
Hgb	9.0	
HCT	27	
MCV	82	80–96 fL/cell
MCH	32	27–33 pg/cell
RDW	12	11.5–14.5%
Platelets	253×10^3	
Neutrophils	70	45–73%
Bands	0	3–5%
Monocytes	2	2–8%
Eosinophils	0	0–4%
Basophils	0	0–4%
Lymphocytes	27	20–40%
Peripheral Smear		
Reticulocyte Count	05	0.5–2.5%
Reticulocyte Index	0.3	1

Which one of the following findings would be consistent with the most likely etiology of her anemia?

(A) Elevated percent (%) iron saturation
(B) Elevated total iron binding capacity
(C) Elevated hepcidin
(D) Decreased ferritin
(E) Decreased creatinine

156. Which of the following would most likely be associated with arterial thrombi?

 (A) Antiphospholipid syndrome
 (B) Factor V Leiden
 (C) Protein C deficiency
 (D) Protein S deficiency
 (E) Coagulation factor X

157. Mr. Smith is a 69-year-old man with dyspnea at rest and productive cough with green sputum containing specks of blood. Vitals are: BP 140/85, temp 101.4°F, RR 18, pulse 112. He reports having shaking and being cold last night. Chest exam reveals crackles but no dullness to percussion on the back. His labs show a white blood cell count of 18,000/mm^3 that is 90% neutrophils. You get a chest X-ray below. What is the most likely pathogen?

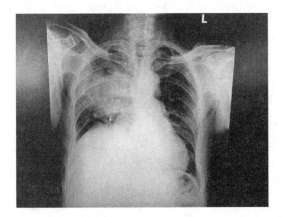

 (A) *Coli*
 (B) *Mycoplasma pneumoniae*
 (C) Bacteroides species
 (D) *Streptococcus pneumoniae*
 (E) *Pseudomonas aurigenosa*

158. A 47-year-old woman is noticed to have the oral exam shown below. The plaques come off when scraped gently. She reports mild odynophagia and no dysphagia. She has used IV heroin, the last time being 4 months ago. Which of the following treatment plans is most appropriate?

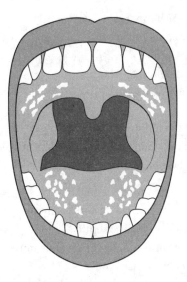

 (A) Admit patient to the hospital for IV antibiotics
 (B) Refer to an oral surgeon for biopsy of the soft palate
 (C) Perform an HIV test and treat with fluconazole
 (D) Reassure the patient and follow in 1 month
 (E) Start oral valacyclovir

159. Which of the following antibiotic regimens is best to use empirically when a hospitalized patient has a severe skin infection? The patient has a history of multiple myeloma and has been in the hospital 3 weeks ago for pneumonia treated with an extended spectrum penicillin.

 (A) Ceftriaxone (cephalosporin) + azithromycin (macrolide)
 (B) Oxacillin (penicillinase-resistant penicillin)
 (C) Ciprofloxacin (quinolone)
 (D) Vancomycin (glycopeptide)
 (E) Ceftriaxone (cephalosporin)

160. A 31-year-old man presents to your clinic with a diffuse macular rash on his trunk, palms, and soles that has been there for 3 days. He reported a painless ulcer on his penis about 4 weeks ago that went away without treatment. What is the most likely agent causing this rash?

(A) Epstein-Barr virus
(B) *Treponema pallidum*
(C) *Haemophilus ducreyi*
(D) *Borrelia burgdorferi*
(E) Parvovirus B19

161. Which of the following antibiotics is the best choice to treat endocarditis caused by methicillin-sensitive *Staphylococcus aureus* (MSSA)?

(A) Ampicillin (aminopenicillin)
(B) Oxacillin (penicillinase-resistant penicillin)
(C) Vancomycin (glycopeptide)
(D) Trimethoprim/sulfa (folate antagonist)
(E) Penicillin G (penicillin)

162. A 24-year-old patient has crampy abdominal pain and watery diarrhea for 4 days. He is afebrile and has not noticed blood or mucus in his stools. The patient just returned from vacation in a developing country. Methylene blue examination of his stool reveals no neutrophils. Which of the following organisms is most likely responsible for this illness?

(A) *Campylobacter jejuni*
(B) Enterotoxigenic *E. coli*
(C) Shigella flexneri
(D) *Salmonella enteritidis*
(E) *Staphylococcus aureus*

163. In which of the following situations should you begin norepinephrine for a patient in septic shock?

(A) Prior to IV fluid resuscitation with 30mL/kg of saline
(B) In a patient with a normal central venous pressure (CVP) of 12 after saline IV fluid replacement
(C) After being unable to maintain mean arterial pressure (MAP) above 65 after saline IV fluid infusion
(D) In a patient recovering from shock to prevent relapse of the inflammatory cascade
(E) In a patient who has received dopamine for high blood pressure

164. A 7-year-old patient with a history of leukemia has come to your clinic with a painful rash on his chest that developed over the last day. He tells you that before the rash developed, he was having a lot of pain in the area. What is the best treatment for this child?

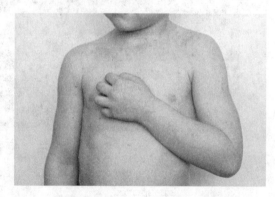

(A) Supportive care
(B) Cefepime (fourth gen cephalosporin)
(C) Acyclovir (antiviral)
(D) Vancomycin (glycopeptide)
(E) Ampicillin (penicillin)

165. Which of the following bacteria produces endotoxin as part of its pathogenicity?

(A) *Streptococcus viridans*
(B) *Listeria monocytogenes*
(C) *Haemophilus influenzae*
(D) *Corynebacterium diphtheriae*
(E) Endotoxin

166. A 54-year-old smoker with mild COPD who is a plumber and currently installing bathrooms at the new local theater presents to your office. She has felt very ill for 2 days, with productive cough, shortness of breath, nausea, and diffuse abdominal pain. Which bacteria is the most likely cause of her pneumonia?

(A) *Staph aureus*
(B) *Klebsiella pneumoniae*
(C) *Chlamydophila pneumoniae*
(D) *Legionella pneumophila*
(E) *Haemophilus influenzae*

167. You are asked to consult on a hospitalized patient with Native Valve Subacute Bacterial Endocarditis. Up to this point, the patient was treated with vancomycin as the blood cultures simply reported that a *Staphylococcus* species was present. Today, updated lab data states the blood cultures are positive for methicillin-sensitive *Staphylococcus aureus* (MSSA). Which treatment is best? Your job is to recommend a cidal antibiotic with a narrow spectrum for an appropriate time course.

(A) Vancomycin 500 mg every 8 hours
(B) Emycin 250 mg every 8 hours
(C) Penicillin G 15 million units daily
(D) Metronidazole 250 mg every 12 hours
(E) Rifampin 1,000 mg IV daily

168. All patients below are currently HIV negative. Based on the information provided, which one is not a candidate to receive pre-exposure prophylaxis for prevention of HIV transmission?

(A) A woman with a history of herpes who is a sex worker
(B) A man who has sex with men who also has end-stage renal failure from hypertension
(C) A man who is beginning a sexual relationship with an HIV+ woman. The woman has sex with men and women
(D) A patient who has a history of injecting heroin and would like to enter a substance abuse treatment program
(E) A patient who is a recovering alcoholic with stable employment

169. A 75-year-old woman presents to the emergency department complaining of a sudden painless unilateral visual loss in her right eye for 2 hours. She has a past medical history of atrial fibrillation, hypertension, type 2 diabetes, and bilateral cataracts. She denies similar symptoms in the past or trauma to the head or eyes. On ophthalmoscopic examination, you note a macular cherry red spot, retinal pallor, and barely visible arteries.

Which of the following is the most likely diagnosis?

(A) Amaurosis fugax
(B) Central retinal artery occlusion
(C) Branch retinal vein occlusion
(D) Optic neuritis
(E) Diabetic retinopathy

170. A 40-year-old man presents to the emergency department with a complaint of pain in the left great toe for 3 days. He has a past medical history of type 2 diabetes. On the physical exam, he has a temperature of 102°F orally. His left great toe is erythematous and tender. White blood cell count is elevated, and radiographs reveal soft-tissue swelling and a periosteal reaction in the great toe. Which of the following is the treatment of choice?

(A) Methotrexate
(B) Prednisone
(C) Ibuprofen
(D) Levofloxicin
(E) Indomethacin

171. A deer hunter from Montana had a fever, weakness, headache, and muscle pain last year. He does not remember what his treating doctor said the infection was, but he has a copy of an old prescription that showed he was on doxycycline (tetracycline) for 6 weeks and gentamicin (aminoglycoside) for 1 week. What infection should you add to his past medical history in his electronic patient record?

    (A) Inhalational anthrax
    (B) Brucellosis
    (C) Schistosomiasis
    (D) Lyme disease
    (E) Psittacosis

172. A patient with a sacral decubitus ulcer that probes to the bone had a fever. Blood cultures were drawn. The aerobic bottle had no bacteria. The anaerobic bottle had Gram-negative bacteria present on Gram stain. Which targeted antibiotic therapy would be best for this infection?

    (A) Metronidazole (Flagyl—nucleic acid synthesis blocker)
    (B) Amoxicillin (penicillin)
    (C) Cefazolin (first gen cephalosporin)
    (D) Gentamicin (aminoglycoside)
    (E) Vancomycin (aminoglycoside)

173. Some bacteria have found ways to "outsmart" antibiotics, like making an enzyme that "cuts penicillin." Which class of antibiotics is most able to counteract this enzymatic activity?

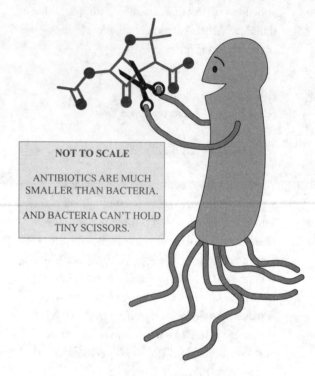

NOT TO SCALE

ANTIBIOTICS ARE MUCH SMALLER THAN BACTERIA.

AND BACTERIA CAN'T HOLD TINY SCISSORS.

    (A) First-generation cephalosporins
    (B) Second-generation cephalosporins
    (C) Carbapenems
    (D) Monobactams
    (E) Aminoglycosides

174. Which statement about the treatment of infective endocarditis is most accurate?

    (A) Beta-lactam drugs should not be used if there is a suitable alternative from another class.
    (B) Bacteriostatic antibiotics may be used as long as the therapy is for 2 weeks.
    (C) Frequently, prosthetic valves can be cleared of *Strep viridans* with antibiotic therapy.
    (D) Typical antibiotic therapy will last for 4 weeks or longer with a bactericidal agent.
    (E) Infection of a prosthetic valve by a staphylococcal organism should be treated with single antibiotic.

175. What is the correct order when performing an orthopedic physical examination?

(A) Inspection, range of motion, neurovascular testing, special tests, palpation

(B) Inspection, neurovascular testing, palpation, range of motion, special tests

(C) Inspection, special tests, range of motion, observation, palpation

(D) Inspection, palpation, range of motion, neurovascular testing, special tests

(E) Special tests, inspection, neurovascular testing, palpation, range of motion

176. A 32-year-old male presents with left knee pain and swelling after playing tennis. He notes the injury occurred while going for a ball, planting his foot, twisting sharply, and the onset of pain over the medial aspect of his left knee. Physical exam notes mild effusion with medial joint line tenderness and a palpable click with flexion. Which of the following imaging studies would be most specific to confirming your suspicions?

(A) Radiographs

(B) Arthroscopy

(C) MRI

(D) CT

(E) Ultrasound

177. Which is most specific question to ask in the history to help focus your physical exam and form your differential diagnosis for an orthopedic injury?

(A) Can you point to the area that hurts?

(B) How are your daily activities affected?

(C) Which movements or activities aggravate the pain?

(D) What was the mechanism of injury?

(E) What time did the injury occur?

178. What is the descriptive term used for a fracture with an unusual pattern or location due to an underlying weakness in the bone?

(A) Pathologic

(B) Avulsion

(C) Subluxated

(D) Fatigue

(E) Extended

179. Normal curvature of the lumbar spine is

(A) kyphosis.

(B) lumbosis.

(C) lordosis.

(D) spondylosis.

(E) forward.

180. A patient that demonstrates a positive apprehension test most likely has a history of which of the following?

(A) Rotator cuff tear

(B) Biceps tendinitis

(C) SLAP lesion

(D) Shoulder dislocation

(E) Acromioclavicular impingement

181. A 34-year-old male presents to the ED complaining of left leg swelling and severe pain after tripping over a curb while running. He is an avid runner, and the injury occurred 6 hours ago. He describes the pain as sharp and a 9/10 on the pain scale. Physical exam reveals a well-developed male in moderate distress. The left leg appears swollen with taut skin. There is pain with passive flexion of the knee and ankle. There is no pitting edema, temperature change, or erythema. The skin appears to be unbroken with no signs of infection. X-rays reveal a high fibular fracture. What is the most likely secondary concern based on the patient's symptoms?

(A) Cellulitis

(B) Deep venous thrombosis

(C) Necrotizing fasciitis

(D) Compartment syndrome

(E) Gravitational dermatitis

182. In the examination of a suspected anterior cruciate ligament tear in the knee, which of the following maneuvers would be the most useful and reliable?

(A) Posterior drawer sign

(B) Lachman test

(C) McMurray test

(D) Apley test

(E) Apprehension test

183. Which of the following is most likely an associated injury in a patient with a recurrent anterior
shoulder dislocation?

(A) Anterolateral humeral head compression
fracture
(B) Tear of the medial labrum
(C) Avulsion of the anteroinferior glenoid
labrum
(D) Glenoid bone loss
(E) Axillary artery occlusion

184. Which of the following terms best describes the
depicted fracture?

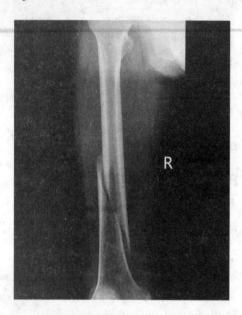

(A) Angulated
(B) Comminuted
(C) Transverse
(D) Spiral
(E) Linear

185. A 45-year-old male comes to clinic with right
heel pain after playing basketball today. He
describes the pain as excruciating. He describes
jumping up and hearing a loud, gunshot-like
sound with immediate pain. Temperature is
98°F (36.6°C), pulse rate is 72/min, and regular
respirations are 16/min unlabored, and blood
pressure is 120/70 mmHg. Exam of the right heel
shows swelling and palpable indentation along
the posterior calcaneus. Which of the following
physical exam tests will assist in the diagnosis?

(A) Homan test
(B) Talar tilt test
(C) Thompson test
(D) Compression test
(E) Haglund test

186. A patient complains of sensory loss in the volar
aspect of the thumb and forefinger. Exam confirms the sensory loss with weakness of wrist
extension. Which nerve root of the spinal cord is
suspected?

(A) C5
(B) C6
(C) C7
(D) T1
(E) T2

187. A 7-year-old male is referred to your orthopedic
clinic after his mother noticed him walking with
a limp. He and his mother deny any history of
trauma. On PE, there is atrophy of the gluteal
muscles and decreased range of motion of the
right hip, particularly with internal rotation and
abduction. Frog-leg X-rays reveal cessation of
growth at the right capital femoral epiphysis and
a smaller femoral head epiphysis with widening of the articular space on the right side. There
is also a linear radiolucency within the right
femoral head epiphysis. CBC, WBC, C-reactive
protein, and ESR are all normal. Which of the
following is the most likely diagnosis?

(A) Slipped capital femoral epiphysis
(B) Legg-Calve-Perthes disease
(C) Developmental dysplasia of the hip
(D) Osteomyelitis of the right hip
(E) Calcaneal deformity

188. Which of the following grades of muscle strength best defines full range of motion against gravity without resistance?

(A) 2

(B) 3

(C) 4

(D) 5

(E) 7

189. A 54-year-old male complains of neck stiffness, especially upon rising, sometimes having numbness and shooting pain in his left arm and hand. Which of the following history questions will best indicate a cervical herniated nucleus pulposus as a diagnosis and NOT thoracic outlet syndrome?

(A) Do you get numbness in your arm when you raise your hand?

(B) Is the pain made worse by coughing, straining, or laughing?

(C) Would you describe the pain as a burning sensation?

(D) Have you noticed your hands feeling colder or changing color with certain head movements?

(E) Do you have a history of blood clots?

190. An obese 12-year-old boy presents to your office with his mother, complaining of pain localized to the front of the tibia. The pain decreases with rest, but is aggravated by running and jumping activities. From the information given, what is the most likely diagnosis?

(A) Chondromalacia patella

(B) Medial meniscus tear

(C) Osgood-Schlatter disease

(D) Legg-Calve-Perthes disease

(E) Patellar tendonitis

191. What is the most common presentation of the limb following a posterior hip dislocation?

(A) Hip flexion, adduction, and internal rotation

(B) Hip flexion, abduction, and external rotation

(C) Hip extension, abduction, and internal rotation

(D) Hip extension, adduction, and external rotation

(E) Hip rotation, abduction, and internal rotation

192. The earliest findings of osteoarthritis of the knee on X-rays is

(A) subchondral bone cysts.

(B) areas of sclerosis.

(C) joint space narrowing.

(D) osteophyte formation.

(E) joint subluxation.

193. The arrow on the diagram below points to which of the following spinal lines?

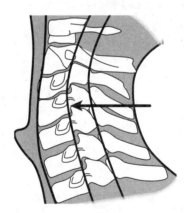

(A) Anterior vertebral line

(B) Posterior vertebral line

(C) Spinolaminal line

(D) Posterior spinous line

(E) Anterior spinal facet

194. A 32-year-old female professional golfer presents with a 3-week history of pain along her thumb and down her wrist. She denies any trauma and states that it is aggravated with any movement of her wrist and thumb. Her physical examination and X-rays are unremarkable. You perform the following test: What is the most likely diagnosis based on this exam finding?

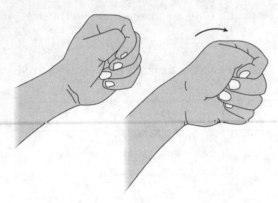

(A) Colle's fracture
(B) De Quervain tenosynovitis
(C) Carpal tunnel syndrome
(D) Ganglion cyst
(E) Cubital tunnel syndrome

195. A 13-year-old male presents to the emergency department with left lower extremity pain after falling off his bike. A plain film of his femur shows the following: Which type of Salter-Harris fracture would this be classified as?

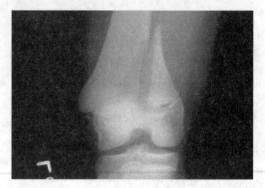

(A) I
(B) II
(C) III
(D) IV
(E) V

196. In a child in whom you suspect abuse, which of the following X-ray findings would highly raise your index of suspicion?

(A) Torus fracture
(B) Salter V fracture
(C) Posterior rib fracture
(D) Spiculated appearance in the distal humerus
(E) Buckle fracture

197. A 32-year-old female presents to your clinic for evaluation of an intermittent tingling sensation in her right arm and leg over the last 3 months. Additionally, she had an episode of decreased vision last month that spontaneously resolved over a few days. Which diagnostic study would be most helpful in confirming your suspected diagnosis?

    (A) Lumbar puncture
    (B) CT with contrast
    (C) EEG
    (D) MRI
    (E) Slit-lamp exam

198. Which of the following is the most prevalent pathogenesis for stroke?

    (A) Intracerebral
    (B) Subarachnoid
    (C) Ischemic
    (D) Aneurysmal
    (E) Neurogenic

199. You are doing rounds in the hospital and enter a room where the patient is not responding to verbal stimuli. You then attempt to awaken the patient and find that they only respond to vigorous persistent stimuli. Their response consists of a mere groan/mumble. What level of consciousness would this patient be classified as?

    (A) Comatose
    (B) Somnolent
    (C) Stuporous
    (D) Obtunded
    (E) REM

200. A 50-year-old male with a long history of poorly controlled hypertension and diabetes has a sudden onset of paralysis to his left arm, left leg, and the right side of his face. He was previously normal 2 hours prior. Increased DTRs and a Babinski sign are present on the left side. He is also unable to move his right eye laterally beyond midline. Sensory examination is normal except for decreased proprioception and vibratory sensation in the left arm and leg. Speech comprehension and production are intact. You order a non-contrast CT scan, and results are shown in the image below. What is the best emergent therapeutic treatment?

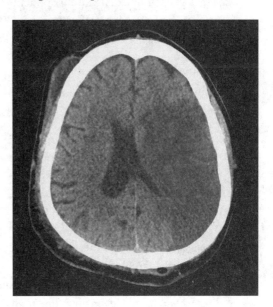

    (A) Aspirin
    (B) tPA
    (C) Coumadin (Warfarin)
    (D) Dabigatran (Pradaxa)
    (E) tTA

201. An 18-month-old is brought to the ER following a 3–5 minute episode of shaking that spontaneously resolved. Mother reports the child has had nasal congestion and a nonproductive cough for the past 3 days but is otherwise healthy. Vitals signs are as follows: temperature 102.7°F (oral), pulse 120 bpm, respirations 20. There are no meningeal signs present. The patient is moving all extremities normally and visually tracks you during the exam. What is the most appropriate management of this patient?

    (A) Order stat EEG
    (B) Prescribe medication for seizure prophylaxis
    (C) Perform an immediate lumbar puncture
    (D) Reassurance and symptomatic care
    (E) IV antibiotics

202. Which of the following is the most important principle to help differentiate seizures from syncopal episodes?

    (A) Total number of episodes
    (B) Type of movement during episode
    (C) Situation or setting of episode
    (D) Duration of episode
    (E) Loss of consciousness

203. A 19-year-old female presents to the ER with complaints of a throbbing headache on the right side. Her symptoms started early this morning and have been present ever since. She tried OTC medications with no relief. She has had similar headaches in the past and says that they usually go away with sleep. Her history is remarkable for photophobia, phonophobia, and nausea. Review of systems is otherwise negative. She is healthy and takes no other medications. Family history is significant for headaches in her mother. Physical exam, including vitals, shows no abnormalities. Urine pregnancy test is negative. Which of the following is the MOST appropriate initial therapy for this patient's condition?

    (A) Acetaminophen
    (B) Butalbital
    (C) Sumatriptan
    (D) Valproic acid
    (E) Naprosyn

204. What is the preferred initial diagnostic study in a patient presenting with a new and progressive cognitive complaint?

    (A) MRI
    (B) Electroencephalogram
    (C) PET scan with fluorodeoxyglucose
    (D) Genetic testing
    (E) Sleep study

205. A 72-year-old male is complaining of a left-sided headache. He also complains of some visual deficits in his left eye with loss of vision intermittently. On the physical exam, you note that the left side of the scalp extending forward to the temple is quite tender. He has a past medical history of diabetes mellitus. What initial test would you order to support your diagnosis?

    (A) Bilateral carotid ultrasound
    (B) Erythrocyte sedimentation rate
    (C) MRI of the brain
    (D) CBC with differential
    (E) Hemoglobin A1C

206. Upon stroking the lateral aspect of the sole from the heel to the ball of the foot, the great toe dorsiflexes and the other toes fan. This is a positive

    (A) Kernig sign.
    (B) Brudzinski sign.
    (C) Gower sign.
    (D) Trousseau sign.
    (E) Babinski sign.

207. A 400-pound patient develops confusion, ataxia, and nystagmus with lateral rectus muscle weakness a week after having gastric bypass surgery. What is the most appropriate initial treatment?

    (A) Glucose
    (B) Niacin
    (C) Thiamine
    (D) Vitamin B12
    (E) Vitamin K

208. The spinal tract responsible for vibration and fine touch intersects at which level?

(A) Midbrain
(B) Medulla
(C) Pons
(D) Spinal cord
(E) Anterior column

209. A 56-year-old female patient presents with symptoms of her legs being jumpy at night. Her husband notes her legs jerk, sometimes kicking him while she is sleeping. Her physical exam is noncontributory. Which of the following lab tests should be assessed to determine the cause of the diagnosis?

(A) AST/ALT
(B) TSH
(C) APOE genotyping
(D) Ferritin
(E) Dilantin level

210. In Parkinson's disease, the diagnostic criteria are bradykinesia and which type of tremor?

(A) Cerebellar
(B) Essential
(C) Intention
(D) Resting
(E) Isometric

211. A 38-year-old female presents with concerns of shaking of her hands when writing. She notes the shaking also occurs if she is stressed involving only her hands and head. She denies disturbance with gait, numbness, or tingling. Family history is significant for her grandmother having similar symptoms. On exam, a tremor is noted in hands which worsens when she writes her name. The most likely diagnosis is which of the following?

(A) Multiple sclerosis
(B) Focal torsion dystonia
(C) Benign essential tremor
(D) Huntington's disease
(E) Anxiety

212. Which of the following is a potential complication of classic Guillain-Barré syndrome?

(A) Dementia
(B) Respiratory failure
(C) Seizures
(D) Urinary incontinence
(E) Fecal incontinence

213. You are seeing a second grader whose mother brings him in to be evaluated for episodes in which he appears dazed and in a trance-like state. He also blinks his eyes in a strange, purposeful way during these episodes. He is doing poorly in school. During the exam, you have him hyperventilate, producing similar symptoms. What is your diagnosis?

(A) Absence seizure
(B) Complex partial seizure
(C) Myoclonic seizure
(D) Tonic-clonic seizure
(E) Atonic seizure

214. You are seeing an obese patient for a complaint of a burning and tingling sensation in the feet. Past medical history is notable for reflux. Family history is unknown. Physical exam reveals an absent vibratory sensation in both feet. Serum chemistry is notable for a fasting glucose of 300. What is the most likely diagnosis?

(A) Brown-Sequard syndrome
(B) Diabetic polyneuropathy
(C) L4-L5 radiculopathy
(D) Charcot-Marie-Tooth
(E) Alcoholism

215. Which of the following is a late complication of Parkinson's disease?

(A) Complex partial seizures
(B) Dementia
(C) Demyelination of the spinal cord
(D) Hydrocephalus
(E) Muscle atrophy

216. Which of the following is tested when you ask a patient to spell the word WORLD backwards?

    (A) Attention
    (B) Language
    (C) Orientation
    (D) Recall
    (E) Cognition

217. Which of the following is defined as a single seizure lasting more than 30 minutes or intermittent seizures lasting for more than 30 minutes in which the patient does not regain normal consciousness?

    (A) Absence seizure
    (B) Complex partial seizure
    (C) Simple partial seizure
    (D) Status epilepticus
    (E) Seizure flurries

218. A 25-year-old female is brought to the ER for a suicide attempt. She reports to you that her boyfriend broke up with her despite her pleading with him to stay. She says that she cut her arm to help numb the pain and loneliness from the breakup. She admits that she has had many "rocky" relationships in her past and that this is not the first time she has cut herself. She tells you that she has always felt "empty" inside. Her mother tells you that her daughter is emotionally labile and has a history of alcohol abuse in addition to the "cutting." What is the most likely diagnosis for this patient?

    (A) Antisocial personality disorder
    (B) Borderline personality disorder
    (C) Generalized anxiety disorder
    (D) Major depressive disorder
    (E) Obsessive-compulsive personality disorder

219. You are following a 23-year-old male with a past medical history significant for the left leg below the knee amputation that was performed after he was wounded in military combat about 9 months ago. He has had difficulty sleeping, frequent nightmares about the events that led to his injury, and flashbacks since the incident. What is the most appropriate treatment for this patient?

    (A) Benzodiazepines
    (B) Mood stabilizers
    (C) Selective serotonin reuptake inhibitors
    (D) Serotonin-norepinephrine reuptake inhibitors
    (E) Cognitive Behavioral Therapy

220. A patient seems preoccupied with concerns of being chased by the "Warner brothers" and tells you that they are calling out to him from "over there" as he points to the air vent. He is 19 y/o and was brought in by his sister who is concerned. She tells you that her brother has been acting "odd" for the last few months, talking about the "Warner brothers," and has mentioned other people being after him as well. She is unaware of anyone being after him. She also reports that her brother has stopped taking care of himself; he has reported hearing voices at home as well. There is no history of substance abuse. His urine drug screen and alcohol screen are negative. What is the most likely diagnosis?

    (A) Depression with psychotic features
    (B) Schizoaffective disorder
    (C) Schizophrenia
    (D) Schizoid personality disorder
    (E) Narcissistic personality disorder

221. The objective evaluation of the psychiatric patient primarily consists of

    (A) laboratory studies.
    (B) physical exam.
    (C) radiology studies.
    (D) brain CT scan.
    (E) mini mental status exam.

222. The treatment of choice for a patient with major depressive disorder and anxiety disorder would be which of the following?

(A) Atypical antipsychotic
(B) Benzodiazepine
(C) TCA
(D) SSRI
(E) Anti-anxiolytic

223. Which of the following is the best treatment of schizoaffective disorder?

(A) Antipsychotic agents
(B) Benzodiazepines
(C) Cognitive behavioral therapy
(D) MAOIs
(E) SSRI

224. Which of the following patients is most likely to be suicidal?

(A) A single 25-year-old female who is depressed
(B) A divorced 62-year-old male with alcohol dependence, recently diagnosed with cancer
(C) A separated 30-year-old male who had an argument with his new girlfriend
(D) A married 65-year-old female who is depressed
(E) A 30-year-old female with unilateral headaches

225. Which of the following disorders is characterized by the presence of two or more distinct personality states that recurrently take control of the individual's behavior?

(A) Factitious disorder
(B) Dissociative amnesia
(C) Dissociative disorder
(D) Dissociative identity disorder
(E) Anxiety-depression

226. The patient is conscious of their behavior and motivation in which of the following disorders?

(A) Body dysmorphic disorder
(B) Factitious disorder
(C) Functional neurological symptom disorder
(D) Somatic symptom disorder
(E) Schizoaffective disorder

227. What is the most commonly recommended treatment for personality disorders?

(A) Antipsychotics
(B) Benzodiazepines
(C) Electroconvulsive therapy
(D) Psychotherapy
(E) SSRIs

228. In a patient with bulimia nervosa, which of the following would be considered purging?

(A) Eating large amounts of food
(B) Fasting
(C) Excessive exercising
(D) Liquid diet
(E) Diuretic use

229. Which of the following would be considered a "negative" symptom in a schizophrenic patient?

(A) Avolition
(B) Delusions
(C) Disorganized speech
(D) Hallucinations
(E) Delusions

230. A patient informs you that she has intrusive thoughts that she has to lock her home repeatedly prior to leaving for work, which causes a significant level of distress. She states knowing this is irrational as she is aware she has already locked her door. What is the most likely diagnosis?

(A) Obsessive-compulsive disorder
(B) Obsessive-compulsive personality disorder
(C) Panic with agoraphobia
(D) Panic without agoraphobia
(E) Avoidant personality disorder

231. A 31-year-old male lost his job 2 weeks ago and according to his wife has become suddenly abusive. He has been sleeping more, withdrawn from friends and activities he previously enjoyed. Which of the following conditions must be considered in your differential diagnosis?

(A) Adjustment disorder
(B) Antisocial personality disorder
(C) Dysthymia
(D) Substance abuse
(E) Obsessive-compulsive personality disorder

232. A 36-year-old woman presents with complaints of muscle tension. She admits to increased stress in her life and sleep disturbances. She reports constant worry about her job and children. Her PMH is significant for an episode of major depressive disorder. She takes no medications. What is the most likely diagnosis?

    (A) Generalized anxiety disorder
    (B) Major depressive disorder
    (C) Panic disorder
    (D) Schizophrenia
    (E) Narcissistic disorder

233. Which of the following side effects is most likely to be reported with SSRIs?

    (A) Blurred vision
    (B) Diarrhea
    (C) Dizziness
    (D) Rash
    (E) Light-headedness

234. A patient has lost her sister and is experiencing intense sadness, insomnia, and difficulty concentrating. Which of the following would be important to differentiate between normal grief and major depression?

    (A) Length of time since loss
    (B) Past medical history
    (C) Presence of anhedonia
    (D) Socioeconomic status
    (E) Previous personal loss

235. In a patient with depressed mood, lack of concentration, and increased sleepiness, which of the following lab tests would be most appropriate in supporting your differential diagnosis?

    (A) LFT
    (B) BMP
    (C) TSH
    (D) Sedimentation rate
    (E) CBC

236. Which of the following patients is the best candidate for ECT?

    (A) A patient with depression and psychotic features and a comorbid history of mild COPD
    (B) A patient with refractory major depressive disorder and a comorbid history of STEMI 2 months ago
    (C) A patient with major depressive disorder and a comorbid history of uncontrolled HTN
    (D) A patient with severe panic disorder and comorbid history of CHF
    (E) A patient with new onset anxiety

237. A 55-year-old female presents with nearly 7 months of hallucinations and (per accompanying family) delusional thinking. In addition, she experienced periods of significant depression over this same time. With thorough questioning, you are able to clarify that for several of these weeks her hallucinations and delusions persisted despite her depression episodes resolving. Given this information, which of the following diagnoses is most likely?

    (A) Schizoaffective disorder
    (B) Schizophreniform
    (C) Schizophrenia
    (D) Major depressive disorder
    (E) Bipolar disorder

238. The set of observations and assessments resulting in a detailed and systematic description of a patient's current cognitive and behavioral state primarily consists of which of the following?

    (A) Laboratory studies
    (B) Mental status exam
    (C) Physical exam
    (D) Radiology studies
    (E) Psychosocial evaluation

239. A 25-year-old recently divorced female with no prior mental health history presents to the ED stating she feels that "she's going crazy" and reports rapid onset of SOB, shakiness, hot and cold sensations, and palpitations. The patient is organized but is clearly in distress. Which of the following pharmacologic interventions would provide the most relief for her acute symptoms?

    (A) Sertraline (Zoloft)
    (B) Alprazolam (Xanax)
    (C) Risperidone (Risperdal)
    (D) Amitriptyline (Elavil)
    (E) Klonopin (Clonazepam)

240. Which of the following is NOT an approved pharmacologic agent for medication-assisted treatment (MAT) in the setting of opioid dependence?

    (A) Buprenorphine
    (B) Clonidine
    (C) Naltrexone
    (D) Methadone
    (E) Alprazolam

241. You are consulted for pharmacologic intervention regarding a 55-year-old female who has been suffering with depressed mood and anxiety. In addition to her mental health concerns, she has past medical history significant for hypertension, hyperlipidemia, and seizure disorder. Which of the following pharmacologic interventions should be avoided in this patient?

    (A) Sertraline (Zoloft)
    (B) Duloxetine (Cymbalta)
    (C) Amitriptyline (Elavil)
    (D) Bupropion (Wellbutrin)
    (E) Alprazolam (Xanax)

242. A 65-year-old male with a history of diabetes and recent knee surgery presents with new onset dyspnea and intense chest pain that worsens with respiration. He has recently returned from a several hour trip to visit family. Which of the following EKG findings most correlates with the suspected condition?

    (A) Wolff-Parkinson-White
    (B) Ventricular premature complex
    (C) AV junctional rhythm
    (D) Sinus tachycardia
    (E) Normal sinus rhythm

243. Which of the following is a classification component in a patient meeting criteria for moderate persistent asthma who is not currently taking long-term control medications?

    (A) Extreme limitation with normal activity
    (B) Awakened > 1 night/week but not nightly
    (C) Short beta agonist use < 2 days/week
    (D) FEV1 > 80%
    (E) Chest pain using high-dose inhaled corticosteroids

244. A patient with an increased FEV1/FVC, FVC less than the lower limit of normal, and reduction in lung volume must suggest which of the following?

    (A) Restrictive pattern
    (B) Obstructive pattern
    (C) Mixed, obstructive, and restrictive
    (D) Normal spirometry study
    (E) Surgically absent lung lobe

245. You are asked to assess a patient with a history of asthma. Upon questioning, the patient reports that within the last 4 weeks, she has experienced daytime symptoms 3 times/week on average and finds herself using her PRN inhaler at roughly the same frequency (3 times/week). She states her symptoms do not interfere with her normal activities nor do they result in any nighttime awakenings. Based on this information, how best would you classify this patient's asthma control?

(A) Persistently controlled
(B) Partly controlled
(C) Not controlled
(D) Well controlled
(E) Intermittent control

246. A 19-month-old child presents with a hoarse, low-pitched barking cough and low-grade fever. Imaging later reveals a tapering of the upper trachea on frontal chest radiograph. What is the most likely diagnosis?

(A) Pertussis
(B) Foreign body aspiration
(C) Influenza
(D) Croup
(E) Bronchitis

247. The severity of ARDS is based on which of the following?

(A) SaO_2
(B) PaO_2/FiO_2
(C) PEEP
(D) DLCOE. Munich criteria

248. Which of the following is the most common cause of bronchiectasis worldwide?

(A) Collagen vascular disease
(B) Alpha1 antitrypsin deficiency
(C) Primary ciliary dyskinesia
(D) Post infectious
(E) Asthma

249. You are seeing a new patient for a physical exam who is generally well except for a chronic cough and some progressive shortness of breath on exertion. He recently retired from his job of 30 years as a stone countertop worker. Which of the following is the most likely diagnosis?

(A) Hypersensitivity pneumonitis
(B) Idiopathic pulmonary fibrosis
(C) Silicosis
(D) Sarcoidosis
(E) Pulmonary fibrosis

250. Which of the following pulmonary physical exam findings is most consistent with a patient presenting with pleural effusion?

(A) Increased breath sounds
(B) Increased tactile fremitus
(C) Dullness to percussion
(D) Symmetric chest expansion
(E) Reduced chest expansion

251. A tall, thin male with no prior PMH is brought to the emergency room with pleuritic chest pain and sudden severe shortness of breath. This occurred while playing a pickup game of basketball. There was no trauma. Physical exam is significant for decreased breath sounds on the right and hyperresonance to percussion. There is a loss of power in the ED and you have no imaging available. How should you manage this patient at this moment?

(A) Obtain an MRI
(B) VATS (Video-assisted thoracoscopic surgery)
(C) Intubate to protect the airway
(D) Place chest tube to decompress
(E) Mask ventilation

252. Prior to treating a person with a biologic medication, such as adalimumab (Humira), a person should be screened for which of the following?

(A) Asthma
(B) Cardiovascular disease
(C) Diabetes mellitus
(D) Tuberculosis
(E) Diabetes

253. In a person with suspected pleural effusion, which of the following standard X-ray views would be best to visualize the effusion?

(A) Apical lordotic view
(B) Lateral decubitus view
(C) Lateral view with full inspiration
(D) PA view with full inspiration
(E) Caudal view

254. A 2-year-old child is brought to the emergency department by his mother for altered mental status, cough, and difficulty breathing. On examination, you note a cyanotic, poorly responsive child, with audible inspiratory stridor, use of accessory muscles, and respirations of 55/minute. Pulse oximetry reveals oxygen saturation of 60%. Which of the following is the most appropriate NEXT step to perform in the management of this child?

(A) Immediate intubation
(B) IV antibiotics
(C) Nebulized albuterol
(D) Nebulized racemic epinephrine
(E) Nasal oxygen

255. A "thumb sign" on a lateral neck X-ray indicates which of the following?

(A) Bronchiolitis
(B) Epiglottitis
(C) Laryngitis
(D) Respiratory distress syndrome
(E) Foreign body

256. Which of the following radiographic features of pulmonary nodule is most commonly associated with malignancy?

(A) Central calcifications
(B) Spiculated appearance
(C) Smooth borders
(D) Presence of hamartoma
(E) Superior location

257. All newly diagnosed patients with COPD should have which of the following tests performed?

(A) Comprehensive metabolic panel
(B) Arterial blood gas
(C) Alpha-1 antitrypsin deficiency
(D) Bronchoprovocation
(E) Pulmonary function tests

258. A 3-month-old is brought into the clinic in January with a 2-day history of cough and increased work of breathing. Her oral intake has decreased. Physical exam reveals a pale infant with tachypnea, dry mouth, and costal retractions. She has diffuse expiratory wheezing. History is significant for prematurity of 34 weeks. What is the most likely cause?

(A) *Haemophilus influenzae*
(B) *Staphylococcus aureus*
(C) *Streptococcus pneumonia*
(D) Respiratory syncytial virus
(E) Collapsed lung

259. A patient who has asthma symptoms daily, awakens 1–2 × monthly and uses their rescue inhaler daily would be classified as having which of the following forms of asthma?

(A) Intermittent
(B) Mild persistent
(C) Moderate persistent
(D) Severe persistent
(E) Mixed persistent

260. A patient who has mild persistent asthma is best treated with which of the following?

(A) As needed short-acting beta 2 agonist
(B) Low-dose inhaled corticosteroid and as needed short-acting beta 2 agonist
(C) Low-dose inhaled corticosteroid/long-acting beta 2 agonist, and as needed short-acting beta 2 agonist
(D) Medium/high-dose inhaled corticosteroid/long-acting beta 2 agonist and as needed short-acting beta 2 agonist
(E) High-dose inhaled corticosteroid

261. A tall, thin male is brought to the emergency room with pleuritic chest pain and sudden, severe shortness of breath. This occurred while playing a pickup game of basketball. There was no trauma. Physical exam is significant for decreased breath sounds on the right and hyper-resonance to percussion. Vital signs as noted below. What is the most appropriate immediate clinical intervention?

BP 138/78 HR 88 RR 20

Pulse oximetry 93% on room air

(A) Obtain an MRI
(B) Place on low flow O2
(C) Intubate to protect the airway
(D) Place chest tube to decompress
(E) Place on inhaled corticosteroids

262. A 24-year-old school secretary presents with 4 days of cough with occasional yellow sputum, headache, nasal congestion, and sore throat. She is afebrile. She notes fatigue and has missed work. Physical exam is significant for minimal erythema in the posterior oropharynx, thin nasal secretions, and some mild lymphadenopathy. She has no rales or rhonchi. She does have bilateral wheezing that decreases after coughing. Which of the following is the most likely organism causing her symptoms?

(A) Legionella
(B) Parainfluenza
(C) *Streptococcus*
(D) Histoplasmosis
(E) *Staphylococcus*

263. You are in the emergency department evaluating a 30-year-old female who complains of dyspnea, nonproductive cough, chest pain, hemoptysis, and syncope. She denies orthopnea and paroxysmal nocturnal dyspnea. On a physical exam, you note jugular venous distention, a sternal heave, a loud P2, and crackles in the lung bases. Given this clinical picture and the following radiograph, what is the most likely diagnosis?

(A) Acute respiratory distress syndrome
(B) Pleural effusion
(C) Pneumonia
(D) Pulmonary nodule
(E) Pulmonary hypertension

264. Tension pneumothorax is associated with which of the following?

(A) Decreased air in the affected hemothorax on CXR
(B) Increased breath sounds on physical examination
(C) Increased tactile fremitus on physical examination
(D) Mediastinal shift to the contralateral side on CXR
(E) Pericarditis

265. The initial diagnostic study of choice for suspected pulmonary embolism is which of the following?

(A) CT-pulmonary angiography
(B) CXR
(C) Ventilation-perfusion scan
(D) Echocardiogram
(E) Chest X-ray

266. You are asked to assess a 13-year-old male, with no prior past medical history, complaining of several months of episodic wheezing and non-productive cough. Following additional history gathering and examination, you obtain PFTs that are consistent with airflow obstruction that is reversible following bronchodilator administration. Which of the following medications is the most appropriate initial scheduled treatment for the patient's condition?

    (A) Short-acting beta agonist (albuterol)
    (B) Low-dose inhaled corticosteroids (budesonide)
    (C) Leukotriene receptor agonist (montelukast)
    (D) Phosphodiesterase inhibitor (theophylline)
    (E) Fasenra (benralizumab)

267. Newly diagnosed symptomatic but stable COPD patients should first be treated with which of the following treatment options?

    (A) Xanthines
    (B) Phosphodiesterase inhibitor
    (C) Inhaled corticosteroids
    (D) Long-acting beta agonist (LABA)
    (E) Bronchodilator

268. What is the most common cause of Acute Respiratory Distress Syndrome?

    (A) Pulmonary contusion
    (B) Inhalational injury
    (C) Massive transfusion of blood
    (D) Sepsis
    (E) Pulmonary mass

269. A 27-year-old female is seen in the ED after witnessing a robbery. She developed chest pain and shortness of breath. Laboratory analysis reveals the following values:

    Na 130 mEq/L (normal 136–145)

    Cl 100 mEq/L (normal 96–106)

    ABG: pH 7.49 (normal 7.36–7.44)

    $PaCO_2$ 32 mmHg (normal 36–44)

    PaO_2 88 mmHg (normal 80–100)

    HCO_3 24 mEq/L (normal 23–30)

    Based on these results, this person has a

    (A) metabolic acidosis.
    (B) metabolic alkalosis.
    (C) respiratory acidosis.
    (D) respiratory alkalosis.
    (E) respiratory hyperventilation.

270. Which of the following is the initial treatment of choice in a person with pulmonary embolism without hemodynamic compromise?

    (A) Warfarin (Coumadin)
    (B) Low-molecular-weight heparin
    (C) Prednisone
    (D) Surgery
    (E) Trendelenburg position

271. Which of the following landmarks, when obscured on an upright chest X-ray, makes one suspect a pleural effusion is present?

    (A) Apex
    (B) Costophrenic angle
    (C) Heart border
    (D) Mediastinum
    (E) Diaphragmatic surface

272. A 58-year-old African-American male comes to your office for follow-up. His PMH is significant for GERD, HTN, and DM. He currently takes metformin, HCTZ, and Prilosec. He tells you that his blood sugar has been about 190 in the mornings. Today, his BP in the office is 136/82. The remainder of his physical exam is unremarkable. His urinalysis is positive for protein. His labs reveal a creatinine of 2.8 and an eGFR of 43. What is the most likely cause of his kidney disease?

    (A) Diabetes
    (B) Hypertension
    (C) Glomerulonephritis
    (D) Polycystic kidney disease
    (E) Sickle cell trait

273. A 62-year-old male presents with lower abdominal discomfort and oliguria × 3 days. On exam, his vitals are WNL. He has significant tenderness to palpation of the lower abdomen without rebound or guarding. A uniformly enlarged nontender prostate is noted on rectal exam, stool is heme negative. The remainder of the physical exam is unremarkable. Labs reveal a creatinine of 4.1, a BUN of 49, and an unremarkable urinalysis. CT exam of the abdomen and pelvis shows bilateral hydronephrosis. What is the most likely cause of his acute kidney injury?

    (A) Acute tubular necrosis
    (B) Acute interstitial nephritis
    (C) Dehydration
    (D) Post renal obstruction
    (E) Trauma

274. A 28-year-old male with a history of tobacco smoking who works in a gasoline distillery presents with dyspnea, hemoptysis, hematuria, reducedrenal function, and positive serum anti-GBM antibodies. Kidney biopsy shows crescentic glomerulonephritis, and immunofluorescence reveals smooth ribbon staining of IgG in the glomerular basement membrane. What is the most likely diagnosis?

    (A) Goodpasture syndrome
    (B) Henoch-Schönlein purpura
    (C) Pauci-immune GN
    (D) Systemic lupus erythematosus
    (E) Chronic kidney disease

275. Which of the following would raise your suspicion for chronic kidney disease?

    (A) BUN:Creatinine ratio of 20:1 once
    (B) GFR of 48 mL/min/1.732 for > 3 months
    (C) Microscopic hematuria for > 2 weeks
    (D) Proteinuria of 27 mg/day once
    (E) Hepatitis A

276. Which of the following statements is true regarding normal potassium homeostasis?

    (A) Approximately 50% of potassium is excreted by the kidney.
    (B) Up to 85% of potassium is reabsorbed in the distal convoluted tubule.
    (C) The majority of potassium is located extracellularly.
    (D) Potassium excretion is regulated by sodium delivery, tubular flow, and aldosterone.
    (E) Diarrhea is a symptom of imbalance.

277. A patient with a PMH of vasculitis presents for evaluation of hematuria and mild proteinuria. Labs are significant for positive ANCA, and kidney biopsy shows a crescentic glomerulonephritis with negative immunofluorescence. Which of the following is most likely the cause of the patient's abnormal urinalysis?

    (A) Henoch-Schonlein purpura
    (B) IgA nephropathy
    (C) Pauci-immune GN
    (D) Postinfectious GN
    (E) Kidney stones

278. A nephrotic syndrome will more likely show which of the following urinalysis findings?

    (A) High pH
    (B) Leukocytes
    (C) Microscopic hematuria
    (D) Dilute urine
    (E) Proteinuria

279. A 62-year-old female with a new diagnosis of type 2 diabetes presents to your clinic for a routine examination. She denies nocturia, dysuria, and hematuria. She takes metformin 500 mg two times per day. Her glucose diary shows good control. Her vital signs on presentation are blood pressure 160/90 mmHg, pulse 82 bpm, respirations 14 per minute, and temperature 98.6°F. Her examination is within normal limits. A urinalysis shows proteinuria. Which of the following is the most appropriate next step for this patient?

    (A) Add an ACE inhibitor to her medication regimen
    (B) Consult endocrinologist for optimal care
    (C) No changes; follow up in 6 months
    (D) Reduce the metformin to 250 mg twice per day
    (E) Check hemoglobin A1C

280. Which of the following diseases is diagnosed with "immunofluorescence" on immunostaining and can cause glomerulonephritis or nephrotic syndrome?

    (A) Pauci-immune GN
    (B) Goodpasture syndrome
    (C) Postinfectious GN
    (D) Systemic lupus erythematosus
    (E) Epididymitis

281. A 17-year-old high school senior is seen in the emergency department for sudden onset of excruciating (L) groin pain, which began 24 hours ago. The patient admits to a recent urinary tract infection. On PE, you note that the patient is sitting very still and the left side of the scrotum is markedly red, tender, swollen, and warm to palpation. There is slight relief from pain with elevation of (L) testicle. Which of the following is the most likely diagnosis?

    (A) Acute epididymitis
    (B) Acute balanitis
    (C) Testicular cancer
    (D) Acute prostatitis
    (E) Testicular torsion

282. A patient has been diagnosed with a category III renal cyst according to the Bosniak Classification System. Which of the following is the most accurate information to provide for the patient?

    (A) Malignancy risk for renal cancer is low and no follow-up is needed.
    (B) Malignancy risk for renal cancer is 50%.
    (C) Malignancy risk for renal cancer is 100%.
    (D) Surgical excision is recommended.
    (E) Cyst will resolve spontaneously.

283. A 41-year-old female presents to the ED with complaints of progressively worsening fever, intractable vomiting, left-sided flank pain, and dysuria × 3 days. Physical exam reveals a temperature of 101.4, heart rate of 109, and moderate CVA tenderness. The remainder of the physical exam is unremarkable. A urinalysis is obtained and shows large leukocytes and trace blood. The microscopy reveals 10–20 WBC per high power field, too numerous to count bacteria, and a few white blood cell casts. The WBC count on CBC is elevated. Pregnancy test is negative. What is the most appropriate treatment plan for this patient?

    (A) Carbapenems and discharge
    (B) Nitrofurantoin and admit
    (C) Penicillins and discharge
    (D) Ampicillin + gentamicin and admit
    (E) Vancomycin

284. A patient presents at 12 weeks gestation. Her BP is 160/110. Repeat blood pressure at the end of the visit is the same. She notes a history of "high bp" but never took medication. She has had sporadic health care her whole life. This is her first pregnancy. Which of the following treatment options is recommended?

(A) Aldomet (an adrenergic blocker)
(B) Lasix (loop diuretic)
(C) Lisinopril (ACE inhibitor)
(D) Hydralazine (vasodilator)
(E) Propranolol (beta-blocker)

285. A patient presents with complaints of a vaginal discharge with odor that worsens with intercourse. Her wet prep is positive for clue cells. Which of the following courses of treatment is most likely to relieve her symptoms?

(A) Oral fluconazole for 3 days
(B) Oral metronidazole for 7 days
(C) Oral tercanazole for 5 days
(D) Oral letrazole for 7 days
(E) Oral valacyclovir for 7 days

286. A patient presents to the office following an episode of painless bright red bleeding after intercourse. She is 28 weeks pregnant. Ultrasound would most likely indicate the presence of which of the following disorders?

(A) Placental abruption
(B) Placenta accreta
(C) Placenta percreta
(D) Placenta previa
(E) Placenta gravidarum

287. A 30-year-old patient presents to the office with complaints of irregular cycles. She has had two cycles in the last 8 months since stopping her oral contraceptives. She has moderate facial hair. Which of the following treatment regimens would be best if this patient does not desire pregnancy?

(A) Clomid plus metformin
(B) Combined oral contraceptive
(C) Letrozole
(D) Metformin alone
(E) Hysterectomy

288. A 22-year-old patient presents to the emergency department complaining of sudden-onset LLQ pain and dizziness that began a few hours ago. The pain is dull and achy, but persistent. She states that her menses are typically regular, but this month, her period is a week late. She is afebrile and hypotensive, and on an abdominal exam she is tender in the LLQ. Her pelvic exam demonstrated left adnexal tenderness. The beta-HCG is positive.

Which of the following is the most likely diagnosis of this patient?

(A) Endometriosis
(B) Ovarian cyst
(C) Ruptured ectopic pregnancy
(D) Pelvic inflammatory disease
(E) Adnexal mass

289. A 30-year-old patient presents with persistently longer than usual periods. Symptoms have been present over the past 6 months. Her past medical history is benign. She has a BMI of 22. Pregnancy test is negative. Initial laboratory workup is normal with exception of elevated TSH and low free T4. Pap is normal. Pelvic exam did not reveal any palpable abnormalities. What is the next best step in the management of this patient?

(A) Combination oral contraceptives
(B) Progesterone only contraceptives
(C) Thyroid replacement
(D) LNG-IUS
(E) Insert IUD

290. Pap smear results on a 36-year-old patient show LSIL (low-grade squamous intraepithelial lesion) with positive HPV (human papillomavirus). Which of the following is indicated in the next step of treatment?

(A) Evaluation with colposcopy
(B) Observation × 3 months
(C) Repeat pap 1 year
(D) Refer for treatment
(E) Hysteroscopy

291. A 19-year-old female presents to the ER with sudden onset severe right lower quadrant pain accompanied by nausea and vomiting. The pain is steadily worsening and radiates into her groin and thigh. Pregnancy test is negative. Bedside ultrasound shows a congested, edematous right adnexa. Which of the following is the appropriate treatment at this time?

(A) Uterine artery embolization/RSO (right salpingo-oophorectomy)
(B) Hysterosalpingogram
(C) Hysterectomy with BSO (bilateral salpingo-oophorectomy)
(D) Laparoscopic BSO (bilateral salpingo-oophorectomy)
(E) Turn to left lateral decubitus position

292. A 27-year-old patient complains of severely painful periods and painful intercourse, and now pelvic pain is occurring in between menstrual cycles as well. On a physical exam, you note nodularity on the uterosacral ligaments as well as a fixed uterus that is normal sized. Which of the following would confirm your diagnosis?

(A) Pelvic ultrasound
(B) Laparoscopy
(C) Pelvic CT
(D) Trial of continuous oral contraceptives
(E) Hysteroscopy

293. A 47-year-old woman presents with heavy menstrual bleeding, postcoital bleeding, and dyspareunia. She is having persistently worsening constipation. Physical exam reveals an enlarged uterus to approximately 15 weeks' size that is minimally tender to palpation. Ultrasound confirms the presence of multiple submucosal fibroids. She has a history of poorly controlled hypertension and migraine. Which of the following therapies would be the best first-line treatment?

(A) Copper containing LNG-IUS
(B) Combined oral contraceptives
(C) Androgens
(D) GnRH agonist
(E) Dilation and curettage

294. Hysterectomy with ovarian preservation may be an option for which of the following types of uterine cancer?

(A) Adenosarcoma
(B) Carcinosarcoma
(C) Endometrial stromal tumor
(D) Leiomyosarcoma
(E) Small cell carcinoma

295. You are seeing a 22-year-old patient for complaints of a mass in the vagina. She is unable to sit or stand comfortably. Your exam reveals a tender, erythematous palpable mass at the 8 o'clock position in the vagina. It feels fluctuant. Which of the following is the most appropriate antibiotic regimen to use post incision and drainage?

(A) Amoxicillin plus clavulanic acid
(B) Doxycycline plus amoxicillin
(C) Metronidazole plus amoxicillin
(D) Metronidazole alone
(E) Erythromycin

296. Which class of medications are indicated for the treatment of erectile dysfunction?

(A) SSRI
(B) Thiazide diuretics
(C) Beta-blockers
(D) Phosphodiesterase type 5 inhibitors
(E) Nitro-Dur

297. An 8-month-old male infant is brought into his pediatrician's office for continued evaluation of undescended testis. The parents were previously advised to wait for 4 months, but have not noted any change to his exam. Physical exam confirms that one of his testis is still undescended. As the provider, what advice would you give the parents for the next course of action in his management plan?

(A) Refer to a pediatric urologist
(B) Advise the parents to wait another 6 months
(C) Order an ultrasound
(D) Attempt to pull the testis down
(E) Order an MRI

298. Which is the most common etiology of organic erectile dysfunction?

    (A) Endocrine
    (B) Neurologic
    (C) Medication
    (D) Vascular
    (E) Psychological

299. A 30-year-old male presents with scrotal swelling over the past several months after being hit with a softball. He denies associated pain, hematuria, and penile discharge. On exam, he has hemiscrotal swelling that is nontender and transilluminates. There is no discrete palpable mass. Which of the following is the most likely diagnosis?

    (A) Hydrocele
    (B) Orchitis
    (C) Spermatocele
    (D) Varicocele
    (E) Hernia

300. The most lethal type of genitourinary cancer is which of the following?

    (A) Bladder cancer
    (B) Renal cell carcinoma
    (C) Prostate cancer
    (D) Testicular cancer
    (E) Penile cancer

ANSWER KEY
Practice Test 1

1. A	39. C	77. C	115. A	153. C	191. A	229. A	267. D
2. B	40. C	78. C	116. C	154. B	192. C	230. A	268. D
3. D	41. A	79. C	117. B	155. C	193. B	231. D	269. D
4. B	42. D	80. A	118. D	156. A	194. B	232. A	270. B
5. B	43. C	81. B	119. A	157. D	195. B	233. B	271. B
6. D	44. B	82. D	120. E	158. C	196. B	234. A	272. A
7. C	45. C	83. A	121. C	159. D	197. D	235. C	273. D
8. B	46. B	84. B	122. C	160. B	198. C	236. A	274. A
9. A	47. E	85. A	123. A	161. B	199. C	237. A	275. B
10. E	48. A	86. C	124. D	162. B	200. B	238. B	276. D
11. B	49. B	87. D	125. B	163. C	201. D	239. B	277. C
12. B	50. A	88. B	126. D	164. C	202. C	240. B	278. E
13. E	51. D	89. C	127. C	165. C	203. C	241. D	279. A
14. B	52. C	90. B	128. D	166. D	204. A	242. D	280. D
15. C	53. E	91. A	129. C	167. C	205. B	243. B	281. A
16. A	54. D	92. B	130. D	168. B	206. E	244. A	282. B
17. A	55. C	93. C	131. B	169. B	207. C	245. B	283. D
18. D	56. B	94. B	132. A	170. E	208. B	246. D	284. A
19. B	57. C	95. B	133. E	171. D	209. D	247. B	285. B
20. D	58. D	96. E	134. B	172. A	210. D	248. D	286. D
21. B	59. A	97. D	135. A	173. C	211. C	249. C	287. B
22. E	60. A	98. A	136. B	174. D	212. B	250. C	288. C
23. C	61. A	99. A	137. B	175. D	213. A	251. D	289. C
24. D	62. D	100. B	138. D	176. C	214. B	252. D	290. A
25. B	63. D	101. A	139. E	177. D	215. B	253. B	291. B
26. A	64. B	102. B	140. E	178. A	216. A	254. A	292. B
27. A	65. A	103. C	141. B	179. C	217. D	255. B	293. D
28. A	66. B	104. A	142. B	180. D	218. B	256. B	294. D
29. D	67. D	105. D	143. A	181. D	219. C	257. C	295. A
30. C	68. A	106. D	144. E	182. B	220. C	258. D	296. D
31. E	69. B	107. A	145. D	183. C	221. E	259. C	297. A
32. A	70. A	108. D	146. B	184. D	222. D	260. B	298. D
33. D	71. D	109. D	147. B	185. C	223. A	261. D	299. A
34. B	72. E	110. B	148. C	186. B	224. B	262. D	300. B
35. A	73. A	111. B	149. D	187. B	225. D	263. E	
36. B	74. D	112. B	150. A	188. B	226. B	264. D	
37. A	75. A	113. D	151. C	189. B	227. D	265. A	
38. A	76. C	114. A	152. B	190. C	228. E	266. B	

Answer Explanations

1. **(A)** The most likely scenario given viral syndrome 3-weeks prior and symptoms of heart failure is myocarditis. The patient does not have ST elevation; therefore, a STEMI is excluded. Pericarditis does not cause elevation in cardiac enzymes. His heart failure is related to myocarditis. Remember myocarditis can cause dilated cardiomyopathy. This patient, given his age, is unlikely to have an NSTEMI even though he has positive cardiac enzymes.

2. **(B)** The bilateral and chronic nature argue against all answers but venous stasis.

3. **(D)** Beta-blockers are not indicated. Understand when to initiate medical therapy for HTN, what the goals of treatment should be, and what drug classes should be considered based on a patient's characteristics, genetics, and medical history. A thiazide diuretic, Ca channel blocker, ACE inhibitor, or ARB is used as a first-line treatment for HTN.

4. **(B)** Hydralazine is not routinely used for the treatment of angina. It may cause tachycardia increasing myocardial demand. Beta-blockers decrease HR, BP, and contractility, which decreases the oxygen demand. Calcium channel blockers also reduce the HR and contractility so oxygen demand is decreased. (E) describes the effect of nitroglycerine.

5. **(B)** The best answer is a CCB to slow AV node conduction and slow the stable, narrow QRS tachycardia. This patient is stable, only the HR is high. Due to stability, cardioversion is not indicated, and amiodarone (antiarrhythmic) is best used on wide QRS tachycardia. Atrial flutter is narrow.

6. **(D)** This is hypertensive emergency. She will need treatment with IV sodium nitroprusside. Beta blockade should not be used because HR is less than 60. Also, a short-acting medication is preferred; metoprolol is not short acting.

7. **(C)** Abdominal ultrasound is useful for documentation of aneurysm size and can be used to screen patients at risk for developing an aortic aneurysm. In one large study, ultrasound screening of men ages 65–74 years was associated with a risk reduction in aneurysm-related death of 42%. For this reason, screening by ultrasound is recommended for men ages 65–75 years who have ever smoked. The child is more likely to have coarctation. Tamponade is associated with thoracic dissection, not an abdominal aneurysm. Women without risk factors do not get routine screening for this condition.

8. **(B)** A young woman with HTN, bruit, and renal failure is typical of renal artery stenosis. Understand who should be evaluated for secondary hypertension, and know potential causes of secondary hypertension.

9. **(A)** Aspirin is indicated for prevention for men with above 7.5% risk of MI in 10 years.

10. **(E)** This scenario of angina pain with increased frequency not relieved by rest or nitroglycerin is typical of either NSTEMI or unstable angina. In light of negative cardiac enzymes and ST depression, this can only be classified, at this point, as unstable angina.

11. **(B)** NSAIDS, including aspirin, are the first-line treatment for acute pericarditis. Steroids can be used if NSAIDS fail, but are not first line due to side effects.

12. **(B)** Diastolic dysfunction is the hallmark of hypertrophic cardiomyopathy. It is due to a genetic protein problem. Beta-blockers are the main treatment and do cause fatigue. BP is reduced while exercising and may result in syncope or arrest.

13. **(E)** This is a Stanford A dissection. 1–2% mortality in 24 hours. Urgent consultation is needed. Other therapies are complementary but would be expected to take a long time for results or for intervention to take effect.

14. **(B)** IV fluids will increase the blood volume resulting in increased preload. High intra-thoracic pressures will decrease the preload as it inhibits venous return to the heart. Nitroglycerin is a venodilator, which will decrease preload to the heart. Diuretics decrease blood volume, which will decrease preload.

15. **(C)** A person would have to have reasonable perfusion with normal BP and renal function to tolerate increase in two medications. The other patients have findings that suggest poor prognosis for CHF asynchrony, arrhythmia and malnutrition.

16. **(A)** Acute STEMI is caused by plaque rupture and total occlusion of a vessel. Fatty streak occurs under the endothelial lining and does not acutely occlude an artery. Triglycerides do not invade the subendothelial space (LDL does), and dissection of a coronary artery can cause MI but the descending aorta should not cause this.

17. **(A)** S4 is caused by pushing blood in during atrial contraction against a stiff left ventricle, as would be seen in HTN and LVH. Pericarditis may result in a rub, and postpartum cardiomyopathy should be dilated and would be associated with an S3.

18. **(D)** AV dissociation is described. Don't panic! Observation is too conservative; death from poor perfusion from bradycardia could result. Adenosine is for supraventricular tachycardias and does not promote resynchronization. Treatment would be a pacemaker as soon as possible.

19. **(B)** Based on the history and presentation, he most likely has a DVT. The first choice for diagnosis is a duplex ultrasound.

20. **(D)** This patient most likely has cardiac tamponade, based on the classic triad of hypotension, JVD, and muffled heart sounds. He also has a drop of greater than 10 mmHg in systolic pressures during inspiration, which is seen with tamponade.

21. **(B)** Stress tests compare rest and stress images of the heart to try and predict areas of ischemia that worsen with increased demand on the heart. In this case, pharmacologic nuclear test is preferred because the patient can't exercise enough to stress the heart adequately and she has ECG changes at baseline.

22. **(E)** S3 comes from extra blood volume "sloshing in" to the LV. Heart failure with low EF is the best answer. Hypertrophic cardiomyopathy is most likely to cause an S4 from pushing against a stiff heart.

23. **(C)** With coarctation of the aorta, the left ventricle works harder to pump blood through the narrowed aorta, and blood pressure increases in the left ventricle.

24. **(D)** Congestive heart failure is the most common serious complication of infective endocarditis and is the leading cause of death among patients with this infection. Roth spots, although classically associated with infective endocarditis, are a nonspecific ophthalmologic finding with multiple etiologies.

25. **(B)** Keeping the same dose will not give relief from muscle pain. Switching to another class is not likely to reduce risk. Diet and exercise alone will unlikely elicit necessary LDL reduction.

26. **(A)** Granulomas and arrhythmia in a young patient with heart failure suggests sarcoidosis, an infiltrative type of nonischemic cardiomyopathy. Chemotherapy and alcohol typically cause dilated type. The patient with ST elevation has ischemic heart disease.

27. **(A)** Transthoracic echo is less expensive, less invasive, and more reliable and gives more information. MRI is the second best choice. Fluid sampling has low sensitivity and specificity. EKG can suggest but not detect effusion, and it cannot determine the degree of the effusion.

28. **(A)** TR comes primarily from heart failure. Its main diagnosis and symptoms (sx) are JVD, ascites, edema in legs, and increased murmur during inspiration. The other choices represent pulmonary stenosis, aortic stenosis, and HOCM (obstructive cardiomyopathy).

29. **(D)** ACE inhibitors can increase potassium. Checking after dosage change in susceptible patients is advisable.

30. **(C)** Right coronary feeds the inferior wall of LV. The objective here is to identify which coronary arteries supply which parts of the heart.

31. **(E)** Atrial flutter (AFl) is a cardiac dysrhythmia characterized by rapid and regular depolarization of the atria that appears as a sawtooth pattern on the electrocardiogram (ECG). The initial treatment for AFl focuses on rate control of the ventricular response with AV nodal blocking agents such as beta-blockers and calcium channel blockers. If rhythm identification is unclear and the patient is stable, adenosine or Valsalva maneuver may be used to slow conduction through the AV node such that the atrial flutter waves are more readily apparent.

32. **(A)** Goal BP 130/90. Patients should have BP more than 20/10 above goal in order to use two drugs at onset of treatment. More than one medication is required in many hypertensive patients to reach blood pressure (BP) goals. Initial treatment with two agents has been recommended for patients whose BP level is > 20/10 mmHg above goal. Calcium channel blockers (CCBs) are effective antihypertensive agents, and evidence suggests that a CCB/ACEI combination is well tolerated and also decreases the risk of cardiovascular and renal disease.

33. **(D)** The 22-year-old with syncope needs an echo and possibly an EP study. He may be at risk for sudden death, and stress test is not best for him; also has an abnormal EKG at baseline. The 68-year-old is having an MI and needs cath. The 43-year-old is not likely able to run on a treadmill and should get a pharmacologic stress test.

34. **(B)** Beta-blockers, ACE, ARB, and mineralcorticoid blockers reduce mortality. Diuretics do not. Create treatment plans for patients with acute and chronic types of heart failure to include medication, diet, and activity.

35. **(A)** The first symptom of pulmonary hypertension is usually shortness of breath with everyday activities. Right ventricular hypertrophy (RVH) is a pathologic increase in muscle mass of the right ventricle in response to pressure overload, most commonly due to severe lung disease. Affected patients will present with symptoms due to pulmonary hypertension and have exertional chest pain, peripheral edema, exertional syncope, and right upper quadrant pain. Ejection clicks are high-pitched sounds that occur at the moment of maximal opening of the aortic or pulmonary valves. The sounds occur in the presence of a dilated aorta or pulmonary artery or in the presence of a bicuspid or flexible stenotic aortic or pulmonary valve.

36. **(B)** Understand when to initiate medical therapy for HTN, what the goals of treatment should be, and what drug classes should be considered. Evaluate which drug classes will reduce the patient's risk of death from a cardiovascular cause. Accomplish trial suggests CCB and ACE are the best combination. Patient needs two drugs since they are more than 20/10 from goal BP.

37. **(A)** A type 2 myocardial infarction (MI) is identified when myocardial necrosis occurs due to imbalance between myocardial oxygen supply and demand. Myocardial supply/demand mismatch without atherothrombosis is characteristic of type 2 MI. The key features to diagnose a type 2 MI include:

   - An elevated and changing troponin value
   - Clinical features inconsistent with type 1 acute MI
   - Clinical conditions known to increase the oxygen demand or decrease the oxygen supply like tachycardia
   - Potentially confounding clinical conditions or comorbidities that are potentially associated or known to be associated with myocardial injury
   - Absence of symptoms and/or signs indicating other nonischemic causes of troponin elevations like myocarditis

38. **(A)** Percutaneous coronary interventions (PCI) are widely accepted as the treatment of choice for STEMI in centers that can perform primary PCI rapidly and effectively. However, very early after the onset of symptoms, when the thrombus in the infarct-related artery is still soft, fibrinolysis may recanalize the artery as quickly as, if not more quickly than, primary PCI. This is true in the first hour and possibly the first 3 hours after symptom onset. Therefore, fibrinolysis is an acceptable treatment in these early time points. However, after 3 hours, primary PCI has a clear benefit over fibrinolysis and should be considered the preferred therapy, and so this patient should be taken to the lab for intervention.

39. **(C)** When an acute thrombotic coronary event causes ST-segment elevation on an ECG, there is a complete and persistent occlusion of blood flow. Coronary atherosclerosis and presence of thin cap fibroatheroma or one with no cap can result in sudden onset plaque rupture.

40. **(C)** Western diet leads to inflammation. Refined carbs are low in cholesterol but are not consistently found to be healthier than meat.

41. **(A)** Major side effects patients should know about when adding a statin are myalgia and LFT elevation.

42. **(D)** The diagnosis of Candida infection is established by visualization of pseudohyphae or hyphae on wet mount (saline and 10% KOH), tissue Gram stain, periodic acid-Schiff stain, or methenamine silver stain in the presence of inflammation.

43. **(C)** Herpes zoster ophthalmicus (HZO) is due to the reactivation of the varicella virus within the trigeminal nerve. Treatment involves use of acyclovir, if it can be started within 48 to 72 hours of the first vesicle appearance. In addition, oral steroids can also be used and have been shown to reduce the duration of the disease. Rapid referral to ophthalmology for confirmation of diagnosis along with early treatment are important.

44. **(B)** Erysipelas is a group A streptococcal cellulitis involving the skin and is more superficial than cellulitis. Commonly affected sites are the face and the lower extremities. Sudden onset of fever, chills, and malaise is typically followed by the appearance of erythematous,

edematous, and painful plaques with sharp and elevated borders. Regional lymphadenopathy may be present. Patients with chronic lymphedema are prone to repeated infections.

45. **(C)** Topical 5% permethrin cream is commonly used to treat scabies. Apply from the neck to the toes overnight and then wash off, repeating treatment in 1 week. Scabies is caused by *Sarcoptes scabiei* var. hominis, a mite within the epidermal layers. Transmission occurs after skin contact with an infected individual or from clothing and bedding.

46. **(B)** Guttate psoriasis, common in children and young adults, presents with an abrupt eruption of 2- to 5-mm erythematous scaly papules on the trunk and extremities. A preceding respiratory infection, usually streptococcal pharyngitis, can be a precipitant of guttate psoriasis.

47. **(E)** Atopic dermatitis presents in three stages: infantile, childhood, and adult. Infantile begins after 2 months of age and is symmetrically distributed on the cheeks, scalp, neck, forehead, and extensor surfaces of the extremities. The lesions begin as erythema or papules, but with persistent itching and rubbing, they become thin plaques, exudative, and crusted. Childhood atopic dermatitis frequently involves the face, neck, antecubital areas, and trunk. The scratching induces plaque lichenification. Adult atopic dermatitis is less specific but can present with a childhood-like distribution, papular lesions that coalesce into plaques.

48. **(A)** Systemic antifungals are required to treat tinea capitis and tinea unguium infections. Due to the long-term treatment requirement and potential side effects, referral to a dermatologist is recommended.

49. **(B)** The indications for Mohs surgery have been defined based on pathologic tumor characteristics, tumor size, clinical tumor characteristics, and certain host characteristics. Tumor location can be subdivided into three areas: high risk, medium risk, and low risk. High-risk areas include eyelids, eyebrows, nose, lips, chin, ear, preauricular skin, temples, genitalia, hands, feet, nail units, ankles, and nipples or areola. Medium-risk areas include the head and neck areas (cheeks, forehead, scalp, neck, and jawline) and pretibial surface. Low-risk areas include the trunk and extremities, excluding the areas included in high- and medium-risk areas.

50. **(A)** A carbuncle is an extremely painful inflammatory abscess based on a hair follicle. *S. aureus* is the causative organism. Predisposing conditions can include diabetes mellitus, HIV, and injection drug use.

51. **(D)** Tinea versicolor is usually asymptomatic. The treatment is mostly for cosmetic reasons. Patients may apply selenium sulfide 2.5% lotion or shampoo or zinc pyrithione shampoo to the involved areas daily for 2 weeks. Specific exposure times are variable and inconclusive.

52. **(C)** Erythema multiforme (EM) begins with symmetric, erythematous, sharply defined extremity or trunk macules and evolves into a target shaped or "bull's eye" morphology. Bullae may appear in the central dusky area (bullous EM). The typical target shaped lesions allow a diagnosis to be made clinically. The rash usually persists for 1 to 4 weeks. Dermatology consult is warranted if bullae are present.

53. **(E)** Cellulitis caused by a dog or cat bite is typically caused by *Pasteurella multocida*. *Pasteurella multocida* is found normally in the respiratory tract of many domestic and wild animals. When humans sustain a penetrating bite or scratch, most often by a cat, a rapidly destructive local soft tissue infection results.

54. **(D)** Oropharyngeal candidiasis (thrush) is usually painful and appears as white curd-like patches overlying erythematous mucosa. Because these white areas are easily rubbed off, only the underlying erythema may be seen. Oral candidiasis is commonly associated with the following factors: use of dentures, poor oral hygiene, diabetes mellitus, anemia, steroid use, antibiotic use, chemotherapy, or local irradiation.

55. **(C)** Syphilis can become the "great imitator" in the secondary and subsequent phases of the disease. **Early infectious syphilis** includes primary lesions (chancre and regional lymphadenopathy). Secondary lesions (commonly involving skin and mucous membranes, occasionally bone and central nervous system) usually appear during secondary syphilis.

    Late (tertiary) syphilis consists of lesions involving skin, bones, and viscera; cardiovascular disease (primarily aortitis); and a variety of CNS and ocular syndromes. Between these stages are symptom-free latent phases. In early latent syphilis, which is defined as the symptom-free interval lasting up to 1 year after initial infection, infectious lesions can recur.

56. **(B)** If a scale is present, scrape it and perform a KOH prep to determine if it is fungal. KOH is reasonably sensitive, easy, and inexpensive. It is preferred in simple cases such as this one. Treating a fungal infection with a corticosteroid will likely cause a severe flare and make the treatment more difficult. Never use a "combination product," such as Lotrisone, when you are unsure of the diagnosis. You are more likely to make diagnosis and further treatment more difficult. Culture takes 1–3 weeks, which would delay care.

57. **(C)** Higher urine calcium excretion increases the likelihood of formation of calcium oxalate and calcium phosphate stones.

58. **(D)** PCOS is characterized by chronic anovulation, polycystic ovaries, and hyperandrogenism. It is associated with hirsutism and obesity, as well as an increased risk of diabetes mellitus, cardiovascular disease, and metabolic syndrome. Unrecognized or untreated PCOS is a risk factor for cardiovascular disease.

59. **(A)** Manifestations of hypocalcemia vary from subtle to life-threatening:

    - Patients may complain of fatigue, irritability, depression, anxiety, cognitive impairment, lethargy, and paresthesias in the perioral area, hands, and feet.
    - More severe manifestations include muscle weakness or cramps, carpopedal spasm, convulsions, tetany, laryngospasm, and stridor.

60. **(A)** The initial step in the diagnostic evaluation for suspected adrenal insufficiency is to perform a rapid ACTH stimulation test to ascertain whether there is adrenal insufficiency. Then, the plasma ACTH level differentiates between primary and secondary adrenal insufficiency. Serum DHEA levels < 1,000 ng/mL (< 350 nmol/L) are found in 100% of patients with adrenal insufficiency.

61. **(A)** The diagnosis of Addison's disease may be delayed, since many early symptoms are nonspecific. Over 90% of patients complain of fatigue, reduced stamina, weakness, anorexia, and weight loss.

62. **(D)** MRI detected prolactinoma, a tumor on the pituitary gland.

63. **(D)** Serum TSH measurement is the most widely employed test to determine whether thyroid dysfunction exists.

64. **(B)** Patients should have an A1C goal of < 7%; less or more stringent goals can be considered in special circumstances.

65. **(A)** ACTH is a 39-amino-acid polypeptide secreted by the anterior pituitary. Its half-life is ~10 minutes. ACTH regulates both the basal secretion of glucocorticoids and increased secretion provoked by stress.

66. **(B)** Typical manifestations in adulthood include short stature, hypogonadism, webbed neck, and high-archedness. Females with Turner syndrome have an increased risk of aortic coarctation, bicupalate, wide-spaced nipples, hypertension, and kidney abnormalities. Cardiac abnormalities are more common in patients with a webbed neck.

67. **(D)** Symptoms of subacute thyroiditis are often overlooked because the symptoms can mimic pharyngitis. The peak incidence occurs at 30–50 years. Women are affected three times more frequently than men.

68. **(A)** Klinefelter syndrome is the most common chromosomal disorder associated with testicular dysfunction and male infertility. Testosterone is decreased and estradiol is increased, leading to clinical features of undervirilization and gynecomastia.

69. **(B)** Syndromes of hormone excess can be caused by growth of endocrine cells, autoimmune disorders, and excess hormone administration.

70. **(A)** Thyroid cancer usually presents as a firm, diffuse nontender nodule in the thyroid. Most thyroid carcinomas are asymptomatic, but large thyroid cancers can cause neck discomfort, dysphagia, or hoarseness.

71. **(D)** Intense thirst, especially for ice water and polyuria (2-20 L) are symptoms of diabetes insipidus.

72. **(E)** Patients with hypothyroidism typically have symptoms that include weight gain, fatigue, lethargy, depression, weakness, dyspnea on exertion, arthralgias or myalgias, muscle cramps, menorrhagia, constipation, dry skin, headache, paresthesias, cold intolerance, carpal tunnel syndrome, and Raynaud syndrome.

73. **(A)** The electrolyte disturbances in Addison's disease are due to diminished secretion of cortisol and aldosterone.

74. **(D)** The symptoms and signs of Cushing's syndrome result directly from chronic exposure to excess glucocorticoids.

75. **(A)** In Graves' thyrotoxicosis, the measurement of TPO antibodies may be useful if the diagnosis is unclear clinically, but not needed routinely. In Graves' disease, the TSH level is suppressed, and total and unbound thyroid hormone levels are increased.

76. **(C)** Symptoms of elevated prolactin levels include irregular or absent menstrual periods, infertility, menopausal symptoms (hot flashes and vaginal dryness), and, after several years, osteoporosis. High prolactin levels can also cause discharge from the breasts.

77. **(C)** PTU is treatment of choice for hyperthyroidism in the first trimester of pregnancy.

78. **(C)** The level of glycated hemoglobin is related to the mean plasma glucose level during the previous 1-3 months. The HbA1c level can be used to estimate the average blood glucose levels.

79. **(C)** These are dendritic lesions consistent with herpes simplex keratitis. This can lead to scarring of the cornea.

80. **(A)** Significant corneal injury, especially if associated with an alkali burn, may lead to scarring and vision loss.

81. **(B)** Hyphemas are characterized by a history of eye trauma or risk factor for nontraumatic hyphema, increased intraocular pressure, and decreased vision. Hyphemas are classified according to the amount of blood in the anterior chamber:

   - Grade 1: Less than one-third of the anterior chamber
   - Grade 2: One-third to one-half of the anterior chamber
   - Grade 3: One-half filled to almost completely filled anterior chamber
   - Grade 4: Completely filled anterior chamber

82. **(D)** The most frequent sites of caries are the occlusal surfaces of the first and second permanent molars.

83. **(A)** Medical treatment is directed toward lowering intraocular pressure. Prostaglandin analog eye drops are commonly used as first-line therapy because of their efficacy, dosing frequency, and lack of systemic side effects. Topical beta-adrenergic blocking agents may be used alone or in combination with a prostaglandin analog.

84. **(B)** A positive Dix-Hallpike test produces a paroxysmal upbeating-torsional nystagmus. The examiner observes the patient's eyes for the characteristic nystagmus that generally lasts for the duration of the patient's vertigo.

85. **(A)** Amoxicillin is a first-choice antibiotic dose: 1 g orally every 8 hours for 5–7 days.

86. **(C)** The image provided in the question shows no evidence of infection or trauma.

87. **(D)** Squamous cell carcinoma of the tongue is the most common site for intraoral cancers.

88. **(B)** Oral candidiasis (thrush) is usually painful and looks like creamy-white curd-like patches overlying erythematous mucosa, and these white areas are easily rubbed off. If so, only the erythematous base will be noted.

89. **(C)** Intranasal examination should be performed to rule out septal hematoma, which appears as a widening of the anterior septum visible just posterior to the columella. An untreated hematoma will result in loss of the nasal cartilage with resultant saddle nose deformity. Septal hematomas may become infected, with *S. aureus* most commonly, and should be drained. The drained fluid should be sent for culture.

90. **(B)** Intranasal corticosteroid sprays are the primary treatment for allergic rhinitis. They are more effective and frequently less expensive than antihistamines. Corticosteroid sprays may also shrink hypertrophic nasal mucosa and nasal polyps, thereby providing improved nasal airway drainage.

91. **(A)** Aphthous ulcers are shallow, painful mucosal ulcers. A prodromal burning sensation may be noted 2 to 48 hours before an ulcer is noted. The initial lesion is a small white papule that ulcerates and enlarges over 48 to 72 hours. Lesions are typically round or ovoid with a raised yellow border and surrounding erythema. Multiple aphthous ulcers may occur on the lips, tongue, buccal mucosa, floor of the mouth, or soft palate. Spontaneous healing occurs in 7 to 10 days.

92. **(B)** Referral to ENT is appropriate to support symptom management and prevent complications. In typical acute mastoiditis, purulent exudate collects in the mastoid producing pressure that may result in erosion of the surrounding bone and formation of abscess-like cavities that are usually evident on CT. Patients typically present with pain, erythema, and swelling of the mastoid process along with displacement of the pinna, usually in conjunction with the typical signs and symptoms of acute middle-ear infection.

93. **(C)** There is a strong familial tendency in primary open-angle glaucoma, and close relatives of affected individuals should undergo regular screening. Prostaglandin analog eye drops are commonly used as first-line therapy.

94. **(B)** *P. aeruginosa* infections of the ears vary from mild swimmer's ear to serious life-threatening infections with neurologic sequelae. Swimmer's ear is common among children and results from infection of moist macerated skin of the external ear canal.

95. **(B)** Conductive hearing loss can occur from obstruction of the external auditory canal by cerumen, debris, and foreign bodies; swelling of the lining of the canal; atresia or neoplasms of the canal; perforations of the tympanic membrane; disruption of the ossicular bones, as occurs with necrosis of the long process of the incus in trauma or infection.

96. **(E)** In central retinal artery occlusion (CRAO), the typical patient experiences a sudden painless monocular loss of vision, either segmental or complete. A cherry-red spot is a finding in the macula of the eye in central retinal artery occlusion.

97. **(D)** Ménière's triad—vertigo, tinnitus, and reduced hearing. Spells typically last for minutes to hours (rarely longer than 4–5 hours) and occasionally up to a day.

98. **(A)** Ear pinna hematomas must undergo incision and drainage or large-needle aspiration using sterile technique, followed by a pressure dressing. After ED drainage, the patient is treated with antistaphylococcal antibiotics and referred to ENT or plastic surgery for follow-up.

99. **(A)** Acute epiglottitis is an infection in which the inflamed epiglottis and surrounding tissues obstruct the airway; *Haemophilus influenzae* type B is one of several causes. Onset is sudden, with fever, sore throat, hoarseness, muffled cough, rapid progression to inspiratory stridor, and use of accessory muscle to breath. The hallmark of the disease is an inflamed, swollen, cherry-red epiglottis that protrudes into the airway.

100. **(B)** Pilonidal cysts develop when hair becomes entrapped within a cyst in the sacrococcygeal region. Next an abscess forms, causing pain, swelling, and erythema. It may be asymptomatic prior to abscess formation. The treatment of a pilonidal abscess is incision and drainage.

101. **(A)** Hepatitis A is commonly linked to consumption of unwashed fruits and vegetables. It has an incubation period of ~4 weeks.

102. **(B)** The typical symptom of gastroesophageal reflux disease (GERD) is heartburn. This typically occurs 30–60 minutes after meals and when reclining. Most reflux episodes occur during transient relaxations of the lower esophageal sphincter that are triggered by gastric distention by a vagovagal reflex. Patients often report relief from taking antacids. Other symptoms of GERD include dyspepsia, dysphagia, belching, chest pain, cough, and hoarseness.

103. **(C)** Testing for IBS should include selected laboratory tests in patients with chronic diarrhea to exclude other diagnoses. A complete blood count should be obtained to screen for

iron deficiency anemia. Serologic testing for celiac disease (TG IgA) should be performed. Consider a fecal calprotectin level is recommended to screen for inflammatory bowel disease; a value of greater than 50 mcg/g may warrant further endoscopic evaluation.

104. **(A)** The diagnosis of Whipple disease requires evidence of infection with *T. whipplei.* Biopsies of multiple areas of the duodenum and jejunum are recommended to avoid sampling error. The tissue should be stained with PAS, and PCR analysis is performed for confirmation of findings.

105. **(D)** Ulcerative colitis with heralding symptoms of bloody diarrhea and fecal urgency. The clinical course is typically one of exacerbations and remissions. Sigmoidoscopy or colonoscopy demonstrates loss of vascular markings, erythema, friability, and exudates in a continuous fashion extending from the rectum proximally.

106. **(D)** Decisions regarding choice of therapy depend on disease location and severity. Distal disease (descending colon and beyond) can often be treated with topical preparations (suppositories or enemas). Options include topical preparations of 5-ASA or corticosteroids (suppositories, enemas, or foams) or oral 5-ASA preparations. More proximal or severe disease requires systemic therapy.

107. **(A)** Achalasia is characterized by progressive dilatation and sigmoid deformity of the esophagus with hypertrophy of the lower esophageal sphincter. Symptoms may include dysphagia, regurgitation, chest pain, and weight loss. Patients frequently report solid and liquid food dysphagia. Regurgitation occurs when food, fluid, and secretions are retained in the dilated esophagus.

108. **(D)** Manifestations of gastroparesis may be chronic or intermittent with symptoms of early satiety, bloating, nausea, and vomiting (1–3 hours after meals). Abdominal radiography shows dilatation of the stomach, esophagus, small intestine, or colon resembling ileus or mechanical obstruction.

109. **(D)** Initial therapy for patients with troublesome reflux symptoms and known complications (e.g., eczema, asthma) includes once-daily oral proton pump inhibitor taken 30 minutes before breakfast for 4–8 weeks. Once-daily proton pump inhibitors achieve adequate control of heartburn in 80–90% of patients.

110. **(B)** An ultrasound will usually show gallstones.

111. **(B)** Infection with *Giardia lamblia* can present as either acute or chronic diarrhea. Giardiasis usually occurs in patients with exposure to infected water supplies, although person-to-person transmission can occur. Symptoms usually include diarrhea, nausea, abdominal cramps, bloating, flatulence, and foul-smelling stools.

112. **(B)** Diarrhea is the most common manifestation caused by *C. difficile.* Stools are almost never grossly bloody and range from soft and unformed to watery or mucoid in consistency, with a characteristic odor. Discontinuation of any ongoing antimicrobial administration is recommended as the first step in treatment of *Clostridium difficile* infection.

113. **(D)** An *H. pylori*–stool antigen (HpSA) test for the detection of *H. pylori* has been suggested as a valuable option with a high-potential role in the diagnosis after eradication therapy. The C-urea breath test in older subjects is also an option.

114. **(A)** Colonoscopy is commonly used to exclude malignancy and make a positive diagnosis in older patients or those with significant and suspicious symptoms.

115. **(A)** Serum amylase and lipase are the principal laboratory tests that aid in the diagnosis of acute pancreatitis. Elevations greater than three times the upper limit of normal are typically used to diagnose acute pancreatitis.

116. **(C)** Choledocolithiais after cholecystecomy is not associated with the development of chronic pancreatitis. Chronic pancreatitis is a syndrome of pancreatic inflammation lasting over 6 months. Until recently, alcohol was considered to be the primary etiology. Potential complications include development of an acute fluid collection and pancreatic ascites from a pancreatic duct disruption. CT scan demonstrates pancreatic structural abnormalities and any of the following: pancreatic ductal dilation, pancreatic parenchymal atrophy, pancreatic fibrosis, inflammatory mass, bile duct structure, pseudocysts, pancreatic calcifications, and absence of any evidence of pancreatic cancer.

117. **(B)** Alarm features include age greater than 50 years at onset of symptoms, male sex, blood mixed in the stool, and blood on the toilet paper. These were all predictors for an organic diagnosis. Key features are abdominal pain or discomfort that is clearly linked to bowel function, either being relieved by defecation or associated with a change in stool form or consistency.

118. **(D)** The incubation period for rotavirus is 1–3 days. Vomiting is the first symptom in 80–90% of patients. Within 24 hours, patients develop low-grade fever and watery diarrhea lasting 4–8 days.

119. **(A)** Early aggressive fluid resuscitation 250–500 mL/h initially may reduce the frequency of systemic inflammatory response syndrome and organ failure in patients with acute pancreatitis. This treatment appears to have the greatest benefit in patients with acute pancreatitis predicted to be mild in severity when started within 4 hours of the patient's arrival at the hospital.

120. **(E)** A colonoscopy is the gold standard for the diagnosis of colorectal cancer.

121. **(C)** Toxic megacolon is characterized by: colon dilation of > 6 cm and signs of toxicity. There is an increased risk for colon perforation.

122. **(C)** The major organic components in bile are bilirubin, bile salts, phospholipids, and cholesterol accounting for the elevated bilirubin. ERCP has become the standard approach for acute presentations of choledocholithiasis and with the overall success of endoscopic bile duct clearance.

123. **(A)** EGD is the best method for examining the upper gastrointestinal mucosa. EGD is superior for detection of gastric ulcers and flat mucosal lesions, such as Barrett's esophagus. It enables directed biopsy and endoscopic therapy.

124. **(D)** The classic presentation for a patient with pancreatic cancer has been abdominal pain and weight loss with or without jaundice. Physical signs include jaundice, weight loss, a palpable gallbladder (Courvoisier sign), hepatomegaly, an abdominal mass, and an enlarged spleen.

125. **(B)** Bowel sounds are hyperactive early in the development of small bowel obstruction. Abdominal distention is often present.

126. **(D)** Inflammatory causes of peritonitis include: perforated stomach or duodenum, bile, ruptured bladder, enzymes released by acute pancreatitis, ruptured ovarian cyst, blood (e.g., bleeding from follicular cyst), recurrent serositis syndromes (e.g., SLE), inflammatory bowel disease (ulcerative colitis, Crohn's disease), and toxic megacolon.

127. **(C)** Neurologic signs predominate in hypocalcemia, including seizure and confusion. Classic physical findings include Chvostek sign (contraction of the facial muscle in response to tapping the facial nerve) and Trousseau sign (carpal spasm occurring with occlusion of the brachial artery by a blood pressure cuff).

128. **(D)** Non-contrast CT is the most accurate imaging modality for evaluating flank pain given its increased sensitivity and specificity. Identified in lecture as "gold standard" for urinary lithiasis imaging.

129. **(C)** Cryptorchidism is a risk factor for a testicular germ cell tumor.

130. **(D)** Patients with pyelonephritis often present toxic, and urine casts are detected. Quinolones are used to treat pyelonephritis.

131. **(B)** The most common organism associated with UTI is *E. coli*, ~80%.

132. **(A)** This scenario represents stress incontinence, which is one of the types of incontinence that should first be addressed with conservative measures. The first-line therapies for stress incontinence are weight loss, behavioral therapy (avoiding caffeinated beverages and timed voiding), and pelvic floor exercises (Kegel exercises). These should be tried prior to cystoscopy or surgery. There is no indication for hormonal therapy in this scenario.

133. **(E)** Vomiting is a cause of chloride depletion alkalosis and is managed with administration of chloride (NaCl, KCl). Patient described is hypovolemic, and NS would be most appropriate.

134. **(B)** An ultrasound with doppler can confirm the suspected diagnosis of testicular torsion.

135. **(A)** Perineal, sacral, or suprapubic pain; fever; and irritative voiding complaints are common. High fevers and a warm and often exquisitely tender prostate are detected on examination.

136. **(B)** Of those listed, hydrocele is the only choice that is nontender. Epididymitis, orchitis, and testicular torsion are painful.

137. **(B)** ECG changes of prolonged PR and tall T-waves associated with absent deep tendon reflexes is seen in hypermagnesemia. Patient has a history of constipation, and laxatives can contain magnesium.

138. **(D)** Dehydration, orthostatic hypotension, hyperosmolality, lethargy, and weakness can all be associated with hypernatremia. His history of dementia with inability to communicate thirst and inability to ambulate independently for easy access to water can contribute to decreased water intake.

139. **(E)** Complicated UTI presents as a symptomatic episode of cystitis or pyelonephritis in a man or woman with an anatomic predisposition to infection, with a foreign body in the urinary tract, pregnancy, or with factors predisposing to a delayed response to therapy.

140. **(E)** Acute glomerulonephritis is defined as the sudden onset of hematuria, proteinuria, and (red blood cell) casts in the urine. Patients experience swelling of hands, feet, and abdomen.

141. **(B)** Fournier gangrene is caused by gram-positive and gram-negative organisms. It is most common in diabetic patients > 60 years old. Fever and signs of sepsis are accompanied by necrotic, foul-smelling, rapidly advancing gangrene of scrotum; crepitation may be present. Emergent wide surgical debridement and antibiotics are essential.

142. **(B)** In iron-deficiency anemia (IDA) % iron saturation is decreased, MCV is low, TIBC is increased, reticulocyte count is low, and ferritin is low.

143. **(A)** Disorders of primary homeostasis can be caused by aspirin. Aspirin irreversibly inhibits platelet function, so the bleeding time effect resolves only as new platelets are made. In contrast, the effect of NSAIDs on platelet function is reversible and resolves as the drug is cleared.

144. **(E)** The NSAIDs are a large group of drugs that inhibit cyclo-oxygenases, thereby preventing the formation of prostaglandins. Traditionally, they have been the drugs most commonly prescribed for pain in the orofacial region and with TMJ.

145. **(D)** Most sickle cell patients experience recurrent attacks of acute pain caused by vaso-occlusion. These episodes account for most of the hospital admissions of sickle cell patients. Pain crises are sporadic and highly unpredictable. Usually, they appear suddenly and are localized to a limited area, particularly the abdomen, chest, back, or joints.

146. **(B)** Thalassemia trait is a common disorder among Asian patients. Clinically, thalassemia trait is manifested by a mild-to-moderate microcytic hypochromic anemia without symptoms. Hemoglobin electrophoresis is the diagnostic test of choice.

147. **(B)** This is consistent with an autoimmune hemolytic anemia.

148. **(C)** This image shows an RBC sickling. Healthy red blood cells appear round, and they move through small blood vessels to carry oxygen to all parts of the body. Patients who have SCD demonstrate red blood cells shaped like the letter "C" and are named after a C-shaped farm tool called a sickle.

149. **(D)** Von Willebrand's disease is the most common inherited bleeding disorder. It is associated with mucocutaneous bleeding (epistaxis, gingival) where women may have menorrhagia. It is inherited in an autosomal dominant pattern so both males and females are affected equally.

150. **(A)** DIC is a complication of a serious condition, often trauma. It manifests with oozing of blood, petechiae, and ecchymosis. Lab abnormalities included thrombocytopenia, prolonged PT and PTT, fragmented RBC on smear, and elevated D-dimer.

151. **(C)** This patient's clinical picture is that of multiple myeloma. Serum protein electrophoresis is the only option listed above that would confirm this diagnosis by showing a peak in the gamma globulin region. Another option would be a urine protein electrophoresis to look for Bence-Jones proteins.

152. **(B)** In almost all blood transfusion reactions, the first step is to stop the transfusion. The next step in this patient having a hemolytic transfusion reaction is to start IV fluids. Dark urine, back pain, fever, chills, and chest tightness are common symptoms.

153. **(C)** This CBC is consistent with iron deficiency anemia. The next best step for this patient is to search for a site of bleeding. Following that, she should be given a trial of oral iron prior to initiating IV iron or blood transfusions.

154. **(B)** In ITP the platelet count is low with large platelets seen on peripheral blood smear; other cell lines are normal. Physical exam, other than the minor bleeding, is normal. A successful clinical trial of corticosteroid therapy may also serve as strong evidence of the correct diagnosis of ITP.

155. **(C)** Hepcidin production is stimulated by inflammatory cytokines, and the overproduction of hepcidin is an important factor in the pathogenesis of the anemia of chronic inflammation.

156. **(A)** Antiphospholipid syndrome is most likely to cause arterial thrombi. The rest of the disorders listed tend to cause venous thrombi.

157. **(D)** Mr. Smith has a lobar pneumonia. Other clues are the rigors, lobar pneumonia, and blood tinged sputum. Mycoplasma should give a non-lobar (atypical appearing) chest X-ray. *E. coli* is uncommon cause of pneumonia. Bacteroides is an anaerobe, and there are no suggestions of an aspiration in the history. This is a middle lobe pneumonia, not lower.

158. **(C)** History suggests HIV risk factor. Nonadherent plaques with erythematous bases are most typical of thrush. Treat with fluconazole.

159. **(D)** Severe infection, empirical therapy, and recent broad-spectrum antibiotics are risks for MRSA. For patients with cellulitis in hospital, vancomycin is the treatment of choice. Oxacilin only treats MSSA. MRSA has resistance to cephalosporins and azithromycin does not cover *S. aureus*. Ciprofloxacin has inadequate gram-positive coverage for a skin infection and is not expected to treat MRSA.

160. **(B)** This patient has a macular rash consistent with secondary syphilis given the history of a painless penile ulcer followed by a rash on his trunk palms and soles—Treponema.

161. **(B)** Endocarditis caused by MSSA should be treated with oxacillin or nafcillin, which is more effective than vancomycin.

162. **(B)** This patient most likely has traveler's diarrhea caused by ETEC, as he just returned from a developing country and his stool has no PMNs. Each of the other bacteria listed would produce an inflammatory diarrhea with leukocytes in the stool. Of the pathogens listed, ETEC and *Salmonella* are most likely to cause a voluminous diarrhea, but *Salmonella* usually has PMNs on the stool smear.

163. **(C)** Norepinephrine is the pressor of choice for inability to maintain goals of CVP and MAP in patients with septic shock. Norepinephrine must be given in the central line. If fluids will maintain normal CVP goal, then a pressor is unnecessary.

164. **(C)** The diagnosis is herpes zoster and the most appropriate treatment is Acyclovir (antiviral). The description of pain over an area a few days before a rash develops is suggestive of zoster. The picture seals the diagnosis, as you see the rash is in a dermatomal distribution and does not cross midline.

165. **(C)** Endotoxin is only produced in gram-negative cell walls and is also called lipopolysaccharide. *H. flu* is the only gram-negative pathogen on this list.

166. **(D)** Legionella fits this description. Patient has water exposure, underlying lung disease, and abdominal complaints.

167. **(C)** Most cases of anaerobic or microaerophilic streptococcal endocarditis can be effectively treated with 12–20 million units of penicillin G intravenously daily for 4–6 weeks. Metronidazole 500 mg every 8 hours IV should be used if bacteroides species is identified.

168. **(B)** HIV-PrEP is contraindicated when creatinine clearance is < 60 mL/min.

169. **(B)** Central retinal artery occlusion occurs when the central retinal artery becomes blocked, usually due to an embolus. It causes sudden, painless, unilateral, and usually severe vision loss. Diagnosis is by history and characteristic retinal findings (cherry-red spot) on fundoscopy.

170. **(E)** Indomethacin is the best choice of treatment. Treatment should start as soon as possible after the patient perceives the beginning of a flare, preferably within several hours of symptom onset. More rapid and complete resolution of symptoms occurs the earlier that treatment is introduced. Monitor temperature for evaluation of additional therapy.

171. **(D)** Stage 2 Lyme disease is characterized by malaise, fatigue, fever, headache, neck pain, and generalized achiness; these are common with the skin lesions. Most symptoms are transient. The most common CNS manifestation is aseptic meningitis with mild headache and neck stiffness.

172. **(A)** Metronidazole is the only choice with anaerobic activity.

173. **(C)** This class of medications is structurally related to beta-lactam antibiotics with a broad spectrum of activity that includes most gram-negative rods (including *P. aeruginosa*), gram-positive organisms, and anaerobes.

174. **(D)** Beta lactams are superior to vancomycin when bacteria is susceptible. Bactericidal antibiotics are preferred. Prosthetic valves are rarely sterilized with an antibiotic.

175. **(D)** The objective here is to outline the components of the musculoskeletal examination including palpation, range of motion, neurovascular testing, and any other further testing.

176. **(C)** Ordering an MRI would help identify patient presentation, solidify physical exam findings, and determine the mechanism of injury. MRI is used to identify meniscal injury.

177. **(D)** Knowing the mechanism of injury may be the key to diagnosing some fractures or dislocations. For example, collision of the knee against the dashboard in a high-speed collision can cause posterior dislocation of the hip.

178. **(A)** The term pathologic (pathological changes in the body) should be used as the descriptive term helping to identify the unusual pattern in the bone.

179. **(C)** This revolves around the spine. Identify the anatomic structures of the entire vertebral column (curvature; sections and number of vertebrae; label vertebrae in coronal and lateral views).

180. **(D)** Positive apprehension test is indicative of shoulder instability and possible dislocation.

181. **(D)** Fractures—recognize potential complications of fractures and dislocations having to do with compartment syndrome.

182. **(B)** Lachman test—a physical examination with certain movements made to the knee. Discuss the following in regards to patient presentation, physical exam findings, and mechanism of injury: Injuries to the collateral and cruciate ligaments.

183. **(C)** When given a clinical scenario, correctly diagnose, order, and interpret the appropriate diagnostic studies, and create a management plan for the following: glenohumeral joint dislocation (anterior vs. posterior).

184. **(D)** This is a type of fracture. Appropriately describe/identify the fracture using proper terms when given the radiograph or picture of a fracture: direction of the fracture line is spiral.

185. **(C)** Foot ankle—understand the physical exam findings, incidence, and etiology of the disorders listed in the question. A Thompson test will identify an Achilles rupture.

186. **(B)** At the C6 level, the key muscles are the wrist extensors. Lateral pinch and active grasp are the functional motor activities.

187. **(B)** Legg-Calves-Perthes disease (LCPD) is an idiopathic condition of osteonecrosis and collapse of the femoral head. Most cases occur between 4 and 8 years of age in boys. Slipped capital femoral epiphysis (SCFE) is defined as the posterior and inferior slippage of the proximal femoral epiphysis on the femoral neck, which occurs through the growth plate. The peak incidence occurs in early adolescence at 12–13 years of age.

188. **(B)** 3—Full active range of motion against gravity, but not against resistance

    Muscle strength grades:

    - 0–No motion, no twitch, complete paralysis
    - 1–Muscle twitch/contraction or fasciculation, no motion
    - 2–Full active range of motion with gravity eliminated
    - 3–Full active range of motion against gravity, but not against resistance
    - 4–Able to overcome gravity and some degree of resistance
    - 5–Normal muscle strength (i.e., symmetric to contralateral side)

189. **(B)** Ask the patient questions that help to compare and contrast cervical disc herniation.

190. **(C)** All of the patient's symptoms identify a condition called Osgood-Schlatter disease. This disease affects mostly children who play sports and other activities, specifically running and jumping. The disease causes a painful lump below the kneecap. There is no specific treatment as it usually resolves on its own, once the child's bones stop growing.

191. **(A)** Hip flexion, adduction, and internal rotation.

192. **(C)** When looking at an X-ray and results of physical examination, a large indication of arthritis would be joint space narrowing.

193. **(B)** The diagram is pointing to posterior vertebral line: curvature; sections and number of vertebrae; label vertebrae in coronal and lateral views.

194. **(B)** When given a clinical scenario, correctly diagnose in regards to physical exam and mechanism of injury, order tests/imaging, and interpret results for the following: De Quervain tenosynovitis, Finkelstein test.

195. **(B)** Discuss the classification of Salter-Harris fractures, and recognize the treatment and possible complications associated with each type.

196. **(B)** Finding a posterior rib fracture is of suspicion and high concern because it can cause issues with a child's breathing and can lead to other internal injuries. Most injuries like these are caused by child abuse.

197. **(D)** Pain and vision loss are early symptoms of multiple sclerosis. An MRI would be the best choice for a diagnostic study to confirm the diagnosis.

198. **(C)** Ischemic: The pathogenic mechanisms of stroke are ischemic, hemorrhage, large vessel, and lacunar infarction.

199. **(C)** Stuporous level of conciousness. A stupor is a level of impaired consciousness in which a patient will only respond minimally to certain stimulation, such as touching a patient's feet or shining a light towards their eyes. Stuporous levels of conciousness can be caused by stroke, drug overdose, lack of oxygen, brain edema, or a heart attack.

200. **(B)** Given a case study, make appropriate treatment decisions in patients with cerebrovascular disease.

201. **(D)** Febrile seizures; outline diagnosis and management of childhood febrile seizures.

202. **(C)** Seizure and syncope are both characterized by transient loss of consciousness and both are associated with abnormal limb jerking. History of the episode is the most important to consider to establish the diagnosis. If there is a fever or sleep deprivation, further studies may be needed (e.g., lumbar puncture or EEG).

203. **(C)** This presentation is most consistent with migraine.

204. **(A)** MRI is the most helpful radiologic tool in the diagnosis of vascular dementias and new onset of cognitive decline. Patients with neurocognitive disorders are often unable to give a reliable history. Clinicians must rely heavily on data obtained from the physical examination and laboratory tests.

205. **(B)** Suspect temporal arteritis in a patient this age with visual deficit and tenderness at the temple.

206. **(E)** This is a normal response in an infant but abnormal response in an adult.

207. **(C)** This patient is not absorbing B1/thiamine.

208. **(B)** The corticobulbar tract is responsible for sensory and voluntary movement at the level of the medulla.

209. **(D)** RLS is treated by treating the underlying cause such as iron deficiency if present. Otherwise, treatment is symptomatic and dopamine agonists may be considered.

210. **(D)** Parkinson's tremor is pronounced at rest. Tremor lessens when body part is active.

211. **(C)** Benign essential tremor worsens with activity, stress, lack of sleep, or caffeine.

212. **(B)** After an insidious onset, paresis and paralysis continue to ascend and cause ventilatory weakness. Management is supportive and incorporates venous thromboembolism prophylaxis, pressure ulcer prevention, and enteral nutrition. Patients are often hospitalized and may require ventilatory assistance.

213. **(A)** Absence seizures are characterized by sudden, brief lapses of consciousness without loss of postural control. The seizure usually lasts for only seconds, consciousness returns quickly, and there is no postictal confusion.

214. **(B)** Diabetic neuropathy can lead to foot ulcerations, infections, and potentially amputations. Foot care is critically important for diabetic patients.

215. **(B)** A late complication of Parkinson's disease is dementia. Other complications include genitourinary and gastrointestinal symptoms and swallowing challenges.

216. **(A)** A mental status exam is an assessment of a patient's cognitive ability, attention, mood, speech, and thought patterns at the time of the evaluation. Spelling WORLD backward tests attention.

217. **(D)** Status epilepticus refers to continuous seizures or repetitive, discrete seizures with impaired consciousness in the interictal period. Status epilepticus has numerous subtypes, including generalized convulsive status epilepticus and nonconvulsive status epilepticus. The duration of seizure activity sufficient to meet the definition of status epilepticus has traditionally been specified as 15–30 min. However, a more practical definition is to consider status epilepticus as a situation in which the duration of seizures prompts the use of anticonvulsant therapy.

218. **(B)** Borderline personality disorder is characterized by unstable and intense relationships, fear of abandonment, impulsivity, recurring suicidal gestures, unstable affect, feelings of emptiness, and difficulty controlling anger.

219. **(C)** SSRIs are considered first-line treatment in PTSD (Sertraline and Paroxetine are FDA approved for PTSD). SNRIs are not currently FDA approved for PTSD, though in some cases they may be considered "second line."

220. **(C)** This patient is displaying features of schizophrenia (auditory hallucinations, paranoid delusions, and lack of self-hygiene). No mood symptoms are noted.

221. **(E)** The mental status exam is the primary focus of the objective evaluation of the psychiatric patient.

222. **(D)** SSRIs are the first line in treatment of depressive disorder and anxiety disorders.

223. **(A)** Atypical antipsychotics are generally used as the mainstay of treatment for schizoaffective disorder as they treat both psychotic symptoms and mood symptoms. Remember that schizoaffective disorder is characterized by depressive or manic episodes (or a mix of the two) in which schizophrenic characteristics are also noted (delusions, hallucinations, etc.). The schizophrenic signs/symptoms last longer than the mood symptoms by definition.

224. **(B)** Patient in (B) has more than one risk factor.

225. **(D)** Dissociative identity disorder is a disruption of identity characterized by two or more distinct personality states. Accompanying symptoms include: alterations in affect, behavior, consciousness, memory, perception, cognition, and/or sensory-motor functioning. Dissociative identity disorder is usually diagnosed in a patient's 20s.

226. **(B)** Patients with factitious disorder are feigning their symptoms to assume the role of a patient; they knowingly create their problem. Conversely, patients with somatization, conversion, and body dysmorphic disorder feel that their condition is real; they are not intentionally faking their symptoms for some type of gain.

227. **(D)** A cognitive-behavioral/psychotherapy approach that focuses on behavioral change while providing acceptance, compassion, and validation of the patient is the most common treatment approach.

228. **(E)** Many of the medical risks associated with bulimia nervosa are a direct consequence of purging, including fluid and electrolyte disturbances and conduction abnormalities. Diuretic use is within this category.

229. **(A)** Avolition is a complete lack of motivation. All others are positive symptoms.

230. **(A)** This scenario most likely describes obsessive-compulsive disorder. OCPD more accurately describes rigidity and perfectionism. OCPD will not come with the same severity of distress.

231. **(D)** Substance abuse should always be included on your differential diagnosis. This man meets some of the criteria for major depressive disorder, but there is not enough information to identify the disorder.

232. **(A)** Generalized anxiety disorder is characterized by subjective reports of excessive worry and increased stress as well as objective findings of sleep disturbances and muscle tension. Agoraphobia is a specific phobia that is associated when a patient is fearful of being away from home, in crowds, or alone in public places. Major depressive disorder would be more likely to present with depressed mood or anhedonia with associated sleep disturbance, feelings of guilt, eating habit changes, etc. Panic disorder is associated with generalized anxiety disorder but is often more severe than generalized anxiety disorder and is associated with episodes of shortness of breath, tachycardia, chest discomfort, nausea, and excessive fear. Schizophrenia would have psychotic symptoms such as hallucinations or delusions.

233. **(B)** GI side effects are commonly reported side effects for SSRIs.

234. **(A)** Time distinguishes differences in MDD and grief.

235. **(C)** Thyroid dysfunction should be considered as a medical reason for depressive symptoms. A TSH can assist in ruling this out. While all other tests can be helpful, they are not likely to yield a diagnosis or rule out anything from the differential that can cause both depressed mood and increased sleepiness.

236. **(A)** Bipolar depression, refractory MDD, and MDD with psychotic features are all potential indications for ECT. Severe COPD, MI within 3 months, and uncontrolled HTN are relative contraindications (conditions that increase risk) with ECT. Panic disorder is not an indication.

237. **(A)** Schizoaffective dx is made when psychotic sx meets criterion A for schizoaffective but the patient is also experiencing mood (depression or manic) episodes. Psychotic sx must be present in absence of mood sx for at least 2 weeks.

238. **(B)** The mental status examination (MSE) is the assessment in question.

239. **(B)** Benzodiazepines are used to relieve acute symptoms. SSRI and TCAs have some role in managing panic disorder, but due to their onset of action (weeks not days), they will not assist with her acute symptoms.

240. **(B)** Buprenorphine, naltrexone, and methadone are approved agents for MAT in opioid dependence. Clonidine is used to assist with symptoms in a setting of opioid withdrawals.

241. **(D)** Wellbutrin should be avoided because it can reduce a patient's seizure threshold.

     Duloxetine and amitriptyline may cause BP elevation and weight gain.

242. **(D)** Sinus tachy, though nonspecific, is the most common EKG finding in pulmonary embolism.

243. **(B)** One of these components within the previous 4 weeks constitutes moderate/persistent asthma:

     Rescue medication needed for asthma symptoms > 2 ×/week, and nighttime awakenings due to asthma.

244. **(A)** This ratio plus decreased FVC would suggest restrictive. Decreased ratio describes obstructive or mixed, depending on FVC.

245. **(B)** This is a patient with two present components of asthma control meeting criteria for only partly controlled.

246. **(D)** Cough and "steeple sign" on imaging are classic for croup.

247. **(B)** PaO_2/FiO_2 ratio is used to rate ARDS severity.

248. **(D)** Infection and cystic fibrosis are the most common causes of bronchiectasis. Less common causes include A1AD, collagen vascular disease, and primary ciliary dyskinesia.

249. **(C)** Symptoms consistent with occupational interstitial lung disease, notably silicosis given his longtime occupation.

250. **(C)** A pleural effusion would more often result in dullness to percussion, decreased breath sounds over effusion, decreased tactile fremitus, and asymmetric chest expansion.

251. **(D)** Waiting for diagnostics in this case delays proper, acute intervention. Placing the chest tube for decompression is the appropriate intervention.

252. **(D)** Immunosuppression association with TB relapse.

253. **(B)** To determine if an effusion is loculated, a decubitus film must be obtained.

254. **(A)** Protecting and securing the airway and assuring adequate ventilation are the first priorities in the resuscitation of any acutely ill or injured patient.

255. **(B)** Epiglottitis should be suspected when a patient presents with a rapidly developing sore throat or when odynophagia is out of proportion to apparently minimal oropharyngeal findings on examination. Lateral plain radiographs may demonstrate an enlarged epiglottis (the epiglottis "thumb sign").

256. **(B)** Spiculated margins are highly suggestive of malignancy.

257. **(C)** All new diagnoses of COPD should have testing for alpha 1 antitrypsin deficiency per *American Journal of Respiratory Critical Care Medicine*. Bronchoprovocation can be used in testing for asthma.

258. **(D)** Acute bronchiolitis is generally caused by RSV and is managed conservatively.

259. **(C)** Patients who use inhalers for rescue daily, have 1×/week but not nightly use of inhalers, and daily symptoms are moderate persistent. This patient left intermittent behind when the symptoms went over 2 days per week. Symptoms are severe if the symptoms were more than once a day.

260. **(B)** Asthma treatment for step 1 management includes a low-dose inhaled corticosteroid and an as needed short-acting beta 2 agonist.

261. **(D)** The most immediate, appropriate step at this time is decompression by chest tube.

Vitals do not warrant intubation. O_2 is possible but symptom severity demonstrates that O_2 is likely too conservative in this case and is not as "immediate."

262. **(B)** The most common pathogens of bronchitis are viruses.

263. **(E)** Patients with pulmonary hypertension will present with dyspnea and/or fatigue, whereas edema, chest pain, presyncope, and syncope are associated with more advanced disease. In early phases of the disease, the physical examination is often unremarkable. As the disease progresses, there may be evidence of right ventricular failure with elevated jugular venous pressure, lower extremity edema, and ascites.

264. **(D)** Diagnosis is made by physical examination showing an enlarged hemithorax with no breath sounds, hyperresonance to percussion, and shift of the mediastinum to the contra-lateral side. Difficulty in ventilation during resuscitation or high peak inspiratory pressures during mechanical ventilation strongly suggest tension pneumothorax.

265. **(A)** Chest CT angiography is the most common imaging modality for PE. This study will identify a clot as a filling defect in contrast-enhanced pulmonary arteries.

266. **(B)** Step 1 recs and step 2 recs remain consistent and prefer using ICS over the other listed choices. CMDT 9-05 also emphasizes ICS use in this case. SABAs are for PRN use.

267. **(D)** A LABA is the best first-line option here. ICS is an option but NOT by itself.

268. **(D)** Although all these conditions may lead to ARDS, sepsis is the most common cause.

269. **(D)** This is a respiratory alkalosis with no attempt at compensation. An elevated Ph leads to alkalosis. The $PaCO_2$ is low and the bicarb is normal.

270. **(B)** In a person without hemodynamic compromise, heparin is the immediate therapy. With hemodynamic compromise, of the options listed, surgery might be the choice. Prednisone has no role in the management of PE. Coumadin is not an initial option but rather a potential long-term anticoagulation option.

271. **(B)** In a pleural effusion, fluid will collect in the costophrenic angles when the person is standing upright. If there is enough fluid, it will obscure the angle. In an upright chest X-ray, a pleural effusion should have no effect on visualizing the apex, heart border, or mediastinum.

272. **(A)** Diabetes is the most common underlying cause of CKD, followed by hypertension (which is also a complication of CKD). Glomerulonephritis and polycystic kidney disease are also causes but occur less frequently than diabetes or hypertension.

273. **(D)** Enlarged prostate and hydronephrosis are suggestive of bladder outlet obstruction from prostate hypertrophy indicating a post renal AKI.

274. **(A)** This is the classic clinical picture and biopsy result of Goodpasture syndrome. Goodpasture syndrome is an autoimmune disorder where the immune system makes anti-bodies that attack the lungs and kidneys.

275. **(B)** CKD is diagnosed when the patient has greater than 3 months of kidney abnormalities and a GFR of < 60 mL/min/1.732.

276. **(D)** Potassium excretion is regulated by sodium delivery, tubular flow, and aldosterone.

277. **(C)** Pauci-immune necrotizing glomerulonephritis is caused by granulomatosis with poly-angiitis, microscopic polyangiitis, eosinophilic granulomatosis with polyangiitis, antineu-trophil cytoplasmic antibody (ANCA). Associated glomerulonephritis can also present as a primary renal lesion without systemic involvement. Renal involvement classically presents as a rapid progressive glomerulonephritis.

278. **(E)** Nephrotic syndromes are characterized by large volumes of protein in the urine.

279. **(A)** The addition of an ACE inhibitor has been shown to slow progression of proteinuria and delay the progression to nephropathy in diabetics.

280. **(D)** Systemic lupus erythematosus can cause glomerulonephritis or nephrotic syndrome because Lupus autoantibodies can deter a patient's body from filtering out waste resulting in the kidneys becoming enflamed. Blood and protein may turn up in the urine, impairing the kidneys.

281. **(A)** Epididymitis is a common cause of acute scrotal pain that must be differentiated from the more severe testicular torsion. The pathophysiology involves the spread of microorganisms from the urethra, prostate, or seminal vesicles causing a painful, parenchymal inflammatory process resulting in epididymal swelling. The swelling may affect the testicle.

282. **(B)** Bosniak rank 3 cysts have up to 50% risk of cancer. Renal cystic lesions are classified according to cyst wall thickness, septations, enhancement, nodularity, calcifications, and fluid density. Higher cyst classification correlates with increased likelihood of renal malignancy. Bosniak I–II lesions do not require additional follow-up, Bosniak IIF lesions require initial short-term (6-month) reimaging with annual imaging for 5 years, and patients with Bosniak III–IV lesions should be counseled about active surveillance or treatment.

283. **(D)** Severe pyelonephritis can manifest as high fever, nausea, vomiting, and flank pain. Symptoms are generally acute in onset and symptoms of cystitis may not be present. Fever is the main feature distinguishing cystitis from pyelonephritis. If the pathogen's susceptibility is not known and TMP-SMX is used, an initial IV 1-g dose of ceftriaxone is recommended. Oral TMP-SMX (one double-strength tablet twice daily for 14 days) also is effective for treatment of acute uncomplicated pyelonephritis if the uropathogen is known to be susceptible.

284. **(A)** This pregnant patient has hypertension. Aldomet is an adrenergic blocker and is safe to use in pregnancy.

285. **(B)** Oral metronidazole is the treatment for bacterial vaginosis. Clue cells are seen on wet prep.

286. **(D)** Placenta previa is a placenta that extends near, partially over, or covering the cervical os. Patients with symptomatic placenta previa present with painless bright-red vaginal bleeding. Risk factors for placenta previa include cesarean delivery, multiple uterine surgeries, advanced maternal age, minority group status, cigarette smoking, and cocaine use.

287. **(B)** Polycystic ovary syndrome (PCOS) is characterized by chronic anovulation, polycystic ovaries, and hyperandrogenism. It is associated with hirsutism and obesity as well as an increased risk of diabetes mellitus, cardiovascular disease, and metabolic syndrome. In obese patients with PCOS, weight reduction and exercise are often effective in reversing the metabolic effects and in inducing ovulation. Combined hormonal contraceptives are first-line treatment to manage hyperandrogenism and menstrual irregularities.

288. **(C)** Ruptured ectopic pregnancy is a potentially life-threatening condition. It is characterized by sudden, severe abdominal or pelvic pain with dizziness or fainting. Pain is due to leakage of blood into the abdomen affecting the diaphragm.

289. **(C)** Primary hypothyroidism—the daily replacement dose of levothyroxine is usually 1.6 µg/kg body weight (typically 100–150 µg), ideally taken at least 30 min before breakfast.

290. **(A)** Colposcopy should be used to evaluate vulvar, vaginal, and cervical cancer. This patient with LSIL should have colposcopy; all patients with cervical abnormalities require careful surveillance. Standards of the American Society for Colposcopy and cervical pathology should be followed.

291. **(B)** Diagnostic studies such as hysterosalpingography can be a treatment modality. It can aid in identifying if the fallopian tube is blocked and treat the etiology.

292. **(B)** Endometriosis is associated with pelvic pain, infertility, and abnormalities of the uterine lining. Laparoscopy is the diagnostic modality of choice as it would allow visualization of the affected areas and may allow surgical restoration of the affected structures.

293. **(D)** Continuous GnRH agonist treatment is used to suppress endogenous gonadotropin secretion in women undergoing ovulation induction with gonadotropins, in women with gynecologic disorders that benefit from ovarian suppression (e.g., endometriosis, uterine leiomyomata).

294. **(D)** Leiomyosarcomas often are > 5 cm in diameter and may be palpable on abdominal examination. Bleeding, obstruction, and perforation are common clinical features.

295. **(A)** Patient has a Bartholin's gland abscess. Amoxicillin with clavulanic acid. If the cyst reoccurs, marsupialization may be indicated.

296. **(D)** Phosphodiesterase type 5 inhibitors have markedly improved the management of ED because they are effective for the treatment of a broad range of causes, including psychogenic, diabetic, vasculogenic, post-radical prostatectomy (nerve-sparing procedures), and spinal cord injury. The onset of action is ~30–120 min; reduced initial doses should be considered for patients who are elderly, patients taking alpha blockers, or patients with renal insufficiency.

297. **(A)** Cryptorchidism occurs when there is incomplete descent of the testis from the abdominal cavity into the scrotum. Cryptorchidism is associated with increased risk of malignancy, infertility, inguinal hernia, and torsion, and for these reasons, referral is appropriate.

298. **(D)** Underlying vascular disorders are the most likely etiology for ED.

299. **(A)** A hydrocele is most consistent with the description provided.

300. **(B)** The presenting signs and symptoms include hematuria, flank or abdominal pain, and a flank or abdominal mass. Other symptoms are fever, weight loss, anemia, and a varicocele. The tumor is most commonly detected as an incidental finding on an X-ray. Surgery has a limited role for patients with metastatic disease. One indication for nephrectomy with metastases at initial presentation is to alleviate pain or hemorrhage of a primary tumor.

ANSWER SHEET
Practice Test 2

1. (A) (B) (C) (D) (E)
2. (A) (B) (C) (D) (E)
3. (A) (B) (C) (D) (E)
4. (A) (B) (C) (D) (E)
5. (A) (B) (C) (D) (E)
6. (A) (B) (C) (D) (E)
7. (A) (B) (C) (D) (E)
8. (A) (B) (C) (D) (E)
9. (A) (B) (C) (D) (E)
10. (A) (B) (C) (D) (E)
11. (A) (B) (C) (D) (E)
12. (A) (B) (C) (D) (E)
13. (A) (B) (C) (D) (E)
14. (A) (B) (C) (D) (E)
15. (A) (B) (C) (D) (E)
16. (A) (B) (C) (D) (E)
17. (A) (B) (C) (D) (E)
18. (A) (B) (C) (D) (E)
19. (A) (B) (C) (D) (E)
20. (A) (B) (C) (D) (E)
21. (A) (B) (C) (D) (E)
22. (A) (B) (C) (D) (E)
23. (A) (B) (C) (D) (E)
24. (A) (B) (C) (D) (E)
25. (A) (B) (C) (D) (E)

26. (A) (B) (C) (D) (E)
27. (A) (B) (C) (D) (E)
28. (A) (B) (C) (D) (E)
29. (A) (B) (C) (D) (E)
30. (A) (B) (C) (D) (E)
31. (A) (B) (C) (D) (E)
32. (A) (B) (C) (D) (E)
33. (A) (B) (C) (D) (E)
34. (A) (B) (C) (D) (E)
35. (A) (B) (C) (D) (E)
36. (A) (B) (C) (D) (E)
37. (A) (B) (C) (D) (E)
38. (A) (B) (C) (D) (E)
39. (A) (B) (C) (D) (E)
40. (A) (B) (C) (D) (E)
41. (A) (B) (C) (D) (E)
42. (A) (B) (C) (D) (E)
43. (A) (B) (C) (D) (E)
44. (A) (B) (C) (D) (E)
45. (A) (B) (C) (D) (E)
46. (A) (B) (C) (D) (E)
47. (A) (B) (C) (D) (E)
48. (A) (B) (C) (D) (E)
49. (A) (B) (C) (D) (E)
50. (A) (B) (C) (D) (E)

51. (A) (B) (C) (D) (E)
52. (A) (B) (C) (D) (E)
53. (A) (B) (C) (D) (E)
54. (A) (B) (C) (D) (E)
55. (A) (B) (C) (D) (E)
56. (A) (B) (C) (D) (E)
57. (A) (B) (C) (D) (E)
58. (A) (B) (C) (D) (E)
59. (A) (B) (C) (D) (E)
60. (A) (B) (C) (D) (E)
61. (A) (B) (C) (D) (E)
62. (A) (B) (C) (D) (E)
63. (A) (B) (C) (D) (E)
64. (A) (B) (C) (D) (E)
65. (A) (B) (C) (D) (E)
66. (A) (B) (C) (D) (E)
67. (A) (B) (C) (D) (E)
68. (A) (B) (C) (D) (E)
69. (A) (B) (C) (D) (E)
70. (A) (B) (C) (D) (E)
71. (A) (B) (C) (D) (E)
72. (A) (B) (C) (D) (E)
73. (A) (B) (C) (D) (E)
74. (A) (B) (C) (D) (E)
75. (A) (B) (C) (D) (E)

76. (A) (B) (C) (D) (E)
77. (A) (B) (C) (D) (E)
78. (A) (B) (C) (D) (E)
79. (A) (B) (C) (D) (E)
80. (A) (B) (C) (D) (E)
81. (A) (B) (C) (D) (E)
82. (A) (B) (C) (D) (E)
83. (A) (B) (C) (D) (E)
84. (A) (B) (C) (D) (E)
85. (A) (B) (C) (D) (E)
86. (A) (B) (C) (D) (E)
87. (A) (B) (C) (D) (E)
88. (A) (B) (C) (D) (E)
89. (A) (B) (C) (D) (E)
90. (A) (B) (C) (D) (E)
91. (A) (B) (C) (D) (E)
92. (A) (B) (C) (D) (E)
93. (A) (B) (C) (D) (E)
94. (A) (B) (C) (D) (E)
95. (A) (B) (C) (D) (E)
96. (A) (B) (C) (D) (E)
97. (A) (B) (C) (D) (E)
98. (A) (B) (C) (D) (E)
99. (A) (B) (C) (D) (E)
100. (A) (B) (C) (D) (E)

101. Ⓐ Ⓑ Ⓒ Ⓓ Ⓔ   126. Ⓐ Ⓑ Ⓒ Ⓓ Ⓔ   151. Ⓐ Ⓑ Ⓒ Ⓓ Ⓔ   176. Ⓐ Ⓑ Ⓒ Ⓓ Ⓔ
102. Ⓐ Ⓑ Ⓒ Ⓓ Ⓔ   127. Ⓐ Ⓑ Ⓒ Ⓓ Ⓔ   152. Ⓐ Ⓑ Ⓒ Ⓓ Ⓔ   177. Ⓐ Ⓑ Ⓒ Ⓓ Ⓔ
103. Ⓐ Ⓑ Ⓒ Ⓓ Ⓔ   128. Ⓐ Ⓑ Ⓒ Ⓓ Ⓔ   153. Ⓐ Ⓑ Ⓒ Ⓓ Ⓔ   178. Ⓐ Ⓑ Ⓒ Ⓓ Ⓔ
104. Ⓐ Ⓑ Ⓒ Ⓓ Ⓔ   129. Ⓐ Ⓑ Ⓒ Ⓓ Ⓔ   154. Ⓐ Ⓑ Ⓒ Ⓓ Ⓔ   179. Ⓐ Ⓑ Ⓒ Ⓓ Ⓔ
105. Ⓐ Ⓑ Ⓒ Ⓓ Ⓔ   130. Ⓐ Ⓑ Ⓒ Ⓓ Ⓔ   155. Ⓐ Ⓑ Ⓒ Ⓓ Ⓔ   180. Ⓐ Ⓑ Ⓒ Ⓓ Ⓔ
106. Ⓐ Ⓑ Ⓒ Ⓓ Ⓔ   131. Ⓐ Ⓑ Ⓒ Ⓓ Ⓔ   156. Ⓐ Ⓑ Ⓒ Ⓓ Ⓔ   181. Ⓐ Ⓑ Ⓒ Ⓓ Ⓔ
107. Ⓐ Ⓑ Ⓒ Ⓓ Ⓔ   132. Ⓐ Ⓑ Ⓒ Ⓓ Ⓔ   157. Ⓐ Ⓑ Ⓒ Ⓓ Ⓔ   182. Ⓐ Ⓑ Ⓒ Ⓓ Ⓔ
108. Ⓐ Ⓑ Ⓒ Ⓓ Ⓔ   133. Ⓐ Ⓑ Ⓒ Ⓓ Ⓔ   158. Ⓐ Ⓑ Ⓒ Ⓓ Ⓔ   183. Ⓐ Ⓑ Ⓒ Ⓓ Ⓔ
109. Ⓐ Ⓑ Ⓒ Ⓓ Ⓔ   134. Ⓐ Ⓑ Ⓒ Ⓓ Ⓔ   159. Ⓐ Ⓑ Ⓒ Ⓓ Ⓔ   184. Ⓐ Ⓑ Ⓒ Ⓓ Ⓔ
110. Ⓐ Ⓑ Ⓒ Ⓓ Ⓔ   135. Ⓐ Ⓑ Ⓒ Ⓓ Ⓔ   160. Ⓐ Ⓑ Ⓒ Ⓓ Ⓔ   185. Ⓐ Ⓑ Ⓒ Ⓓ Ⓔ
111. Ⓐ Ⓑ Ⓒ Ⓓ Ⓔ   136. Ⓐ Ⓑ Ⓒ Ⓓ Ⓔ   161. Ⓐ Ⓑ Ⓒ Ⓓ Ⓔ   186. Ⓐ Ⓑ Ⓒ Ⓓ Ⓔ
112. Ⓐ Ⓑ Ⓒ Ⓓ Ⓔ   137. Ⓐ Ⓑ Ⓒ Ⓓ Ⓔ   162. Ⓐ Ⓑ Ⓒ Ⓓ Ⓔ   187. Ⓐ Ⓑ Ⓒ Ⓓ Ⓔ
113. Ⓐ Ⓑ Ⓒ Ⓓ Ⓔ   138. Ⓐ Ⓑ Ⓒ Ⓓ Ⓔ   163. Ⓐ Ⓑ Ⓒ Ⓓ Ⓔ   188. Ⓐ Ⓑ Ⓒ Ⓓ Ⓔ
114. Ⓐ Ⓑ Ⓒ Ⓓ Ⓔ   139. Ⓐ Ⓑ Ⓒ Ⓓ Ⓔ   164. Ⓐ Ⓑ Ⓒ Ⓓ Ⓔ   189. Ⓐ Ⓑ Ⓒ Ⓓ Ⓔ
115. Ⓐ Ⓑ Ⓒ Ⓓ Ⓔ   140. Ⓐ Ⓑ Ⓒ Ⓓ Ⓔ   165. Ⓐ Ⓑ Ⓒ Ⓓ Ⓔ   190. Ⓐ Ⓑ Ⓒ Ⓓ Ⓔ
116. Ⓐ Ⓑ Ⓒ Ⓓ Ⓔ   141. Ⓐ Ⓑ Ⓒ Ⓓ Ⓔ   166. Ⓐ Ⓑ Ⓒ Ⓓ Ⓔ   191. Ⓐ Ⓑ Ⓒ Ⓓ Ⓔ
117. Ⓐ Ⓑ Ⓒ Ⓓ Ⓔ   142. Ⓐ Ⓑ Ⓒ Ⓓ Ⓔ   167. Ⓐ Ⓑ Ⓒ Ⓓ Ⓔ   192. Ⓐ Ⓑ Ⓒ Ⓓ Ⓔ
118. Ⓐ Ⓑ Ⓒ Ⓓ Ⓔ   143. Ⓐ Ⓑ Ⓒ Ⓓ Ⓔ   168. Ⓐ Ⓑ Ⓒ Ⓓ Ⓔ   193. Ⓐ Ⓑ Ⓒ Ⓓ Ⓔ
119. Ⓐ Ⓑ Ⓒ Ⓓ Ⓔ   144. Ⓐ Ⓑ Ⓒ Ⓓ Ⓔ   169. Ⓐ Ⓑ Ⓒ Ⓓ Ⓔ   194. Ⓐ Ⓑ Ⓒ Ⓓ Ⓔ
120. Ⓐ Ⓑ Ⓒ Ⓓ Ⓔ   145. Ⓐ Ⓑ Ⓒ Ⓓ Ⓔ   170. Ⓐ Ⓑ Ⓒ Ⓓ Ⓔ   195. Ⓐ Ⓑ Ⓒ Ⓓ Ⓔ
121. Ⓐ Ⓑ Ⓒ Ⓓ Ⓔ   146. Ⓐ Ⓑ Ⓒ Ⓓ Ⓔ   171. Ⓐ Ⓑ Ⓒ Ⓓ Ⓔ   196. Ⓐ Ⓑ Ⓒ Ⓓ Ⓔ
122. Ⓐ Ⓑ Ⓒ Ⓓ Ⓔ   147. Ⓐ Ⓑ Ⓒ Ⓓ Ⓔ   172. Ⓐ Ⓑ Ⓒ Ⓓ Ⓔ   197. Ⓐ Ⓑ Ⓒ Ⓓ Ⓔ
123. Ⓐ Ⓑ Ⓒ Ⓓ Ⓔ   148. Ⓐ Ⓑ Ⓒ Ⓓ Ⓔ   173. Ⓐ Ⓑ Ⓒ Ⓓ Ⓔ   198. Ⓐ Ⓑ Ⓒ Ⓓ Ⓔ
124. Ⓐ Ⓑ Ⓒ Ⓓ Ⓔ   149. Ⓐ Ⓑ Ⓒ Ⓓ Ⓔ   174. Ⓐ Ⓑ Ⓒ Ⓓ Ⓔ   199. Ⓐ Ⓑ Ⓒ Ⓓ Ⓔ
125. Ⓐ Ⓑ Ⓒ Ⓓ Ⓔ   150. Ⓐ Ⓑ Ⓒ Ⓓ Ⓔ   175. Ⓐ Ⓑ Ⓒ Ⓓ Ⓔ   200. Ⓐ Ⓑ Ⓒ Ⓓ Ⓔ

ANSWER SHEET
Practice Test 2

201. Ⓐ Ⓑ Ⓒ Ⓓ Ⓔ	226. Ⓐ Ⓑ Ⓒ Ⓓ Ⓔ	251. Ⓐ Ⓑ Ⓒ Ⓓ Ⓔ	276. Ⓐ Ⓑ Ⓒ Ⓓ Ⓔ
202. Ⓐ Ⓑ Ⓒ Ⓓ Ⓔ	227. Ⓐ Ⓑ Ⓒ Ⓓ Ⓔ	252. Ⓐ Ⓑ Ⓒ Ⓓ Ⓔ	277. Ⓐ Ⓑ Ⓒ Ⓓ Ⓔ
203. Ⓐ Ⓑ Ⓒ Ⓓ Ⓔ	228. Ⓐ Ⓑ Ⓒ Ⓓ Ⓔ	253. Ⓐ Ⓑ Ⓒ Ⓓ Ⓔ	278. Ⓐ Ⓑ Ⓒ Ⓓ Ⓔ
204. Ⓐ Ⓑ Ⓒ Ⓓ Ⓔ	229. Ⓐ Ⓑ Ⓒ Ⓓ Ⓔ	254. Ⓐ Ⓑ Ⓒ Ⓓ Ⓔ	279. Ⓐ Ⓑ Ⓒ Ⓓ Ⓔ
205. Ⓐ Ⓑ Ⓒ Ⓓ Ⓔ	230. Ⓐ Ⓑ Ⓒ Ⓓ Ⓔ	255. Ⓐ Ⓑ Ⓒ Ⓓ Ⓔ	280. Ⓐ Ⓑ Ⓒ Ⓓ Ⓔ
206. Ⓐ Ⓑ Ⓒ Ⓓ Ⓔ	231. Ⓐ Ⓑ Ⓒ Ⓓ Ⓔ	256. Ⓐ Ⓑ Ⓒ Ⓓ Ⓔ	281. Ⓐ Ⓑ Ⓒ Ⓓ Ⓔ
207. Ⓐ Ⓑ Ⓒ Ⓓ Ⓔ	232. Ⓐ Ⓑ Ⓒ Ⓓ Ⓔ	257. Ⓐ Ⓑ Ⓒ Ⓓ Ⓔ	282. Ⓐ Ⓑ Ⓒ Ⓓ Ⓔ
208. Ⓐ Ⓑ Ⓒ Ⓓ Ⓔ	233. Ⓐ Ⓑ Ⓒ Ⓓ Ⓔ	258. Ⓐ Ⓑ Ⓒ Ⓓ Ⓔ	283. Ⓐ Ⓑ Ⓒ Ⓓ Ⓔ
209. Ⓐ Ⓑ Ⓒ Ⓓ Ⓔ	234. Ⓐ Ⓑ Ⓒ Ⓓ Ⓔ	259. Ⓐ Ⓑ Ⓒ Ⓓ Ⓔ	284. Ⓐ Ⓑ Ⓒ Ⓓ Ⓔ
210. Ⓐ Ⓑ Ⓒ Ⓓ Ⓔ	235. Ⓐ Ⓑ Ⓒ Ⓓ Ⓔ	260. Ⓐ Ⓑ Ⓒ Ⓓ Ⓔ	285. Ⓐ Ⓑ Ⓒ Ⓓ Ⓔ
211. Ⓐ Ⓑ Ⓒ Ⓓ Ⓔ	236. Ⓐ Ⓑ Ⓒ Ⓓ Ⓔ	261. Ⓐ Ⓑ Ⓒ Ⓓ Ⓔ	286. Ⓐ Ⓑ Ⓒ Ⓓ Ⓔ
212. Ⓐ Ⓑ Ⓒ Ⓓ Ⓔ	237. Ⓐ Ⓑ Ⓒ Ⓓ Ⓔ	262. Ⓐ Ⓑ Ⓒ Ⓓ Ⓔ	287. Ⓐ Ⓑ Ⓒ Ⓓ Ⓔ
213. Ⓐ Ⓑ Ⓒ Ⓓ Ⓔ	238. Ⓐ Ⓑ Ⓒ Ⓓ Ⓔ	263. Ⓐ Ⓑ Ⓒ Ⓓ Ⓔ	288. Ⓐ Ⓑ Ⓒ Ⓓ Ⓔ
214. Ⓐ Ⓑ Ⓒ Ⓓ Ⓔ	239. Ⓐ Ⓑ Ⓒ Ⓓ Ⓔ	264. Ⓐ Ⓑ Ⓒ Ⓓ Ⓔ	289. Ⓐ Ⓑ Ⓒ Ⓓ Ⓔ
215. Ⓐ Ⓑ Ⓒ Ⓓ Ⓔ	240. Ⓐ Ⓑ Ⓒ Ⓓ Ⓔ	265. Ⓐ Ⓑ Ⓒ Ⓓ Ⓔ	290. Ⓐ Ⓑ Ⓒ Ⓓ Ⓔ
216. Ⓐ Ⓑ Ⓒ Ⓓ Ⓔ	241. Ⓐ Ⓑ Ⓒ Ⓓ Ⓔ	266. Ⓐ Ⓑ Ⓒ Ⓓ Ⓔ	291. Ⓐ Ⓑ Ⓒ Ⓓ Ⓔ
217. Ⓐ Ⓑ Ⓒ Ⓓ Ⓔ	242. Ⓐ Ⓑ Ⓒ Ⓓ Ⓔ	267. Ⓐ Ⓑ Ⓒ Ⓓ Ⓔ	292. Ⓐ Ⓑ Ⓒ Ⓓ Ⓔ
218. Ⓐ Ⓑ Ⓒ Ⓓ Ⓔ	243. Ⓐ Ⓑ Ⓒ Ⓓ Ⓔ	268. Ⓐ Ⓑ Ⓒ Ⓓ Ⓔ	293. Ⓐ Ⓑ Ⓒ Ⓓ Ⓔ
219. Ⓐ Ⓑ Ⓒ Ⓓ Ⓔ	244. Ⓐ Ⓑ Ⓒ Ⓓ Ⓔ	269. Ⓐ Ⓑ Ⓒ Ⓓ Ⓔ	294. Ⓐ Ⓑ Ⓒ Ⓓ Ⓔ
220. Ⓐ Ⓑ Ⓒ Ⓓ Ⓔ	245. Ⓐ Ⓑ Ⓒ Ⓓ Ⓔ	270. Ⓐ Ⓑ Ⓒ Ⓓ Ⓔ	295. Ⓐ Ⓑ Ⓒ Ⓓ Ⓔ
221. Ⓐ Ⓑ Ⓒ Ⓓ Ⓔ	246. Ⓐ Ⓑ Ⓒ Ⓓ Ⓔ	271. Ⓐ Ⓑ Ⓒ Ⓓ Ⓔ	296. Ⓐ Ⓑ Ⓒ Ⓓ Ⓔ
222. Ⓐ Ⓑ Ⓒ Ⓓ Ⓔ	247. Ⓐ Ⓑ Ⓒ Ⓓ Ⓔ	272. Ⓐ Ⓑ Ⓒ Ⓓ Ⓔ	297. Ⓐ Ⓑ Ⓒ Ⓓ Ⓔ
223. Ⓐ Ⓑ Ⓒ Ⓓ Ⓔ	248. Ⓐ Ⓑ Ⓒ Ⓓ Ⓔ	273. Ⓐ Ⓑ Ⓒ Ⓓ Ⓔ	298. Ⓐ Ⓑ Ⓒ Ⓓ Ⓔ
224. Ⓐ Ⓑ Ⓒ Ⓓ Ⓔ	249. Ⓐ Ⓑ Ⓒ Ⓓ Ⓔ	274. Ⓐ Ⓑ Ⓒ Ⓓ Ⓔ	299. Ⓐ Ⓑ Ⓒ Ⓓ Ⓔ
225. Ⓐ Ⓑ Ⓒ Ⓓ Ⓔ	250. Ⓐ Ⓑ Ⓒ Ⓓ Ⓔ	275. Ⓐ Ⓑ Ⓒ Ⓓ Ⓔ	300. Ⓐ Ⓑ Ⓒ Ⓓ Ⓔ

Practice Test 2

DIRECTIONS: Find a quiet place to take this practice test. For each question, select the choice that best answers the question and mark that answer on the sheet provided. There are 300 questions and a review of the correct answers suggested upon test completion. You have a total of 5 hours to complete this test. Allow 1 minute per question and take breaks. Good luck!

1. You are seeing a 6-year-old girl who has bilateral leg pain when running. You note decreased pulses and blood pressure in both lower extremities and a blowing systolic murmur in the left infrascapular area. What is the most likely diagnosis?

   (A) Coarctation of the aorta
   (B) Transposition of the great arteries
   (C) Patent ductus arteriosus
   (D) Ventricular septal defect
   (E) Bicuspid aortic valve

2. Which of the following is true when discussing the use of CK (Creatinine Kinase), CK-MB, and Troponin enzymes when evaluating a patient for acute coronary syndromes?

   (A) Troponin is metabolized within 6 hours, so checking CK-MB may be the only way to catch a myocardial infarct (MI) more than 6 hours after it has occurred.
   (B) CK-MB is the most sensitive marker for cardiac injury, but Troponin, when checked serially every 6 hours, raises the false positive rate of testing.
   (C) CK is only released from cardiac muscle, so it would differentiate between heart muscle and skeletal muscle injury.
   (D) Troponin remains elevated in blood for 5–10 days. It is very specific for cardiac muscle injury, but it may not indicate re-infarction of cardiac muscle.
   (E) CK-MB is cardiac specific.

3. An 82-year-old woman has COPD and hypertension. She has dyspnea at 100 ft of walking for 2 months. Six months ago she could walk for 30 minutes without symptoms. BP 120/75, HR 85, Sat 94%, RR 16. Exam shows jugular venous distention, a diastolic decrescendo murmur at the left, upper sternal border, and there is pitting edema of both shins. There are no crackles and a chest X-ray shows no lung infiltrates or effusion. An echocardiogram shows a normal left ventricle ejection fraction of 60%. The right ventricle systolic pressure is elevated to 55 mmHg (normal is 20–30). What diagnosis best explains her clinical picture?

   (A) Diastolic left heart failure from an acute coronary syndrome
   (B) Systolic left heart failure from hypertension
   (C) Right heart failure as a result of COPD
   (D) Right heart failure caused by systolic left heart failure from mitral regurgitation
   (E) Left heart failure following a URI

4. A 65-year-old man has dyspnea that has gotten worse over the past 2 days. He has diabetes and hypertension. Exam: BP is 135/85, HR-105, RR-26, and O_2 saturation of 87% on room air. He is sitting in bed, coughing pink sputum. Cardiac: tachycardia, regular rhythm, and there is an extra heart sound just after S2. You note jugular venous distention (JVD). Extremities are warm to the touch with pitting edema in both legs. Lung: diffuse crackles. His creatinine and potassium are normal. What is the most appropriate medical management?

   (A) Dobutamine (inotrope) and furosemide (loop diuretic)
   (B) Furosemide (loop diuretic) and ACE-inhibitor
   (C) Metoprolol (beta-blocker) and dobutamine (inotrope)
   (D) Metoprolol (beta-blocker) and chlorthalidone (thiazide diuretic)
   (E) Verapamil (calcium channel blocker)

5. Which of the following is true about atrial septal defects (ASD)?

   (A) Adults with ASDs are protected from development of pulmonary hypertension.
   (B) They are one of the four defects making up Tetralogy of Fallot.
   (C) Large ASDs do not need closure because equalization of pressures between the atria will occur.
   (D) Due to flow from the left side of the heart to the right, they cause a fixed and wide-split S2.
   (E) They develop in pediatric patients after 1 year of age.

6. Which of the following is associated with an increased risk for myocardial infarction from vasospasm?

   (A) Cocaine
   (B) Ecstasy
   (C) Marijuana
   (D) Opiates
   (E) Nicotine

7. Which of the following medications is a best choice for patients with hypertension who also have had previous myocardial infarction?

   (A) Furosemide (diuretic)
   (B) Hydralazine (vasodilator)
   (C) Clonidine (alpha 2 agonist)
   (D) Cardizem (calcium channel blocker)
   (E) Metoprolol (beta-blocker)

8. Which of the following represents normal electrical conduction through the heart?

   (A) AV node, SA node, bundle of His, bundle branches, and Purkinje fibers
   (B) SA node, AV node, bundle of His, bundle branches, and Purkinje fibers
   (C) SA node, AV node, bundle branches, bundle of His, and Purkinje fibers
   (D) SA node, bundle of His, AV node, bundle branches, and Purkinje fibers
   (E) AV node, SA node, bundle branches, bundle of His, and Purkinje fibers

9. A 40-year-old woman is in your clinic for dyspnea and orthopnea that has gotten worse over 3 years. She has severe mitral stenosis. Which treatment is most likely to improve both her quality of life and life expectancy?

   (A) Enrollment in a cardiac rehabilitation program
   (B) Placing clips to treat mitral regurgitation
   (C) Increasing her dose of a beta-blocker
   (D) Opening the stenotic valve with a balloon
   (E) Surgical valve replacement

10. Which of the following is most likely to cause only right-sided, systolic heart failure?

   (A) Obstructive sleep apnea
   (B) Aortic regurgitation
   (C) Viral myocarditis
   (D) Occlusion of the left circumflex coronary artery
   (E) Sarcoidosis

11. A patient is in intensive care after an ST Elevation MI (STEMI). He has reduced left ventricular function (EF 20%). You find: BP 65/40, HR 128, RR 26, O_2 saturation of 78%. General: drowsy and hard to arouse. Chest: crackles in all lung fields. Cardiovascular: tachycardia with regular rhythm, S1 and S2 normal, S3 present, no murmurs. Extremities: cool, cyanotic. Pulses decreased in radial arteries. You have placed him on a ventilator. What would be the next intervention?

   (A) Furosemide (loop diuretic)
   (B) Lisinopril (ace inhibitor)
   (C) Dobutamine (inotrope)
   (D) Nitroglycerin (vasodilator)
   (E) Metoprolol (beta-blocker)

12. A 62-year-old man comes to your clinic to address his leg pain. He is a smoker and has a history of stable angina. His pain worsens when he walks for more than 5 minutes or upstairs. On exam, he has normal S1 and S2 with no murmur and a decreased pulse in the posterior tibial artery on the left. What is the best diagnostic study and treatment plan?

   (A) Troponin, lifestyle modification, treadmill stress-test
   (B) Fasting lipid panel, suggest smoking cessation, ankle-brachial index (ABI)
   (C) D-dimer, CT angiogram, compression stockings
   (D) High density lipoprotein (HDL), physical therapy, angiography
   (E) CK-MB, exercise

13. A patient is brought into your ED with palpitations. On exam: HR-135, BP-135/70, oxygen saturation 98%, and RR-16. She is alert and behaving normally. Peripheral pulses are 2+; extremities are warm. EKG shows an irregularly-irregular rhythm with no P-waves and an HR of 135. What is the next step in the management of this patient?

   (A) Synchronized cardioversion
   (B) Atropine (anticholinergic)
   (C) Diltiazem drip IV (calcium channel blocker)
   (D) Nitroglycerin drip IV (vasodilator)
   (E) Cardizem (calcium channel blocker)

14. Mr. T has diaphoresis, confusion, BP of 70/45, and weak radial pulses. What is the most appropriate immediate management for this patient in sustained, monomorphic, ventricular tachycardia with a rate of 140 bpm?

   (A) IV adenosine (AV nodal blocker)
   (B) Carotid sinus massage
   (C) IV magnesium
   (D) Synchronized cardioversion
   (E) Nitroglycerin drip IV (vasodilator)

15. Which valvular disease is represented by a diastolic, decrescendo murmur located along the lower left sternal border, often associated with wide pulse pressures, and best heard by having the patient lean forward while sitting?

   (A) Aortic regurgitation
   (B) Aortic stenosis
   (C) Mitral regurgitation
   (D) Tricuspid stenosis
   (E) Bifid tricuspid valve

16. A patient with which of the following conditions is most likely to have a fourth heart sound (S4)?

   (A) Left ventricular hypertrophy from hypertension
   (B) Postpartum cardiomyopathy
   (C) Myocarditis from parvovirus
   (D) Patent foramen ovale in a patient with a deep vein thrombosis
   (E) Mitral valve prolapse

17. You are called at 1:00 A.M. to a patient's room to evaluate dyspnea, hypotension, and confusion. The EKG shows bradycardia (HR 39) and no relationship between the P-waves and QRS complexes. What would be the best course of action?

   (A) Intubate the patient to maintain the airway.
   (B) Draw a basic metabolic panel (BMP) and troponin. Observe for any worsening in condition.
   (C) Place a cardiac pacer on the patient's chest, and call a cardiologist.
   (D) Give adenosine IV to temporarily block the AV node.
   (E) Order a 12 lead EKG.

18. All of the following patients got a cardiac echo to evaluate dyspnea on exertion and some chest pressure. Choose the patient most likely to have heart failure with preserved ejection fraction (HFpEF) as the cause of their symptoms?

    (A) A 55-year-old man who smokes has an aneurysm of the ascending aorta 5 cm in diameter.
    (B) A 65-year-old man has COPD. His echocardiogram shows normal left ventricle systolic function; there is severe pulmonic regurgitation.
    (C) A 75-year-old woman with diabetes has a normal left ventricle EF of 60%; R and L ventricular walls look thicker than average.
    (D) A child being treated for lymphoma has a large pericardial effusion. R and L ventricles have the same systolic pressure.
    (E) A 70-year-old female patient has a recent history of pulmonary embolism.

19. A 60-year-old man is in the emergency department with substernal chest pain starting 30 minutes ago. He has radiation to the left arm, diaphoresis, and nausea. He had a stroke after a ruptured cerebral aneurysm 1 year ago. Vitals: blood pressure 162/95 mmHg, heart rate 110 bpm. Physical exam has no murmurs on the heart exam and no crackles on the lung exam. EKG revealed sinus tachycardia with frequent PVC and ST elevation in the anterior leads. You have drawn labs, given the patient aspirin, clopidogrel (anti-platelet) and sublingual nitroglycerin, but he continues to have pain. What is the best care plan for this patient?

    (A) Administer morphine for sedation, then complete a synchronized cardioversion
    (B) Administer IV nitroglycerin (vasodilator) and TPA (thrombolytic) to relieve ischemia, then observe in the ED
    (C) Administer beta-blocker and arrange for cardiac catheterization within 90 minutes
    (D) Await troponin high sensitivity blood test result 1 hour after arrival, and if elevated arrange for a cardiologist consultation
    (E) Order CK-MB

20. A 74-year-old male patient is seen in your clinic for leg swelling and shortness of breath, which is worse over 6 months. Six months ago, he was walking 1.5 miles most days; now he has dyspnea at 50 feet. He has hyperlipidemia and smokes two packs daily. Lungs have crackles in both bases. Heart shows regular rate and rhythm, no murmurs or rubs. Jugular vein pressure is estimated at 9 cm. There is hepatomegaly. His pretibial areas both have edema and red-brown discoloration. Which category of heart failure fits best?

    (A) Right heart failure—cor pulmonale
    (B) Left and right ventricle failure—can't tell if ejection fraction is preserved or not
    (C) Acute right diastolic heart failure—with preserved ejection fraction
    (D) Left ventricle systolic heart failure—with reduced ejection fraction
    (E) Mitral regurgitation—with preserved ejection fraction

21. Mr. Noble is 73 and presents to your ED with sudden-onset tearing chest pain. He reports nausea and pain radiating to his back. He is constantly moving in bed, appearing very anxious. BP-165/85, HR-100, RR-25. He has a diastolic murmur along the left lower sternal border. Abdominal exam reveals a non-tender abdomen that is not distended. You note normal pulses in the right arm and decreased pulses in the left arm. Lower extremities are without edema. What is the most likely diagnosis?

    (A) Aortic dissection
    (B) Left femoral artery pseudoaneurysm
    (C) Coarctation of the aorta
    (D) Arterial embolism
    (E) Pneumothorax

22. Mr. R is a 71-year-old man in your office with pain on the back of his right hand. You find out that he donated plasma for research about 5 days ago. He has no fever or chills. What would be the best management?

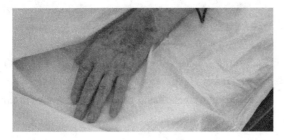

(A) Antibiotic orally and topical on the hand for 7 days

(B) Heparin anticoagulation and ultrasound looking for deep vein thrombosis

(C) Surgical debridement and wound care measures

(D) Drainage

(E) Warm compress and ibuprofen (NSAID)

23. Which of the following cases describing chest pain best represent acute pericarditis?

(A) Progressive dyspnea over several hours with pink sputum production

(B) Elevated troponin blood levels, but no coronary artery blockages on catheterization

(C) Recent cough, fever, and muscle aches resulting in pain relieved by sitting forward

(D) Burning sensation in the central chest and back of throat, belching relieves pain

(E) Chest pain and somnolence

24. Which patient is most likely to be having an acute exacerbation of heart failure when these labs are drawn?

	Brain Natriuretic Peptide (Norm Below 120)	High Sensitivity Troponin I (Norm Below 14)
Patient A	100	13
Patient B	71	6
Patient C	216	12
Patient D	89	27

(A) Patient A

(B) Patient B

(C) Patient C

(D) Patient D

(E) None

25. Which of the following would result in a fixed split S2 heart sound?

(A) Mitral regurgitation

(B) Atrial septal defect

(C) Left bundle branch block

(D) Deep inspiration

(E) Congestive heart failure

26. A patient presents with a unilateral swollen leg 48 hours after returning to the US from Japan. Her BP is 120/80 and HR is 80. Which treatment strategy is best to begin for this condition immediately?

(A) Unfractionated heparin IV

(B) Tissue plasminogen activator (TPA, thrombolytic treatment) IV

(C) Warfarin orally

(D) Inferior vena cava filter

(E) Administer oxygen

27. An infarction in the inferior wall of the left ventricle should correlate to a blockage of which coronary artery? (All other sections of the heart appear to be squeezing normally on echo.)

(A) Right main
(B) Left main
(C) Left anterior descending
(D) Circumflex artery
(E) Posterior descending artery

28. At what percentage of cross-sectional, luminal narrowing would you expect a patient to have angina symptoms due to a significant reduction in blood flow to the myocardium?

(A) 10%
(B) 25%
(C) 45%
(D) 55%
(E) 75%

29. Name a medical condition that you would suspect in a patient who has right ventricle enlargement with moderate systolic pressure elevation estimated at 40–45 mmHG. The right ventricular ejection fraction appears normal. The left atrium and ventricle are of normal size, pressure, and function, with ejection fraction of 55%.

(A) Aortic valve prolapse
(B) Pulmonary valve stenosis
(C) Pulmonary embolism
(D) Mitral valve prolapse
(E) Amyloidosis

30. Which is true regarding the effect of alcohol on the myocardium?

(A) It is toxic when used in excess, resulting in a major cause of non-ischemic cardiomyopathy.
(B) It is a cause of septal hypertrophy that can obstruct flow out of the left ventricle.
(C) It is the alcohol in red wine that is proposed to reduce heart disease risk in those who consume it in moderation.
(D) It causes ballooning dilation of the left ventricle that is reversible.
(E) It elevates systolic blood pressure.

31. Which of the following cardiac conditions is associated with the development of atrial fibrillation?

(A) Hypertension
(B) Hyperthyroidism
(C) Pericarditis
(D) Aortic dissection
(E) Foramen ovale

32. A patient has a blood pressure that is consistently 35/20 mmHg above her goal BP. Which medication regimen is best at reducing her risk of death from a cardiovascular cause?

(A) Benazepril (ACE inhibitor) + valsartan (angiotensin receptor blocker)
(B) Chlorthalidone (diuretic) + amlodipine (calcium channel blocker)
(C) Amlodipine (calcium channel blocker) + benazepril (ACE inhibitor)
(D) Chlorthalidone (diuretic) + benazepril (ACE inhibitor)
(E) Furosemide (diuretic)

33. Which of the following patients most likely has had a Type 2 myocardial infarction? A high sensitivity troponin I normal range is less than 14.

(A) A 72-year-old woman has angina. EKG shows sinus tachycardia and acute ischemia. Troponin levels are elevated and rising rapidly over 3 hours.
(B) Earlier, a 58-year-old man had ventricular tachycardia, rate 140 bpm, as a result of hyperkalemia. His heart rate is controlled now at 90 bpm. Troponin levels (21, 21, 17) at 0, 1, and 3 hrs.
(C) A man in the cardiac cath lab has chest pain while having a stent placed. After opening the artery, pain is resolved. The first troponin after the procedure is 88.
(D) A woman has ST elevations on an EKG done in an ambulance. She smokes. She reports symptoms of classic angina. The medic draws blood, but troponin results are not back yet.
(E) A male patient with a history of diabetes and recent coronary artery bypass graft presents with shortness of breath.

34. All patients below are having a non-ST elevation myocardial infarction (NSTEMI). Which should go to the cath lab as soon as possible for a coronary revascularization?

    (A) Woman has ST segment depression persisting after starting six drugs appropriate for NSTEMI
    (B) Man has troponin levels that peak then begin to decline after 8 hours of medical therapy
    (C) Woman has a TIMI risk score of 2 (1 point for risk factors and 1 for EKG changes)
    (D) Man has a history of heart failure with preserved ejection fraction (HFpEF); EF right now is 55%
    (E) Woman with ejection fraction of 70%

35. A patient with a 27% chance of having a coronary event in the next 10 years is taking a high intensity statin (HMGcoA inhibitor). She begins to have muscle aching after walking, which her PA says is due to the drug. Her lab testing shows the statin has been effective and there is no liver or muscle inflammation. What is the best recommendation for this patient?

    (A) Keep the statin dose the same, no change in therapy
    (B) Lower the statin dose to a moderate intensity and monitor closely
    (C) Stop taking statin; no other interventions warranted
    (D) Stop taking statin; maintain her reduced LDL with diet and exercise; no medication
    (E) Advise patient to continue exercising without change in medication

36. Your patient had a viral-like illness, and you suspect there is now pericarditis. You want a test that will see if there is a pericardial effusion and, if present, find out its impact on the heart. Which test is the best first test for this indication?

    (A) Transthoracic echocardiogram
    (B) Fluid sampling of the pericardium
    (C) Cardiac MRI
    (D) Electrocardiogram
    (E) Chest X-ray

37. Which patient with a systolic murmur most likely has tricuspid regurgitation?

    (A) A 60-year-old woman with a dilated right ventricle has JVD and a new murmur that gets louder with inspiration.
    (B) A child with a history of a "heart defect" has a systolic, crescendo-decrescendo murmur at the left upper sternal border.
    (C) An 80-year-old man has dyspnea on exertion attributed to calcifications that significantly narrowed one of his heart valves.
    (D) A teenager learns their murmur represents a condition that lowers blood pressure when exercising and can cause syncope or death.
    (E) A thin 25-year-old athlete experiences dyspnea on exertion

38. A man with multiple myeloma is undergoing chemotherapy. He presents to his oncology clinic with fatigue, cough, and shortness of breath. His carotid pulse is fast and regular.

    Vitals:

    - Temperature 102°F (40°C)
    - Heart rate 124 bpm
    - Blood pressure 130/70 mmHg
    - Resp rate 16 rpm, unlabored
    - O_2 saturation 96% on room air

    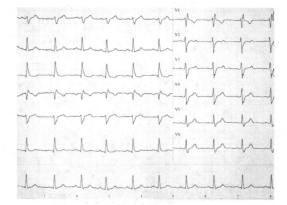

    Which is the best therapy for the patient's sinus tachycardia?

    (A) Infusion of a beta-blocker
    (B) Treat his fever
    (C) Transcutaneous pacemaker
    (D) Administer atropine (antimuscarinic)
    (E) Reverse trendelenburg position

39. A 32-year-old female comes to the clinic for evaluation of dyspnea on exertion. She notes she no longer can walk a block without becoming extremely winded and tired. Medical history is significant for rheumatic heart disease as a child. Temperature is 36.6°C (98°F), pulse rate is 64/min and regular, respirations are 12/min and unlabored, and blood pressure is 100/60 mmHg. Cardiac exam shows a prominent "a" wave of the jugular pulse, a diastolic murmur heard in the left fifth intercostal space, increasing with inspiration, and bilateral lower extremity peripheral edema. ECG shows regular rate and rhythm with tall peaked P-waves in lead II. Which of the following Is the most likely diagnosis?

    (A) Mitral stenosis
    (B) Tricuspid stenosis
    (C) Pulmonary regurgitation
    (D) Aortic regurgitation
    (E) Tension pneumothorax

40. You are seeing a fair-skinned 75-year-old male patient for a routine wellness exam. Numerous rough, poorly defined papules are visible on his forehead, along with an irregularly shaped nonhealing nodule. If left untreated, these may develop into which of the following lesions?

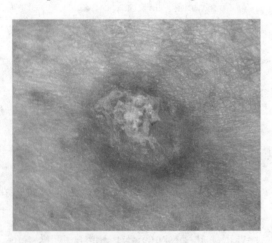

    (A) Basal cell carcinoma
    (B) Lentigines
    (C) Malignant melanoma
    (D) Squamous cell carcinoma
    (E) Sarcoma

41. A patient presents to your clinic complaining of severe sunburn over the last week. She states she remembers being in the sun for her morning walk at sunrise and some light gardening in the late afternoon. In the chart, you note her medication list and find that she is currently taking a sulfonamide antibiotic to treat a urinary tract infection. What is the most likely diagnosis?

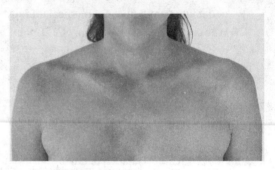

    (A) Contact dermatitis
    (B) Atopic dermatitis
    (C) Photosensitive drug reaction
    (D) Toxic drug reaction
    (E) Xanthelasma

42. Which of the following dermatophyte infections should always be treated using systemic antifungals?

    (A) Tinea capitis
    (B) Tinea corporis
    (C) Tinea cruris
    (D) Tinea pedis
    (E) Tinea versicolor

43. An adult patient seen in your clinic one week ago for an adverse skin reaction to an antibiotic presents again with complaints of persistent pruritic pink macules over the trunk and extremities, despite cessation of antibiotic. He states the rash has not spread to other areas, and he has not had oral lesions or pain. Which of the following would be the most appropriate recommendation?

    (A) Low potency topical steroids
    (B) Perform a bunch biopsy to identify cause of rash
    (C) Oral antihistamine for symptomatic treatment
    (D) Antibiotic ointment to apply over rash
    (E) Ultraviolet light therapy

44. Which of the following forms of dermatitis occurs principally on the legs as a result of vascular compromise with noted edema and progression to ulcerations on the tibia and ankles?

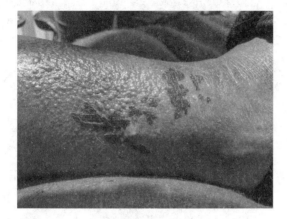

(A) Irritant contact dermatitis
(B) Stasis dermatitis
(C) Atopic dermatitis
(D) Cellulitis
(E) Diabetic dermatitis

45. A patient presents to the clinic with complaints about changes in her skin coloration, which she noticed 1 month ago. On examination, you note non-scaly, depigmented patches on the hands and lower extremities. The patient has a history of thyroid disease but no other pertinent medical history. What is the most likely diagnosis?

(A) Tinea versicolor
(B) Vitiligo
(C) Neurofibromatosis
(D) Albinism
(E) Eczema

46. A 21-year-old avid outdoor enthusiast reports to the clinic because of a gradual expansion of what first started as a red papule on his neck 5 days ago. You note that the redness is now seen around his entire neck. The patient recently returned from a camping trip 1 week ago. He reports that over the last 5 days, he has experienced fatigue, a low-grade fever of 100.9°F, headaches, joint pains, and swollen glands. The appropriate next step is

(A) amoxicillin (oral penicillin-based antibiotic).
(B) doxycycline (oral tetracycline-based antibiotic).
(C) topical hydrocortisone cream (topical corticosteroid).
(D) to perform a skin biopsy and wait for treatment.
(E) Lotrimin (clotrimazole, antifungal).

47. A 5-year-old patient comes in with a chief complaint of crusted lesions around his mouth. His mother notes that several days earlier he had a couple of mosquito bites that he persistently scratched. He has no fever and is not looking ill or debilitated. The most likely diagnosis for these lesions is

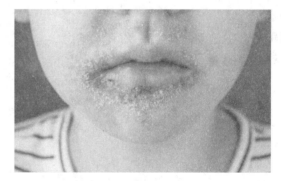

(A) folliculitis.
(B) pityriasis rosea.
(C) ecthyma.
(D) rosacea.
(E) impetigo.

48. A patient is seen with a rash that has been present intermittently for 2 months. The rash usually lasts less than 24 hours and goes away for a few days to a week. It is pruritic and usually on her trunk and upper extremities. She denies recent medication changes or changes in soaps or detergents. She denies urgent symptoms of angioedema or joint pain. What is the likely diagnosis?

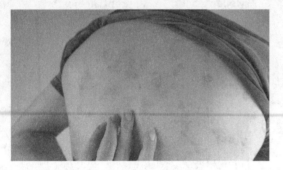

(A) Acute urticaria

(B) Systemic lupus erythematosus

(C) Chronic urticaria

(D) Psoriasis

(E) Ringworm

49. A 36-year-old male develops inflammatory streaks with widespread blisters on both legs and around his eyes 24 hours following a hunting trip. He sees you in the office immediately upon his return and states that his rash is "continuing to spread" and he is unable to sleep due to the extreme itching. His legs are swollen with a large number of vesicles. The diagnosis is contact dermatitis. Which of the following is the most appropriate treatment?

(A) Oral antibiotic

(B) Topical antibiotic

(C) Oral corticosteroid

(D) Topical corticosteroid

(E) Valacyclovir (antiviral)

50. You are called to the hospital on a dermatology consult for a blistering rash on a 61-year-old female patient's trunk. On exam you note widespread painful erosions, bullae, crusts, and skin sloughing of the skin on her back and chest. You also note she has oral erosions on the mucosa of the mouth. She reports she has had mouth sores for a few months. What is the most likely diagnosis?

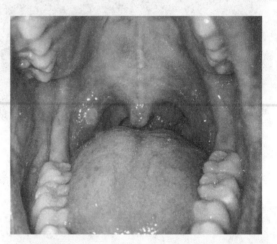

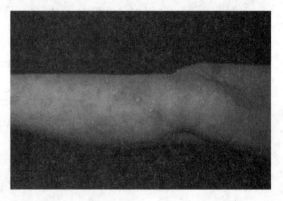

(A) Erythema multiforme

(B) Herpes simplex

(C) Bullous impetigo

(D) Pemphigus vulgaris

(E) Tinea corporis

51. What is a common, acute, self-limited dermatosis that typically affects children and young adults and presents as shown below?

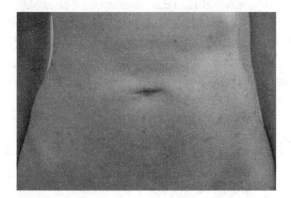

(A) Erysipelas
(B) Lichen planus
(C) Pityriasis rosea
(D) Secondary syphilis
(E) Sarcoidosis

52. A 25-year-old man returned from a camping trip in North Carolina 5 days ago and now presents to your office with a 3-day history of fevers to 102°F, severe headaches, myalgias, nausea, and generalized abdominal tenderness. He started developing a macular rash around his wrists and ankles yesterday and it appears to be spreading with lesions on his buttocks, arms, and legs but has spared his face. He recalls removing a tick that was embedded on his ankle. What is the most probable organism causing his symptoms?

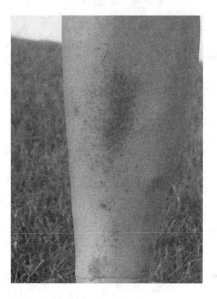

(A) *Rickettsia rickettsii*
(B) *Borrelia burgdorferi*
(C) *Rickettsia typhi*
(D) *Treponema pallidum*
(E) *Pasteurella multocida*

53. A 55-year-old male presents to the clinic with complaints of a red, burning rash on the face intermittently for 5 years. Recently it has become worse, and he notes he is breaking out like an adolescent. He complains that his nose has changed shape and is very oily. You perform an exam and note the appearance on his face. Which is the most likely diagnosis?

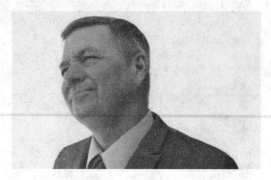

(A) Acne vulgaris

(B) Erysipelas

(C) Psoriasis

(D) Rosacea

(E) Herpes zoster

54. What is a sexually transmitted disease with an eroded, crusted papule that may appear 18–21 days after infection? If left untreated, this disease can have other skin manifestations, as well as potentially serious, systemic manifestations and is often referred to as the "great imitator."

(A) Herpes simplex

(B) Herpes whitlow

(C) Syphilis

(D) Herpes gladiatorum

(E) *Neisseria gonorrhoeae*

55. What test is recommended for routine screening for peripheral neuropathy in a person with diabetes?

(A) Ankle-brachial index

(B) Hemoglobin A1C

(C) Monofilament testing

(D) Nerve conduction study

(E) Skin biopsy

56. A 24-year-old man presents to your clinic complaining of several months of episodic headaches, sweating, and palpitations. He says that he started graduate school recently and is not sure if these episodes are associated with stress. His medical history includes surgical repair of ankle injuries sustained in a fall while ice skating 3 months ago. The anesthesiologist noted that the patient's blood pressure fluctuated during the procedure and advised him to be evaluated for possible hypertension, but he has not followed up yet. On the physical exam, pulse is 90, BP is 142/86. He has no exophthalmos, lid lag, or goiter. Labs: normal thyroid function tests, electrolytes, and creatinine. Which of the following is the best laboratory evaluation to order on this patient?

(A) Cosyntropin stimulation test

(B) Metanephrine assay (plasma fractionated/ urine fractionated)

(C) Serum cortisol level at 8 A.M.

(D) Thyroid-stimulating immunoglobulin antibodies

(E) Urinalysis

57. A 43-year-old female is found to have a 2 cm solitary thyroid nodule on chest CT. Her exam is remarkable for palpable, firm anterior cervical nodes. Which of the following is the best method to further evaluate the nodule for thyroid cancer?

(A) Fine needle aspiration biopsy

(B) Thyroid ultrasound

(C) PET scan

(D) RAI scan

(E) Monitor

58. Where is vasopressin (ADH) produced?

(A) Zona reticularis

(B) Zona glomerulosa

(C) Posterior pituitary

(D) Anterior pituitary

(E) Thyroid gland

59. Which of the following is the corticosteroid replacement of choice in a person with acute adrenocortical insufficiency?

   (A) DHEA
   (B) Prednisone
   (C) Hydrocortisone
   (D) Lotrisone
   (E) Betamethasone

60. Which of the following lab findings, if elevated, would be contraindicated to prescribing Metformin?

   (A) Creatinine
   (B) WBC
   (C) Triglycerides
   (D) TSH
   (E) Cholesterol

61. Which of the following complications of diabetes may be the initial presentation of type 1 DM?

   (A) DKA
   (B) HHS
   (C) Peripheral neuropathy
   (D) Pancreatitis
   (E) Folliculitis

62. A 45-year-old gentleman presents to your clinic reporting he has had to purchase larger shoes and can no longer wear his wedding ring due to the markedly increased soft tissue bulk of his fingers. He also complains of fatigue and coarsening of his facial features over time. Which of the following is the most likely diagnosis?

   (A) Acromegaly
   (B) Cretinism
   (C) Hyperandrogenism
   (D) Klinefelter syndrome
   (E) Obesity

63. A 57-year-old female with type 1 diabetes presents to the clinic because of increased swelling in her feet for the past several weeks. She has no cardiac history. She denies shortness of breath, chest pain, or abdominal pain. Vitals are: HR 68, BP 148/92, RR 10.2+ peripheral edema of her feet and ankles. The rest of her physical exam is unremarkable. A1c level is 9%. What would be an expected finding on a urinalysis?

   (A) Bilirubinuria
   (B) Proteinuria
   (C) Hematuria
   (D) Leukocytes
   (E) White blood cells

64. Patient presents for follow-up to review annual labs and perform physical exam. He has a history of hypertension, and BP today is 190/100. Labs reveal hypokalemia and hypernatremia. Suspicion of an adenoma causing overproduction of the hormone that is produced in the

   (A) zona glomerulosa.
   (B) zona fasciculata.
   (C) zona reticularis.
   (D) adrenal medulla.
   (E) adrenal cortex.

65. The dawn phenomenon is caused by what?

   (A) Reduced tissue sensitivity to insulin in the early morning
   (B) Surge of counter-regulatory hormones that produce hyperglycemia
   (C) Refractory hypoglycemia in the early morning
   (D) Nocturnal hypoglycemia causing hyperglycemia
   (E) Somogyi effect

66. A 60-year-old female with type 2 DM presents to the office with complaints of "not feeling well" for 2 days. While talking to the patient, you notice that she seems confused and lethargic. The patient's son is accompanying her and has said that his mother has not been drinking any water for the past several days. Her BP is 80/50 with a HR of 120. Urinalysis reveals specific gravity of 1.035 (1.010-1.030), no ketones. What associated lab finding would further help to confirm the diagnosis?

    (A) Lactic acid 3.0 mmol/L (0.5–2.2 mmol/L)
    (B) pH of 7.2 (7.35–7.45)
    (C) Glucose of 800 mg/dL (65–99 mg/dL)
    (D) Potassium of 3 mEq/L (3.5–5 mEq/L normal)
    (E) Brain MRI

67. A 58-year-old male presents to the office with concerns of "getting bigger" and general fatigue for the past year and brought in pictures to prove it. He has also noted a decreased libido in addition to mood swings, increased appetite, anxiety, and sleep disturbances. The only medication he is on is 40 mg lisinopril once daily. The change of facial features to a moon face appearance, along with central obesity, is representative of which disorder?

    (A) Pheochromocytoma
    (B) Acromegaly
    (C) Cushing's syndrome
    (D) Addison's disease
    (E) Diabetes

68. Peripheral resistance to the action of insulin and decreased insulin secretion in spite of elevated serum glucose levels is most indicative of which disease/process?

    (A) Type I diabetes mellitus
    (B) Type II diabetes mellitus
    (C) Diabetes insipidus
    (D) Reactive hypoglycemia
    (E) Tumor of pancreas

69. The most common adverse consequence of treating Graves' disease with thyroid ablation using radioactive iodine (RAI) is

    (A) hypothyroidism.
    (B) increased WBC count.
    (C) thyroid cancer.
    (D) thyroiditis.
    (E) elevated blood pressure.

70. Which lab test or exam is most important to monitor in routine care for patients with diabetes mellitus?

    (A) Blood pressure
    (B) Blood glucose
    (C) Lipid profile
    (D) Fundoscopy
    (E) All of the above

71. A 45-year-old female presents with complaints of milky discharge from her breast and menstrual irregularity for about 6 months. She is quite concerned because she has also been having loss of her peripheral vision. What is her most likely diagnosis?

    (A) Pregnancy
    (B) Pituitary adenoma
    (C) Polycystic ovary
    (D) Breast cancer with metastasis
    (E) Uterine cancer with metastasis

72. Which of the following disorders is most likely to present with these laboratory abnormalities: increased alkaline phosphatase, decreased vitamin D, elevated parathyroid hormone (PTH), and low serum calcium?

    (A) Paget's disease
    (B) Osteoporosis
    (C) Osteogenesis imperfecta
    (D) Osteomalacia
    (E) Diabetes insipidus

73. Patients with suspected Turner's syndrome should have which of the following as part of their initial workup?

 (A) Karyotyping
 (B) Buccal smear
 (C) Chest ultrasound
 (D) Uterine ultrasound
 (E) MRI of c-spine

74. Primary hyperparathyroidism is diagnosed initially by which of the following?

 (A) Elevated PTH (parathyroid hormone level)
 (B) Hypocalcemia
 (C) Parathyroid premalignant syndrome
 (D) Bone density testing
 (E) Hypercalciuria

75. Intraocular pressures are normally between

 (A) 5–9 mm Hg.
 (B) 10–20 mm Hg.
 (C) 30–40 mm Hg.
 (D) 40–50 mm Hg.
 (E) 50–60 mm Hg.

76. A patient presents with sudden painless loss of vision in the left eye. The patient has a past medical history for hyperlipidemia and carotid stenosis. Visual acuity is 20/20 in the right eye and light perception only in the left eye. Fundoscopic exam of the right eye is normal. The left eye shows a pallid retinal swelling with a cherry red spot in the area of the fovea. What is the most likely diagnosis?

 (A) Central retinal artery occlusion
 (B) Central retinal vein occlusion
 (C) Giant cell arteritis
 (D) Retinal detachment
 (E) Acute angle closure glaucoma

77. Which of the following is a staphylococcal infection characterized by an acutely tender lump, redness, and swelling of the gland(s) of the eyelid margin?

 (A) Blepharitis
 (B) Chalazion
 (C) Dacryocystitis
 (D) Hordeolum
 (E) Herpes zoster

78. Mrs. Smith is a 65-year-old female who presents with worsening of her peripheral vision. She states that it feels like she is driving in a tunnel. On her exam, her visual acuity is 20/30 bilaterally, but her visual fields are reduced. Her intraocular pressures are 35 in both eyes, and a fundoscopic exam reveals cupping of the optic disc. What is the most likely diagnosis?

 (A) Acute angle closure glaucoma
 (B) Cataracts
 (C) Central retinal artery occlusion
 (D) Open angle glaucoma
 (E) Amaurosis fugax

79. Mr. Smith is a 44-year-old male who reports a 2-week history of left eye irritation, burning, foreign body sensation, and mattering of the eyelids. He also reports blurred vision that improves with blinking. On exam you note scales around the base of the eyelashes and erythema at the lid margins as shown below. What is the most likely diagnosis?

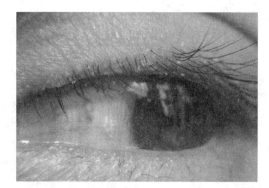

 (A) Blepharitis
 (B) Chalazion
 (C) Dacrocystitis
 (D) Hordeolum
 (E) Ptosis

80. Mr. Jones is a 70-year-old male who presents with blood in his left eye. He states that his wife mentioned there was blood; he wasn't aware of it. He denies pain, vision loss, or trauma. He does report 3–4 episodes of vomiting this morning prior to his wife noticing the blood covering the "whites" of his left eye. What is the most likely diagnosis?

    (A) Acute angle closure glaucoma
    (B) Conjunctivitis
    (C) Episcleritis
    (D) Subconjunctival hemorrhage
    (E) Ocular cancer

81. A patient presents with right eye pain, blurred vision, redness, and photophobia for 3 days. The patient is a contact lense wearer and admits to sleeping in the contacts for 2–3 nights before the symptoms began. On examination, you note circumcorneal injection. Slit lamp exam reveals a hazy cornea with hypopyon. A central ulceration is noted with fluorescein. What is the most likely diagnosis?

    (A) Acute glaucoma
    (B) Anterior uveitis
    (C) Bacterial keratitis
    (D) Viral keratitis
    (E) Dacryocystitis

82. Which of the following is the most appropriate treatment for the patient in the previous question?

    (A) Topical antiviral (Viroptic)
    (B) Topical steroids (Pred Forte)
    (C) Topical antibiotics (Fluoroquinolone/ Vigamox)
    (D) Topical beta-blocker (Timolol)
    (E) Artificial tears

83. A 68-year-old male with a history of myopia and prior cataract extraction presents to the ER with complaints of sudden visual loss in the left eye that he describes as a curtain moving across his eye. The patient also reports that he saw bright flashing lights before losing his vision. The fundoscopic exam is shown. What is the most appropriate diagnosis?

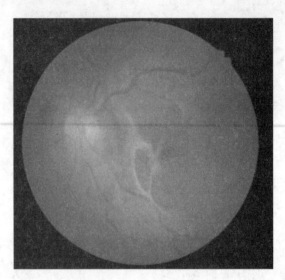

    (A) Age-related macular degeneration
    (B) Central retinal artery occlusion
    (C) Central retinal vein occlusion
    (D) Retinal detachment
    (E) Amaurosis fugax

84. A patient presents to the emergency department with complaints of sudden onset right eye pain while watching TV in a dark room. He also reports blurred vision with halos around lights, headache, abdominal pain, and nausea/vomiting. On the exam, you see a steamy cornea, circumcorneal injection, and a nonreactive mid dilated pupil. What is the most likely diagnosis?

    (A) Acute angle closure glaucoma
    (B) Acute anterior uveitis
    (C) Bacterial keratitis
    (D) Chronic open angle glaucoma
    (E) Retinal detachment

85. Which of the following is an appropriate treatment for a dental abscess without cellulitis?

    (A) Gingival biopsy
    (B) Incision and drainage
    (C) Oral antibiotics
    (D) Topical antibiotics
    (E) Peroxide treatments

86. Which of the following is a common site for squamous cell carcinoma in the oral cavity?

    (A) Buccal mucosa
    (B) Hard palate
    (C) Soft palate
    (D) Tonsillar pillars
    (E) Tongue

87. Which of the following drugs has been found to cause gingival hyperplasia?

    (A) Acyclovir
    (B) Morphine
    (C) Penicillin
    (D) Phenytoin
    (E) Diltiazem

88. Which of the following would be most likely to cause conductive hearing loss?

    (A) Acoustic neuroma
    (B) Drug toxicity
    (C) Labyrinthitis
    (D) Otitis media
    (E) Trigeminal neuralgia

89. Which of the following is the most common etiology of laryngotracheobronchitis or "croup"?

    (A) Parainfluenza
    (B) Adenovirus
    (C) Rhinovirus
    (D) Streptococcal
    (E) Respiratory syncytial virus

90. A patient presents to the emergency room and is suspected of having acute epiglottitis. To help confirm the diagnosis, a lateral radiograph of the neck was obtained. What is the name of the "sign" presented on this radiograph?

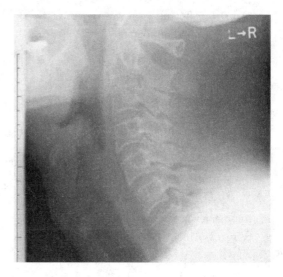

    (A) Battle's
    (B) Steeple
    (C) Sail
    (D) Thumbprint
    (E) Chimney

91. A patient presents to your clinic with white plaques on the tongue, palate, and buccal mucosa for 3 days. The patient can wipe the plaques off, but they keep coming back. The patient is currently undergoing chemotherapy for colon cancer. What is the most likely diagnosis?

    (A) Herpes stomatitis
    (B) Oral candidiasis
    (C) Oral lichen planus
    (D) Oral leukoplakia
    (E) Verrucous leukoplakia

92. An 18-year-old male comes to your office with complaints of hearing loss. You place a tuning fork firmly on the patient's head, and the sound lateralizes to the right ear. The test you performed is called the

   (A) Dix-Hallpike.
   (B) electronystagmography.
   (C) Rinne.
   (D) pneumatic otoscopy.
   (E) Weber.

93. A patient presents to your office complaining of recurrent spells of dizziness lasting less than a minute over the last 5 days. The patient tells you the episodes seem to be brought on when laying down and turning the head. She denies head trauma, fever, ringing in her ears, or hearing changes. Which of the following is the most likely diagnosis?

   (A) Acoustic neuroma
   (B) Benign paroxysmal positional vertigo
   (C) Ménière's disease
   (D) Vestibular neuronitis
   (E) Basilar skull fracture

94. A toddler presents to the ED with a loud deep cough and fever. These symptoms began early yesterday, but mom states that they have progressively worsened. The patient had rhinorrhea and a mild cough in the days preceding these symptoms. On exam, there is a fever of 102°F, tachypnea, tachycardia, and inspiratory stridor is audible without a stethoscope with associated nasal flaring. Radiograph of the neck shows a steeple sign. Which of the following is the most appropriate management?

   (A) Admit to the hospital for treatment
   (B) Discharge home with oral antibiotics
   (C) Observe in the ED for a short period after a dose of IV antibiotics
   (D) Prescribe nebulizer treatments every 2–4 hours
   (E) Intubate

95. The most common area involved in anterior nasal epistaxis is

   (A) anterior nasal floor.
   (B) inferior turbinate.
   (C) Kiesselbach's plexus.
   (D) superior turbinate.
   (E) nasal septum.

96. A patient is brought to the emergency department after a family member came home and found them difficult to rouse. The patient remains very drowsy during the exam. Mental status exam is abnormal, and the patient is not able to verbalize person, place, or time. You note asterixis on the neurologic exam. Chart is significant for past admissions to the hospital in the last several months for draining of ascites. What is the best treatment for this patient?

   (A) Administer dextrose
   (B) Administer glucose
   (C) Administer lactulose
   (D) Administer xylose
   (E) Administer Narcan

97. A patient is being evaluated for the development of the findings below. He also has icteric sclera. What laboratory studies would give you a MELD score in this patient?

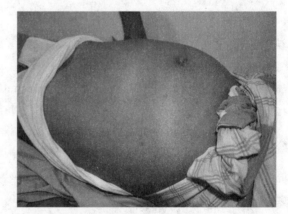

   (A) Creatinine, INR, total bilirubin
   (B) Creatinine, INR, AST
   (C) Creatinine, INR, total protein
   (D) Creatinine, INR, alk phosphatase
   (E) Creatinine, PTT, BUN

98. A patient is seen by primary care following a terminal ileum resection of 120 centimeters. The patient is reporting diarrhea that has orange streaks and has developed symptoms consistent with biliary colic. While waiting on abdominal imaging, what treatment would you start the patient on?

(A) Iron and zinc supplements
(B) Fat soluble vitamins
(C) Prescription enzymes
(D) Vitamins with added triglycerides
(E) Bismuth

99. Patients living in overcrowded conditions with inadequate sanitation may have development of the following stools. Which of the following agents is most likely responsible?

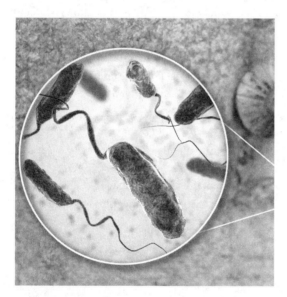

(A) Campylobacter
(B) Shigella
(C) Cholera
(D) Salmonella
(E) *C. difficile*

100. A patient returns from a 3-month trip abroad and reports progressive nausea, vomiting and diarrhea, abdominal pain, fatigue, and fever over the last month. Physical exam is positive for mild hepatosplenomegaly, generalized lymphadenopathy, and abdominal tenderness. There is no significant past medical history, and the patient is not taking any medication. What is the first line of treatment?

(A) Oral antivirals (ribavirin)
(B) Begin vaccination series
(C) Immunoglobulins
(D) Supportive care
(E) Azithromycin (macrolide)

101. A patient diagnosed with irritable bowel syndrome, constipation subtype, could be treated with all of the following except

(A) a bulking agent (e.g., psyllium).
(B) antispasmodics (e.g., hyoscyamine).
(C) selective serotonin reuptake inhibitors (e.g., fluoxetine).
(D) non-steroidal anti-inflammatory (e.g., mesalamine).
(E) antidiarrheal (e.g., Imodium).

102. In which of the following locations is a pancreatic cancer most commonly found?

(A) Head
(B) Body
(C) Tail
(D) Duct
(E) Inferior

103. Which of the following diagnostic criteria is most associated with irritable bowel syndrome?

(A) Disease of males
(B) Symptoms for less than 3 months
(C) Related to defecation
(D) Related to meals
(E) Dawn phenomenon

104. A 24-year-old female undergoes a colonoscopy. The results demonstrate colonic mucosal inflammation that spares the rectum. She has had weight loss, persistent abdominal pain, and frequently misses work due to diarrheal episodes. A recent CBC shows mild microcytic anemia. Which of the following treatments should be initiated?

    (A) Corticosteroids and 5-ASA
    (B) Corticosteroids, immunomodulators, and an anti-TNF
    (C) Corticosteroids and antibiotics
    (D) Corticosteroids, anti-TNF, and anti-integrins
    (E) Immunomodulators and antibiotics

105. A patient returns from hiking in South America and complains of watery diarrhea for the last 2 weeks. There is no blood or associated mucus in the stool. Which of the following organisms is most likely responsible?

    (A) Norovirus
    (B) Shigella
    (C) *E. coli*
    (D) Campylobacter
    (E) *Clostridium sp.*

106. What is the number one cause of acute pancreatitis in the United States?

    (A) Alcohol abuse
    (B) Blockage of the pancreatic duct
    (C) Hypertriglyceridemia
    (D) Cholelithiasis
    (E) Cancer

107. A 44-year-old female presents with colicky right upper quadrant pain that has occurred previously and is currently very intense, rated 8/10 in severity. Transabdominal ultrasound demonstrates a thickened gallbladder wall at 6 mm. Vitals are 100.6, p 104, r18, BP 130/88. She has no significant PMH. What is your first-line management?

    (A) IV Fluids, pain control, and schedule for cholecystectomy in the morning
    (B) IV Fluids, pain control, and schedule for cholecystectomy in 6–8 weeks
    (C) IV Fluids, pain control, and antibiotics
    (D) IV Fluids, pain control, drain gallbladder
    (E) Oral antibiotics

108. Mr. G. Tritis has just completed a 2-week course of therapy for an *H. pylori* infection. Which of the following is the best course of action to determine if he has cleared his infection?

    (A) *H. pylori* IgG serum screening
    (B) *H. pylori* stool antigen
    (C) *H. pylori* breath test
    (D) *H. pylori* rapid screen
    (E) White blood cell count

109. Which of the following may initially be treated with an nasogastric tube for decompression?

    (A) Intussusception
    (B) Diverticular abscess
    (C) Small bowel obstruction
    (D) Volvulus
    (E) None of the above

110. Which of the following polyps would be classified as neoplastic?

    (A) Haematoma
    (B) Tubular adenoma
    (C) Lymphoid
    (D) Hyperplastic
    (E) Lipoma

111. A patient presents complaining of black, tarry stools that have a strong smell. Which of the following tests would be indicated in the primary evaluation of this patient?

     (A) Capsule endoscopy
     (B) Colonoscopy
     (C) EGD (esophagogastroduodenoscopy)
     (D) ERCP (endoscopic retrograde cholangiopancreatography)
     (E) Urea breath test

112. A 24-year-old patient presents with reflux symptoms that have not responded well to using over the counter Prilosec (a PPI). He is well known to the practice for his poorly controlled asthma, multiple environmental allergens, and eczema. He is concerned because he is now having an increased difficulty swallowing his food and has vomited several times after eating. What finding on endoscopy would confirm your diagnosis?

     (A) Bird's beak (tapering of lower esophageal sphincter)
     (B) Chain of beads (alternating strictures and dilation)
     (C) Feline esophagus (multiple esophageal rings)
     (D) Nutcracker (high amplitude contractions)
     (E) Normal endoscopic finding

113. This rash is found on a physical exam of your patient. It has been present for several days. Which of the following tests should be performed next?

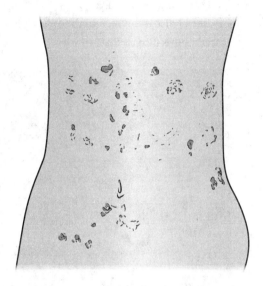

     (A) Colonoscopy with biopsy of terminal ileum
     (B) Endoscopy with biopsy of duodenum
     (C) Capsule endoscopy without biopsy
     (D) Push enteroscopy
     (E) Sigmoidoscopy

114. This image is most reflective of the chronic inflammatory process of the biliary tree that results in fibrosis, cirrhosis, and liver failure. It may be an initial manifestation of ulcerative colitis but can also be seen outside of inflammatory bowel disease. Which of the following best describes this disease?

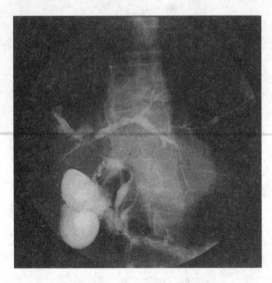

(A) Autoimmune hepatitis
(B) Biliary colic
(C) Choledocholithiasis
(D) Cholangiocarcinoma
(E) Primary sclerosing cholangitis

115. A patient presents with a persistent cough, progressive hoarseness, and dysphagia over the last 6 months. He has a history of gastroesophageal reflux disease. He has lost 15 lbs unintentionally. Social history is significant for prior smoking 1 pack per day × 14 years. HPI is also significant for an increase in heartburn that is not responsive to a proton pump inhibitor. Laboratory findings are significant for anemia. Which of the following is the most likely cause of these symptoms?

(A) Gastroesophageal reflux disease
(B) Barrett's esophagitis
(C) *H. pylori* infection
(D) Carcinoma of the esophagus
(E) Erosive esophagitis

116. A healthcare worker presents for evaluation following a needle stick. The worker has never been vaccinated against hepatitis B. Which of the following regimens should be offered?

(A) One dose of HBIG (hepatitis B immunoglobulin) followed by a repeat dose in 7 days
(B) One dose of HBIG (hepatitis B immunoglobulin) followed by initiation of HBV vaccine series
(C) Start the HBV (hepatitis B vaccination) series
(D) Draw blood for possible natural immunity to HBV (hepatitis B virus)
(E) Administer second and third HBIG doses, skipping first dose

117. Which of the following forms of hepatitis is most likely to be complicated by hepatocellular carcinoma?

(A) Hepatitis A
(B) Hepatitis G
(C) Hepatitis B
(D) Hepatitis E
(E) Hepatitis F

118. Using the following table, select the interpretation letter that best indicates a patient recently experiencing acute hepatitis B.

HBsAg	Anti-HBs	Anti-HBc	HBeAg	Anti-HBe	Interpretation
+	–	IgM	+	–	A
+	–	IgG	+	–	B
+	–	IgG	–	+	C
+	+	IgG	–	–	D
–	+	–	–	–	E

(A) A
(B) B
(C) C
(D) D
(E) E

119. Using the following, choose the correct interpretation letter for a patient demonstrating a chronic state of HBV infection.

HBsAg	Anti-HBs	Anti-HBc	HBeAg	Anti-HBe	Interpretation
+	−	IgM	+	−	A
+	−	IgG	+	−	B
+	−	IgG	−	+	C
+	+	IgG	+/−	−	D
−	+	−	−	−	E

(A) A
(B) B
(C) C
(D) D
(E) E

120. A middle-aged man has a year-long history of nonbilious emesis consisting of saliva and undigested food. He has lost 12 pounds in 3 months. He has more difficulty with solid food, but liquids also cause chest pain within minutes of swallowing. He has no heartburn or GERD symptoms. Which diagnostic test result would be expected for a patient with this type of dysphagia and medical history?

(A) A biopsy at the pyloric valve shows an ulcer caused by *H. pylori*
(B) 24-hour esophageal pH monitoring
(C) The lower esophageal sphincter has low pressure on esophageal manometry
(D) A narrow caliber esophagus with erythema and proximal strictures on endoscopy
(E) A barium swallow with tight narrowing at the lower esophageal sphincter

121. A middle-aged woman has vomiting, diarrhea, and abdominal cramps which started 2 hours ago. She had lunch about 4 hours ago. She ate at a buffet restaurant where she sampled eight different items. She looks ill but not yet dehydrated. She has no fever and her BP and pulse are within normal limits. What is the most likely pathogen causing her illness?

(A) Campylobacter
(B) *S. aureus*
(C) *Salmonella*
(D) Norwalk virus
(E) Vibrio

122. A 30-year-old man has persistent epigastric pain and heartburn despite adequate treatment with a proton pump inhibitor. In the next step of diagnosing this patient, a serum gastrin level is checked and is well above the upper limits of a normal test. Which of the following procedures is the single best test to localize the root cause of this man's heartburn?

(A) CT scan of the abdomen
(B) MR colangiopancreatography (MRCP)
(C) Somatostatin receptor scintigraphy
(D) Ultrasound of the abdomen
(E) Endoscopy

123. A 32-year-old man presents to the clinic for an annual health maintenance visit. His mother was diagnosed with colorectal cancer at 50 years of age. The patient reports no rectal bleeding or other symptoms. His medical history consists of hypercholesterolemia, and his physical examination is normal. When should this patient undergo colorectal cancer screening?

(A) Now
(B) At age 40 years
(C) At age 45 years
(D) At age 49 years
(E) At age 50 years

124. A patient is consistently getting right upper quadrant abdominal pain following rich or caloric meals. Immediately following a "7/10" painful episode she goes to an urgent care center. Based on her presenting history, which blood test is most likely to be elevated today?

    (A) Alkaline phosphatase (ALP)
    (B) Aspartate aminotransferase (AST)
    (C) Prothrombin time (PT)
    (D) Prealbumin
    (E) Cholesterol (chol)

125. Which of the following is true regarding prostate-specific antigen (PSA) testing?

    (A) PSA has a lower accuracy rate in detecting prostate cancer than digital rectal examination.
    (B) PSA is specific for cancer detection.
    (C) PSA is an excellent tool for assessing response to therapy in prostate cancer treatment.
    (D) PSA level of below 4.0 ng/mL essentially rules out prostate cancer.
    (E) PSA level is not impacted by medications.

126. A 46-year-old mother of three children complains of small amounts of urine leaking when she coughs or laughs. Her physical examination reveals no remarkable findings of the genitourinary system. Urinalysis is normal. Which of the following is the most appropriate first step in management of her condition?

    (A) Recommend pelvic floor therapy
    (B) Recommend hormonal replacement therapy
    (C) Refer for cystoscopy
    (D) Pessary placement
    (E) Urinalysis

127. You are evaluating a patient with complaints of a recent rash and new hematuria. The hematuria has been present and worsening over the last 2 days. Chemical urinalysis shows large blood and moderate protein. Microscopic urinalysis results note RBC that are too numerous to count, many are noted to be dysmorphic and RBC casts. Which of the following disorders does this suggest?

    (A) Glomerulonephrosis
    (B) Glomerulonephritis
    (C) Nephrotic syndrome
    (D) Wilm tumor
    (E) Kallmann disorder

128. A patient with SIADH with complications of confusion is best treated with which of the following?

    (A) Free water
    (B) Hypertonic saline
    (C) Lactated ringers
    (D) Normal saline
    (E) 0.45% NaCl

129. A 28-year-old male gas station attendant with a history of tobacco smoking presents with dyspnea, hemoptysis, hematuria, declining renal function, and positive serum anti-GBM antibodies. Kidney biopsy shows a crescentic GN when examined under a light microscope, and immunofluorescence reveals smooth ribbon staining of IgG in the glomerular basement membrane. What is the most likely diagnosis?

    (A) Goodpasture syndrome
    (B) Henoch-Schönlein purpura
    (C) Pauci-immune GN
    (D) Systemic lupus erythematosus
    (E) Amyloidosis

130. A 73-year-old male presents to the clinic with complaints of a weak urinary stream, nocturia, straining, and hesitancy with urinating for the past year. He notes his symptoms are getting worse. Digital rectal exam reveals an enlarged, non-tender prostate with no nodularity. Which of the following classes of medications is indicated in this patient?

    (A) ACE inhibitors
    (B) Alpha-blockers
    (C) Beta-blockers
    (D) Diuretics
    (E) Quinolones

131. Which of the following is a well-established risk factor for development of bladder cancer?

    (A) Cigarette smoking
    (B) Diabetes mellitus
    (C) Family history
    (D) Testosterone therapy
    (E) Kidney cancer history

132. The most common etiology of organic erectile dysfunction is

    (A) endocrine.
    (B) neurologic.
    (C) medication.
    (D) vascular.
    (E) cancer.

133. A patient who reports voiding small amounts every 1–2 hours, gets up frequently at night to void, and wears adult bladder control pads to avoid accidents is seen and evaluated. There is no infection and no physical abnormality. This patient would best be treated by

    (A) placement of sling.
    (B) pelvic floor physical therapy.
    (C) medications.
    (D) self-catheterization.
    (E) management of hemoglobin A1C.

134. In a patient with urinary incontinence, medication management is indicated for

    (A) urinary urgency, small and frequent voids, and 3–4 overnight voids.
    (B) urinary incontinence with activity, and occasional "dribbling."
    (C) large cystoceles with elevated post void residuals.
    (D) incontinence that causes elevated post void residuals.
    (E) postoperative incontinence.

135. You are seeing a 22-year-old patient for complaints of a mass in the vagina. She is unable to sit or stand comfortably. Your exam reveals a tender, erythematous palpable mass at the 8 o'clock position in the vagina. It feels fluctuant. Which of the following is the most appropriate antibiotic regimen to use post incision and drainage?

    (A) Amoxicillin plus clavulanic acid
    (B) Doxycycline plus amoxicillin
    (C) Metronidazole plus amoxicillin
    (D) Metronidazole alone
    (E) Azithromycin

136. A patient presents with complaints of a vaginal discharge with odor that worsens with intercourse. Her wet prep is positive for clue cells. Which of the following courses of treatment is most likely to relieve her symptoms?

    (A) Oral fluconazole for 3 days
    (B) Oral metronidazole for 7 days
    (C) Oral terconazole for 5 days
    (D) Oral letrozole for 7 days
    (E) Oral doxycycline for 7 days

137. A 26-year-old female patient presents with a 24-hour history of dysuria, urinary hesitancy, and urgency. She has some associated suprapubic pressure as well. She denies fever, chills, nausea, and vaginal symptoms. A urinalysis reveals positive nitrites and large leukocyte esterase. The remainder of the urinalysis is unremarkable. What is the most likely infectious organism?

(A) Enterobacter
(B) *Escherichia coli*
(C) *Staphylococcus*
(D) Proteus
(E) Chlamydia

138. Which of the following dietary changes can affect the absorption of sildenafil (Viagra)?

(A) High fat diet
(B) High carb diet
(C) Low carb diet
(D) Low fat diet
(E) No dietary impact

139. A 37-year-old African American woman is referred to you for refractory iron-deficiency anemia. She has been treated with oral iron intermittently for the last 10 years. She denies menorrhagia or melena. Her physical exam is normal.

Her CBC shows:

Test	Result	Reference Range
WBC	5.5	
Hgb	12	
HCT	36	
RBC	4.5	$4.0–4.9×10^6$/ml
MCV	72	80–96 fL/cell
RDW	12	11.5–14.5%
Platelets	172	

Which chromosome is affected in this patient, causing this hematologic disorder?

(A) X chromosome
(B) Chromosome 6
(C) Chromosome 10
(D) Chromosome 16
(E) Chromosome 18

140. A 32-year-old African American woman is seen for anemia. Her menstrual bleeding is described as normal. She has no other chronic illnesses. Her mother and sister are anemic. She has no obvious toxin, travel, or pet exposures. The following laboratory data are obtained.

Laboratory studies:	Patient result	Reference range
Hemoglobin	11.1 g/dL	
Hematocrit	33%	
MCV	73 fL	80–100 fL
WBC count	9,900/uL	
Platelet count	461,000/uL	
Reticulocyte count:	1.7%	0.5–1.8%
RDW	elevated	

(A) Alpha thalassemia minor
(B) Anemia of chronic disease/inflammation
(C) Lead poisoning
(D) Iron-deficiency anemia
(E) Pernicious anemia

141. A 15-year-old female comes into your office for a visit. She had a severe cold last week, and though her sore throat and runny nose have resolved, her mother is concerned because in the last few days she has noted that her daughter bruises easily, has had a bloody nose twice, and has some mild bleeding from her gums when she brushes her teeth. Her past medical history is negative for bleeding, including no heavy or abnormal menstrual cycles. Her family history is also negative. What is the most likely diagnosis for this patient?

(A) Idiopathic thrombocytopenic purpura (ITP)
(B) Thalassaemia
(C) Aplastic anemia
(D) Hereditary sideroblastic anemia
(E) Von Willebrand disease

142. Which material is obtained by centrifuging thawed, previously frozen plasma and may be used to treat bleeding patients with documented coagulation factor deficiencies?

    (A) Platelets
    (B) Cryoprecipitate
    (C) Packed RBC
    (D) Factor VII
    (E) Factor X

143. A 72-year-old female underwent an elective total knee arthroplasty to treat degenerative joint disease. Post-operatively, she is taking Coumadin (warfarin) orally for prophylaxis against development of a deep venous thrombosis. Which of the following blood tests would be most useful to monitor her anticoagulation?

    (A) Bleeding time
    (B) PT/INR
    (C) PTT
    (D) Platelet count
    (E) Vitamin K agonist

144. You are following a patient with acute myelogenous leukemia. She started induction chemotherapy yesterday. Today you note hyperkalemia, hyperphosphatemia, hyperuricemia, and renal failure in her lab work. The most likely diagnosis is

    (A) leukostasis.
    (B) paraneoplastic syndrome.
    (C) tumor lysis syndrome.
    (D) hemophilia.
    (E) normal chemotherapy effect.

145. What type of reaction is anaphylaxis due to penicillin?

    (A) Type I hypersensitivity reaction
    (B) Type II hypersensitivity reaction
    (C) Type III hypersensitivity reaction
    (D) Type IV hypersensitivity reaction
    (E) Type V hypersensitivity reaction

146. Which of the following markers is the earliest and most sensitive indicator of iron deficiency?

    (A) Ferritin
    (B) Hemoglobin
    (C) RDW
    (D) TIBC
    (E) Vitamin D

147. Which finding would be a diagnostic indicator for multiple myeloma?

    (A) Auer rods
    (B) Bence-Jones proteins
    (C) Philadelphia chromosome
    (D) Reed Sternberg cells
    (E) Normal plasma cells

148. Replicated cells mature, enter a nondividing period in their life cycle, perform their function for a prescribed period of time, and then die and are replaced. This process of programmed life expectancy is called

    (A) proto-oncogenic.
    (B) apoptosis.
    (C) anaplasia.
    (D) paraneoplastic.
    (E) hybridosis.

149. A 45-year-old man is admitted for intravenous antibiotics for pyelonephritis. On admission, his labs reveal an elevated PTT. He has no prior history of bleeding disorders and has had multiple prior surgeries. He has no current bleeding. There is no family history of bleeding. PT and CBC are normal except for WBC of $14 \times 103/$ mm3. His PTT 1:1 mix reveals a lack of correction of his aPTT. FVIII and FIX activity is normal. Three months ago, coagulation studies were normal. The specimen was drawn from a peripherally inserted central catheter (PICC line). What is the most likely cause of his incidentally discovered prolonged aPTT?

    (A) Congenital hemophilia
    (B) Fibrinogen deficiency or dysfibrinogenemia
    (C) Contamination of lab draw with heparin
    (D) Unrecognized warfarin usage from prior to his hospitalization
    (E) Amyloidosis-associated factor IX deficiency

150. An 18-year-old woman with hemoglobin SS presents after being discharged from the hospital, where she was treated for a sickle cell pain episode. She has been admitted to the hospital at least five times this year and was diagnosed with acute chest syndrome during a previous hospital admission. She takes folic acid daily and is up to date on all of her health maintenance. Which one of the following medications should you consider prescribing at this time?

    (A) Aspirin
    (B) Multivitamin
    (C) Vitamin D
    (D) Hydroxyurea
    (E) Vitamin B12

151. Which of the following genetic markers is consistent with hereditary hemochromatosis?

    (A) BCR/ABL translocation
    (B) H63D mutation of the HFE gene
    (C) JAK2 mutation
    (D) Tyrosine kinase marker
    (E) TSAT

152. Which granulocytes contain histamine and heparin and play a role in hypersensitivity reactions?

    (A) Basophils
    (B) Eosinophils
    (C) Neutrophils
    (D) Monocytes
    (E) Cytophils

153. You have been treating your patient for AML. She has received induction chemotherapy. Fortunately, her bone marrow biopsy following induction chemotherapy comes back with no evidence of leukemia. What is the next step?

    (A) She is cured. Continue to monitor for signs of relapse.
    (B) This is remission. She needs maintenance chemotherapy for 2–3 years.
    (C) This is primary induction failure. Move to salvage chemotherapy.
    (D) This represents primary treatment failure. Move to autologous hematopoietic cell transplantation.
    (E) This is remission. She needs consolidation chemotherapy for four to five cycles.

154. Which method is the most sensitive and specific for diagnosis of pulmonary tuberculosis?

    (A) Sputum culture
    (B) RNA amplification on blood
    (C) Quantiferon assay on blood
    (D) Sputum acid-fast smear
    (E) Urine LAM test

155. Which genetic phenomena is most likely to result in an influenza pandemic?

    (A) Alanine to lactate point mutation in the hemagglutinin gene
    (B) Inefficient use of host RNA transcriptase
    (C) Mixing of two viral genomes in a common host species
    (D) Plasmid transfer during conjugation
    (E) Detachment of surface glycoproteins

156. An 18-year-old boy has clusters of vesicles that form on the lip. He has had them before and they tend to recur after a test or after a day at the beach. What is the most likely cause of this condition?

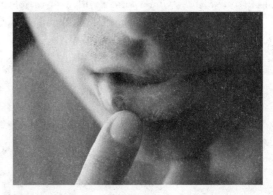

    (A) Human herpesvirus 8
    (B) Epstein-Barr virus
    (C) Herpes simplex virus 1
    (D) Cytomegalovirus
    (E) Syphilis

157. Which of the following pathogens secrete an exotoxin that blocks the release of acetylcholine at the neuromuscular junction and results in flaccid paralysis?

    (A) *Clostridium botulinum*
    (B) *Clostridium tetani*
    (C) *Corynebacterium diphtheriae*
    (D) *Vibrio cholerae*
    (E) *Streptococcus viridans*

158. Which HIV test should be completed first in a patient recently diagnosed with *Pneumocyctis jirovacii* pneumonia (PJP)?

    (A) CD4 count
    (B) HIV genotype
    (C) HIV viral load
    (D) HIV 1 and 2 antibody/antigen combo
    (E) Western blot for HIV 1 and 2

159. Based on the modified Duke criteria, which of the following is a major criterion for the diagnosis of endocarditis?

    (A) Two Janeway lesions on the left hand, present for 5 days
    (B) Pulmonic stenosis with a murmur, unchanged since the patient was an infant
    (C) Two blood cultures positive for *E. coli*, drawn at the same time
    (D) Two blood cultures positive for *Streptococcus viridans*, drawn 1 hour apart
    (E) Dental work completed in the previous 48 hours

160. An ambulance brings in a 73-year-old woman for confusion and fever. She has had a fever and headache since yesterday. Two days prior she was on a farm and had fresh dairy products. Temp 103°F, RR 20, BP 100/85, HR 105. She is in moderate distress. Neuro exam: drowsy, pupils are 6 mm and reactive. No papilledema. Lumbar puncture: opening pressure high, CSF = WBCs 400/mm3; 90% neutrophils, glucose low & protein high. Gram stain has gram-positive bacilli. Which antibiotic is the most targeted choice for the bacteria causing this infection?

    (A) Ampicillin (aminopenicillin)
    (B) Cefazolin (cephalosporin 1st gen)
    (C) Ceftriaxone (cephalosporin 3rd gen)
    (D) Aztreonam (monobactam)
    (E) Azithromycin (macrolide)

161. An adult patient was recently treated for lung cancer. Ten days after receiving chemotherapy, he was admitted to the hospital with a fever of 102°F. Which of the following antibiotics would be the best single agent for treating infection caused by pseudomonas and methicillin-sensitive *Staph aureus* (MSSA)?

    (A) Cefazolin (1st-generation cephalosporin)
    (B) Cefoxitin (2nd-generation cephalosporin)
    (C) Ceftriaxone (3rd-generation cephalosporin)
    (D) Cefepime (4th-generation cephalosporin)
    (E) Ceftaroline (5th-generation cephalosporin)

162. Which of the following is true about viral replication?

    (A) Both DNA and RNA viruses use host cell ribosomes to translate RNA to proteins.
    (B) DNA viruses produce their own DNA and RNA polymerase.
    (C) The viral envelope is derived from viral DNA.
    (D) The viral capsid is a location for energy storage.
    (E) The viral capsid is uncoated.

163. Dr. L is a 35-year-old woman from Nigeria with "flu" symptoms for 1 week. Upon further questioning, you find out that she has fevers, "bone pain," headache, and loss of appetite. You notice her eyes appear yellow and that her urine is darker than normal. Which diagnostic test result fits best with this patient's illness presentation?

    (A) An antibody/antigen combo test on blood is positive for a virus.
    (B) An early morning sputum sample has acid fast bacilli.
    (C) A blood smear after a fever spike has signet ring forms.
    (D) An MRI reveals destruction in a long bone, most likely from bacteria.
    (E) A thick blood smear shows visible parasites.

164. A 57-year-old man has a 2-day history of bloody diarrhea, abdominal pain, and lethargy. Some families that ate at his house are also ill. Temp-98.9°F, HR 92, BP 150/88, RR 18. Chest and cardiac exam normal. Abdomen: increased bowel sounds, diffuse tenderness, and patient groans when you press. Extremities: 1+ pitting edema and warm to touch. The patient is drowsy but answers your questions appropriately. There is a petechial rash over his trunk. Fecal studies show a few WBCs and many RBCs. CBC shows anemia and thrombocytopenia. Metabolic profile shows elevated creatinine and BUN that was not noted on labs last month. Which therapy is best for this condition?

    (A) Azithromycin (macrolide)
    (B) Ciprofloxacin (quinolone)
    (C) No antibiotics; supportive care
    (D) Trimethoprim-sulfamethoxazole (folate inhibitor)
    (E) Ceftriaxone (cephalosporin)

165. You are evaluating a 55-year-old patient with diarrhea. She has been treated twice for sinusitis in the last month. The second course of antibiotics had an expanded spectrum due to fear that there was a beta-lactamase producing strain. The diarrhea has been present for 3 days, and she has to go about eight times daily. Which of the following statements would be incorrect advice when educating the patient about this condition?

    (A) Your condition is transmittable; you should wash hands frequently.
    (B) Your therapy for the diarrhea will be extended to 14 days to eradicate bacterial spores.
    (C) If this diarrhea does not go away, antidiarrheals and IV vancomycin will be the therapy of choice.
    (D) Using antibiotics with a broad spectrum likely caused this condition, so we will need to stop this as soon as possible.
    (E) A candida infection may occur following antibiotic therapy.

166. A deer hunter from Montana had a fever, weakness, headache, and muscle pain last year. He does not remember what his treating doctor said the infection was, but he has a copy of an old prescription that showed he was on doxycycline (tetracycline) for 6 weeks and gentamicin (aminoglycoside) for 1 week. What infection should you add to his past medical history in his electronic patient record?

    (A) Inhalational anthrax
    (B) Brucellosis
    (C) Schistosomiasis
    (D) Lyme disease
    (E) COPD

167. A new animal owner is bitten on the hand by a frightened large dog. Which antibiotic therapy would be best for the patient?

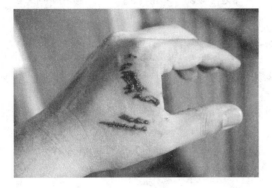

    (A) Ampicillin/sulbactam (penicillin)
    (B) Vancomycin (glycopeptide)
    (C) Tetracycline
    (D) Aztreonam (monobactam)
    (E) Azithromycin (macrolide)

168. You are treating a patient who has an ulcer on her heel. You can place a probe in the ulcer and touch bone. The patient had a debridement of the ulcer. Antibiotics were targeted at the bacteria found in the biopsy of this wound. You are now seeing the patient after 2 weeks of antibiotic therapy, and they are still having pain, fever, and redness around the ulcer site. You are convinced that the antibiotic selected is proper. What would be the best next step in this patient's treatment?

    (A) Request a surgical consultation to assess for an abscess
    (B) Stop antibiotics; a long antibiotic course is complete
    (C) Continue antibiotics for 2 more weeks
    (D) Swab the wound to see if any additional organisms are present
    (E) Check a calcaneus X-ray to confirm osteomyelitis

169. Which statement about the treatment of infective endocarditis is most accurate?

    (A) Beta-lactam drugs should not be used if there is a suitable alternative from another class.
    (B) Bacteriostatic antibiotics may be used as long as the therapy is for 2 weeks.
    (C) Frequently, prosthetic valves can be cleared of *Strep viridans* with antibiotic therapy.
    (D) Typical antibiotic therapy will last for 4 weeks or longer with a bactericidal agent.
    (E) It commonly affects two or more valves prior to diagnosis.

170. A young patient has a skin lesion of 2 days duration without fever or white blood cell count elevation. Which bacteria is the most likely cause of the infection in this picture?

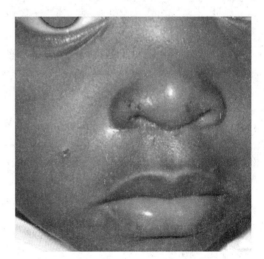

    (A) *Pseudomonas*
    (B) *Streptococcus*
    (C) *Enterococcus*
    (D) *Mycobacterium*
    (E) *Staphylococcus*

171. Which statement about urethritis is most accurate?

    (A) Diagnosis is primarily made by use of DNA probes run on the purulent discharge.
    (B) Chlamydia and *Neisseria gonorrhoeae* infections are distinguishable by physical examination.
    (C) Ciprofloxacin (quinolone) is the best treatment.
    (D) *Neisseria gonorrheae* is difficult to transmit via sexual intercourse.
    (E) Azithromycin is the treatment of choice.

172. Pain from an acute fracture is often described as

    (A) crampy and achy.
    (B) sharp and burning.
    (C) throbbing and diffuse.
    (D) stabbing and hot.
    (E) tearing and localized.

173. A 32-year-old male presents with left knee pain and swelling after playing tennis. He notes the injury occurred while going for a ball, planting his foot, twisting sharply, and feeling pain over the medial aspect of his left knee. PE significant for mild effusion with medial joint line tenderness and a palpable click with flexion. Which of the following imaging studies would be most specific to confirming your suspicions?

    (A) Radiographs
    (B) Arthroscopy
    (C) MRI
    (D) CT
    (E) Ultrasound

174. A 39-year-old female presents to your clinic complaining of left ankle pain. She was doing jump kicks at her karate class last night when she landed on the outside of her left foot, which was plantar flexed. She heard a "pop" and experienced a sharp pain. On PE there is visible swelling of the lateral aspect of her left ankle (see picture) and an anterior drawer test shows a difference of 8 mm between the injured and non-injured ankles. Talar tilt test shows no instability and she has only minimal restriction of weight-bearing ability. Which ligament is most likely affected?

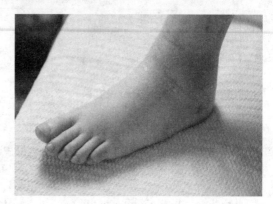

    (A) Syndesmosis
    (B) Delta ligament
    (C) Anterior talofibular ligament
    (D) Superficial talotibial ligament
    (E) Calcaneofibular ligament

175. A 7-year-old male is referred to your orthopedic clinic after his mother noticed him walking with a limp. He and his mother deny history of trauma. On PE there is atrophy of the gluteal muscles and decreased range of motion of the right hip, particularly with internal rotation and abduction. Frog-leg X-rays reveal cessation of growth at the right capital femoral epiphysis and a smaller femoral head epiphysis with widening of the articular space on the right side. There is also a linear radiolucency within the right femoral head epiphysis. CBC, WBC, C-reactive protein, and ESR are all normal. Which of the following is the most likely diagnosis?

(A) Slipped capital femoral epiphysis
(B) Legg-Calvé-Perthes disease
(C) Developmental dysplasia of the hip
(D) Osteomyelitis of the right hip
(E) Osgood Schlatter disease

176. Which of the following grades of muscle strength best defines full range of motion against gravity without resistance?

(A) 2
(B) 3
(C) 4
(D) 5
(E) 6

177. A 54-year-old male complains of neck stiffness, especially upon rising, sometimes having numbness and shooting pain in his left arm and hand. Which of the following history questions will best indicate a cervical herniated nucleus pulposus as a diagnosis and NOT thoracic outlet syndrome?

(A) Do you get numbness in your arm when you raise your hand?
(B) Is the pain made worse by coughing, straining, or laughing?
(C) Would you describe the pain as a burning sensation?
(D) Have you noticed your hands feeling colder or changing color with certain head movements?
(E) Is there pain in the shoulder when hands are at your side?

178. A patient presents with complaints of sharp medial heel pain that occurs when he first steps onto his foot in the morning or after prolonged periods of rest. The pain improves after walking for short periods of time. He experiences severe, dull-achy pain in his foot with prolonged weight bearing. A tight Achilles tendon is noted on examination with a negative Thompson's sign. From the information given, what is the most likely diagnosis?

(A) Achilles tendonitis
(B) Morton's neuroma
(C) Plantar fasciitis
(D) Metatarsalgia
(E) Paget's disease of bone

179. A 16-year-old male presents with right hand swelling and pain after getting into a fight at school. He states that when trying to punch another kid, he missed and struck the wall. On imaging, you identify a non-displaced distal fracture of the fifth metacarpal with 10 degrees of angulation. With physical examination, you note all nerves to be intact and palpate strong pulses. Based on your diagnosis from the imaging, mechanism of injury, and physical examination, what is the best treatment plan?

(A) Thumb spica splint
(B) Short-arm ulnar gutter splint
(C) Radial gutter splint
(D) Refer for surgical intervention
(E) Rest and ice

180. Which of the following should be considered as a surgical emergency when it is associated with acute onset of back pain?

(A) Night sweats, fever, chills
(B) Bowel and bladder dysfunction
(C) History of cancer
(D) History of spondylolisthesis
(E) History of compression syndrome

181. A patient that demonstrates a positive apprehension test most likely has a history of

(A) rotator cuff tear.
(B) biceps tendinitis.
(C) SLAP lesion.
(D) shoulder dislocation.
(E) anxiety.

182. The most important complication of a posterior dislocation of the knee is

(A) instability of the joint.
(B) ligament damage.
(C) inability to reduce the joint.
(D) arterial injury.
(E) patellar tendon rupture.

183. Normal curvature of the cervical spine is

(A) kyphotic.
(B) lumbotic.
(C) lordotic.
(D) spondylosis.
(E) military neck.

184. A 25-year-old man sustains a FOOSH injury of his left wrist falling from his bicycle. There is tenderness to palpation in the radial fossa. The X-ray below shows the following. Which of the following is the most likely course of action for this presentation?

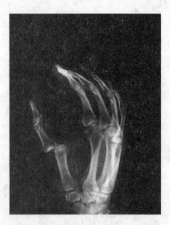

(A) Ace wrap wrist and ice to area for 1 week
(B) Thumb spica splint and repeat X-ray in 4 weeks
(C) Send for a bone scan
(D) Apply radial gutter cast
(E) Refer patient for surgical repair

185. Which of the following grades of muscle strength best defines full range of motion with gravity eliminated?

(A) 2
(B) 3
(C) 4
(D) 5
(E) 6

186. A golfer comes in complaining of pain along the radial aspect of their thumb, wrist, and forearm. They tell you it is exacerbated whenever they try grabbing onto something like a door handle. What physical exam test would confirm your suspicions?

(A) Tinel test
(B) Finkelstein test
(C) Phalen test
(D) Allen test
(E) Faber test

187. A mother brought her 14-month-old son to your clinic after he stopped moving his left arm. Earlier today, she lifted her son by "grabbing him by the wrists and pulling him up off the floor." The child is sitting in his mother's lap with his left forearm flexed and refusing to move his left arm, forearm, or wrist. The arm and joints appear normal with no noted deformities, edema, or erythema. Distal pulses and capillary refill are normal, and he moves his fingers well. The most likely diagnosis is

(A) lateral epicondylitis.
(B) subluxation of the radial head.
(C) anterior shoulder dislocation.
(D) Galeazzi fracture.
(E) ulnar fracture.

188. The primary reason hip dislocations should be reduced as soon as possible is to

(A) make the person more comfortable.
(B) avoid complications of avascular necrosis.
(C) prevent rupture of the muscle-tendon unit.
(D) help reduce femur fractures.
(E) enable continuation of activities of daily living.

PRACTICE TEST 2

189. In a child who you suspect abuse, which of the following X-ray findings would highly raise your index of suspicion?

(A) Torus fracture
(B) Salter V fracture
(C) Posterior rib fracture
(D) Spiculated appearance in the distal humerus
(E) Foreign bodies in trachea

190. A 42-year-old right-hand dominant male presents complaining of right elbow pain. The pain is aggravated by extension of the wrist against resistance. X-rays of the elbow and forearm are normal. The most likely diagnosis is

(A) arthritis.
(B) lateral epicondylitis.
(C) occult radial head fracture.
(D) extensor carpi ulnaris tendonitis.
(E) scaphoid fracture.

191. The initial treatment of choice for torticollis is

(A) passive stretching.
(B) surgical release of the sternocleidomastoid muscle.
(C) Botox injection.
(D) muscle relaxants, such as low-dose Flexeril.
(E) lateral manipulation of the c-spine.

192. A fracture in the mid-portion of the fifth metatarsal metadiaphyseal junction is called a

(A) Dancer's fracture.
(B) Jones fracture.
(C) fifth metatarsal avulsion fracture.
(D) Lisfranc injury.
(E) greenstick fracture.

193. Tenderness during palpation of the anatomic snuffbox should raise the suspicion of what disorder?

(A) Boxer's fracture
(B) Ulnar collateral ligament tear
(C) Ganglion cyst
(D) Scaphoid fracture
(E) Comminuted fracture

194. Normal curvature of the lumbar spine is

(A) kyphosis.
(B) lumbosis.
(C) lordosis.
(D) spondylosis.
(E) scoliosis.

195. A 60-year-old woman is brought to the ER. Her husband reports that upon rising this morning his wife had difficulty speaking and could not move her right arm. Neurologic examination reveals that the patient is alert, but she cannot speak well. She seems to be trying hard to speak, with occasional appropriate words. She understands commands. With the exception of paralysis of and decreased sensation over the right side of her face, no other cranial nerve deficits are found. What type of aphasia is most consistent with this patient's presentation?

(A) Wernicke's
(B) Broca's
(C) Receptive
(D) Sensory
(E) Conduction aphasia

196. Which of the following is suggestive of an upper motor neuron lesion?

(A) Negative Babinski
(B) Decreased deep tendon reflexes
(C) Muscle atrophy
(D) Spasticity
(E) Ipsilateral weakness

197. A 26-year-old patient is being evaluated for bilateral lower extremity weakness. The symptoms started 2 days ago with pins and needles in the shins. The patient is now unable to bear weight due to weakness. The patient has no chronic medical problems. Physical exam findings include absence of deep tendon reflexes in bilateral knees and ankles. What is the most likely diagnosis?

(A) Amyotrophic lateral sclerosis
(B) Multiple sclerosis
(C) Guillain-Barré Syndrome
(D) Myasthenia gravis
(E) Bell's palsy

198. In Parkinson's disease, the diagnostic criteria are bradykinesia and which type of tremor?

    (A) Cerebellar
    (B) Essential
    (C) Intention
    (D) Resting
    (E) Dystonic

199. What physical examination abnormality would you expect in a patient with pseudotumor cerebri?

    (A) Confusion and altered mental status
    (B) Low blood pressure and tachycardia
    (C) Muscle weakness, hyperactive DTRs, and a Babinski sign
    (D) Blurred/decreased vision and papilledema
    (E) Polyphagia

200. You are evaluating a patient with a suspected stroke. On exam, you note hemiplegia, hemi-sensory deficits, homonymous hemianopsia with global aphasia. Which artery is most likely affected by occlusion?

    (A) Anterior cerebral
    (B) Posterior inferior cerebral
    (C) Middle inferior
    (D) Vertebral
    (E) Middle cerebral

201. A 76-year-old man presents with his 40-year-old daughter who describes recent memory loss episodes by her father. The man acknowledges his problems but assigns no importance to them. However, he describes a recent episode when he was driving home and suddenly lost his way, although he was taking the usual route. The patient has been under chronic treatment for hypertension and high cholesterol for 20 years. He is otherwise healthy. Physical examination is unremarkable. Neuropsychological tests are inconclusive, showing only some borderline memory alterations, with a MoCA score of 24. What is the most likely preliminary diagnosis?

    (A) Cortical basal degeneration
    (B) Benign memory loss
    (C) Early Alzheimer's
    (D) Brain tumor
    (E) syphilis

202. Upon stroking the lateral aspect of the sole from the heel to the ball of the foot, the great toe dor-siflexes and the other toes fan. This is a positive

    (A) Kernig's sign.
    (B) Brudzinski's sign.
    (C) Babinski's sign.
    (D) Gower's sign.
    (E) striatal toe sign.

203. Which of the following dystrophies has a rapid progression of symptoms with death about 15 years after onset?

    (A) Becker
    (B) Myotonic
    (C) Facioscapulohumeral
    (D) Duchenne
    (E) Distal

204. You are seeing a second grader whose mother brings him in to be evaluated for episodes in which he appears dazed and in a trance-like state. He also blinks his eyes in a strange, purposeful way during these episodes. He is doing poorly in school. During the exam, you have him hyperventilate producing similar symptoms. What is your diagnosis?

(A) Absence seizure
(B) Complex partial seizure
(C) Myoclonic seizure
(D) Tonic-clonic seizure
(E) Simple seizure

205. This PE finding is noted in which of the following types of headache?

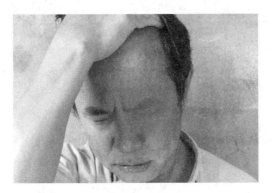

(A) Cluster
(B) Migraine
(C) Pseudotumor cerebri
(D) Tension
(E) Sinus headache

206. A 66-year-old male presents to the emergency department with a history of right temporal headache and blurred vision of the right eye for 3 days. On physical examination, he is tachycardic and has a visual acuity 20/100 OD. There is tenderness over the right temporal region. The remainder of his neurologic exam is noncontributory. Laboratory studies show an ESR of 96. Which of the following is the most appropriate management?

(A) Prednisone
(B) Hydrocodone
(C) Imitrex
(D) Acetaminophen
(E) Augmentin

207. You are seeing a patient with a complaint of diplopia. On a physical exam, you notice that the patient is tilting his head to the side. When examining the extraocular movements, you notice that the patient cannot move the right eye laterally. You suspect a problem with which of the cranial nerves?

(A) CN III
(B) CN IV
(C) CN V
(D) CN VI
(E) CN IX

208. A patient is transported to the ED after suffering a head injury in an automobile accident. She is comatosed and responds to painful stimuli by flexing her arms at the elbow and extending her hips and knees. Blood pressure is 160/100, pulse is 52/min, and respirations are irregular. The pupillary reflex is pictured. This clinical picture is consistent with what potential complication of head trauma:

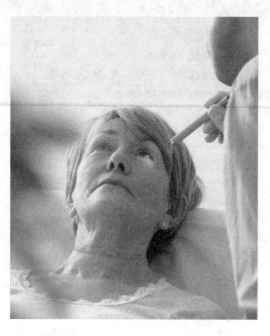

(A) Brain herniation
(B) Basilar artery occlusion
(C) Brainstem lesion
(D) Abscess
(E) Coup-contrecoup brain injury

209. A 43-year-old data entry clerk presents with a 1-month history of pain and tingling in the right thumb, index finger, and middle finger. The pain is interfering with her daily work. Tinel's sign and Phalen's maneuver are positive. What is the most appropriate initial intervention?

(A) Methylprednisolone steroid pack
(B) Splint in neutral position
(C) Observation
(D) Surgery
(E) Cortisone injections

210. A 63-year-old male presents to the clinic with a sudden onset of right-sided facial droop and inability to close his right eye or raise his right eyebrow. He reports that his face feels stiff. What additional complaint would be consistent with this patient's disorder?

(A) Facial pruritus
(B) Hearing loss
(C) Periauricular pain
(D) Scalp tenderness
(E) Impaired vision

211. A 50-year-old male presents with complaint of 1-month history of brief attacks of intense, shooting pain in his left cheek. He notes that the pain is triggered by touching his face and chewing. What is the most likely diagnosis?

(A) Cluster headache
(B) Sinus headache
(C) Temporal arteritis
(D) Trigeminal neuralgia
(E) Herpes zoster

212. A 30-year-old male presents with complaints of headache for the last week. He describes the headache as sharp, severe pain around his left eye. It is associated with tearing and nasal congestion on the left side. The pain lasts for 20 minutes before resolving, but recurs during the day. He had a similar presentation about 4 years ago. What is the most appropriate treatment for prevention of his headaches?

(A) Dihydroergotamine
(B) Naproxen
(C) Sumatriptan
(D) Verapamil
(E) Oxygen

213. You are evaluating a 30-year-old female with complaints of a headache with vision changes. Which of the following clinical presentations is most consistent with diagnosis of migraine headache?

    (A) Flashing lights in left eye lasting for ten minutes followed by onset of throbbing headache
    (B) Progressively worsening throbbing headache with unilateral vision loss and generalized myalgias
    (C) Severe retro-orbital headache associated with unilateral ptosis and rhinorrhea
    (D) Unilateral headache followed by persisting vision loss in left eye
    (E) Unilateral headache radiating to the maxilla

214. What is the best diagnostic study for evaluating changes in a patient's chronic headache pattern?

    (A) CT without contrast
    (B) CT with contrast
    (C) MRI
    (D) PET
    (E) Sleep EEG

215. Along with memory loss, what other signs/symptoms are typically present at diagnosis of mild (early) Alzheimer's disease?

    (A) Delirium
    (B) Loss of spontaneity and personality changes
    (C) Tremor
    (D) Weight loss
    (E) Impared sleep

216. Which clinical presentation is most important in making the diagnosis of epilepsy in a patient presenting with seizure activity?

    (A) Age of patient
    (B) Generalized versus focal
    (C) Loss of consciousness
    (D) Recurrence or risk of recurrence
    (E) Vital signs

217. A 25-year-old female is brought to the ED for a suicide attempt. She reports to you that her boyfriend broke up with her despite her pleading with him to stay. She says that she cut her arm to help numb the pain and loneliness from the breakup. She admits that she has had many "rocky" relationships in her past and that this is not the first time she has cut herself. She tells you that she has always felt "empty" inside. Her mother tells you that her daughter is emotionally labile and has a history of alcohol abuse in addition to the "cutting." What is the most likely diagnosis for this patient?

    (A) Antisocial personality disorder
    (B) Borderline personality disorder
    (C) Generalized anxiety disorder
    (D) Major depressive disorder
    (E) Psychotic disorder

218. You are following a 23-year-old male with a past medical history significant only for left below the knee amputation that was performed after he was wounded in military combat about 9 months ago. He has had difficulty sleeping, frequent nightmares about the events that led to his injury, and flashbacks since the incident. What is the most appropriate treatment for this patient?

    (A) Benzodiazepines
    (B) Mood stabilizers
    (C) Selective serotonin reuptake inhibitors
    (D) Serotonin-norepinephrine reuptake inhibitors
    (E) Prazosin (minipress)

219. A 33-year-old female is seeing you with complaints of anxiety. She worries that she may lose her job because her coworkers are talking about her and laughing behind her back. She admits that she has very few friends because "people cannot be trusted." She refuses to give any additional history because she is afraid that the information will be "used against her." The most likely diagnosis is

(A) borderline personality disorder.
(B) narcissistic personality disorder.
(C) paranoid personality disorder.
(D) schizotypal personality disorder.
(E) histrionic personality disorder.

220. Following the unexpected death of her husband, a 65-year-old patient has seizures with no medical explanation. Which of the following is correct regarding this patient's condition and treatment?

(A) Functional neurological symptom disorder, treat with antiepileptic medications
(B) Functional neurological symptom disorder, reassurance, and regular follow-up
(C) Somatization (complex somatic symptom) disorder, treat with antiepileptic medications
(D) Somatization (complex somatic symptom) disorder, reassurance, and regular follow-up
(E) Complex focal seizure disorder, treat with diet therapy

221. A 32-year-old female patient presents reporting having become increasingly depressed over the last 2–3 months. She has a history of major depressive disorder and had previously been treated with SSRIs but was tapered off medications approximately 1 year ago in the setting of symptom improvement at that time. She now has thoughts of suicide and is refusing to eat. She has no other significant past medical history and takes no current medications. Which of the following treatment options would be best initial treatment in this case?

(A) ECT
(B) SNRI
(C) SSRI
(D) TMS
(E) EEG

222. An 18-year-old female is in your office for evaluation of dizziness. The mother notes that, over the last 4–6 months, her daughter eats very little and exercises an extraordinary amount. The patient tells you that she has to stay in shape for ballet and just isn't hungry. On exam, you note that the patient is 5'7" tall and weighs 100 lbs. What is the most likely diagnosis?

(A) Anorexia nervosa
(B) Bulimia nervosa
(C) Bipolar disorder I
(D) Major depression
(E) Plant-based diet

223. A 46-year-old man presents with a long-standing belief that his thoughts are being taken from his head by alien spies. He is certain that the government is involved because they often communicate with him through a microchip that they implanted in his brain. Ultimately, he tells you that they are planning to utilize him in their efforts to take over the world; he will be the "human sacrifice." He appears very nervous and is easily excitable. What is the most likely diagnosis?

    (A) Catatonic schizophrenia
    (B) Disorganized schizophrenia
    (C) Paranoid schizophrenia
    (D) Residual schizophrenia
    (E) Undifferentiated schizophrenia

224. A 36-year-old is brought into the ER by EMS for evaluation of severe abdominal pain and diarrhea. On exam, you note a pulse rate of 115 bpm, a blood pressure of 188/102, and dilated pupils. On previous ER records, you note that the patient has a PMH of anxiety and chronic back pain following a motor vehicle accident. His medication list includes Zoloft (SSRI), Xanax (benzodiazepine), and MS Contin (opioid). Which of the following is the most likely diagnosis?

    (A) Benzodiazepine overdose
    (B) Benzodiazepine withdrawal
    (C) Opioid overdose
    (D) Opioid withdrawal
    (E) Aortic dissection

225. A 36-year-old man has essentially no friends, except for a cousin with whom he has been close since childhood. He has never had a sexual encounter and works from home for a computer programming company. He expresses no desire to have friends or intimate relationships. He enjoys playing computer games, such as solitaire, and surfing the Internet. What is the most likely diagnosis?

    (A) Avoidant personality disorder
    (B) Borderline personality disorder
    (C) Schizotypal personality disorder
    (D) Narcissistic personality disorder
    (E) Schizoid personality disorder

226. Agoraphobia is most frequently associated with

    (A) bipolar disorder.
    (B) generalized anxiety disorder.
    (C) obsessive-compulsive disorder.
    (D) schizotypal personality disorder.
    (E) panic disorder.

227. Which of the following factors is indicative of alcohol tolerance?

    (A) Twelve-year history of daily alcohol use
    (B) Conviction of driving while intoxicated
    (C) Marital discord due to the alcohol use
    (D) Requirement of more alcohol to become intoxicated
    (E) None of the above

228. A pregnant woman believes that she is carrying musician John Lennon's child. This is an example of

    (A) delirium.
    (B) delusion.
    (C) dementia.
    (D) hallucination.
    (E) narcissistic personality.

229. A 30-year-old man presents to your office for "anxiety." He reports that he has an intense fear of heights but is very interested in overcoming this fear so that he can take his wife on a mountain hiking trip for their anniversary next year. What is the treatment of choice for this man's condition?

    (A) Exposure therapy
    (B) Benzodiazepines
    (C) Electroconvulsive therapy
    (D) Selective serotonin reuptake inhibitors
    (E) Light therapy

230. In a patient with depressed mood, lack of concentration, and increased sleepiness, which of the following lab tests would be most appropriate in supporting your differential diagnosis?

    (A) LFTs
    (B) BMP
    (C) TSH
    (D) Sedimentation rate
    (E) BUN

231. Which of the following patients is the best candidate for ECT?

    (A) A patient with depression and psychotic features and a comorbid history of mild COPD
    (B) A patient with refractory major depressive disorder and a comorbid history of STEMI 2 months ago
    (C) A patient with major depressive disorder and a comorbid history of uncontrolled HTN
    (D) A patient with severe panic disorder and comorbid history of CHF
    (E) A patient with bipolar disorder and hypertension

232. A 55-year-old female presents with nearly 7 months of hallucinations and (per accompanying family) delusional thinking. In addition, she endorses periods of significant depression over this same time. With thorough questioning, you are able to clarify that for several of these weeks her hallucinations and delusions persisted despite her depression episodes resolving. Given this information, which of the following diagnoses is most likely?

    (A) Schizoaffective disorder
    (B) Schizophreniform
    (C) Schizophrenia
    (D) Major depressive disorder
    (E) Schizotypal disorder

233. The set of observations and assessments resulting in a detailed and systematic description of a patient's current cognitive and behavioral state primarily consists of

    (A) laboratory studies.
    (B) mental status exam.
    (C) physical exam.
    (D) radiology studies.
    (E) MOCA.

234. Which of the following is NOT an approved pharmacologic agent for medication-assisted treatment (MAT) in the setting of opioid dependence?

    (A) Buprenorphine
    (B) Clonidine
    (C) Naltrexone
    (D) Methadone
    (E) Fentanyl

235. Which of the following antibiotics is first-line treatment for an infant presenting with a severe hacking cough that is followed by a high-pitched, gasping intake of breath?

    (A) Amoxicillin (penicillin)
    (B) Ciprofloxacin (fluoroquinolone)
    (C) Doxycycline (tetracycline)
    (D) Azithromycin (macrolide)
    (E) Cephalexin (cephalosporin)

236. Which of the following is the hallmark finding of ARDS (adult respiratory distress syndrome) on a chest X-ray?

    (A) Bilateral fluffy infiltrates
    (B) Blunting of the costophrenic angles
    (C) Coin lesions
    (D) Hilar lymphadenopathy
    (E) Aortic arch prominence

237. Which of the following is the initial treatment of choice in a person with pulmonary embolism without hemodynamic compromise?

    (A) Warfarin (Coumadin)
    (B) Low-molecular-weight heparin
    (C) Prednisone
    (D) Surgery
    (E) Compression stockings

238. A 45-year-old male nonsmoker presents to your clinic with a recent chest X-ray that shows a solid solitary pulmonary nodule 5 mm in size. He just moved to the area. The X-ray was done because he fell off a ladder and was suspected to have a rib fracture (no fractures found). Of the following options, which is the best choice?

    (A) Perform spirometry
    (B) Obtain a MRI scan
    (C) Obtain a PET scan
    (D) Request old chest X-rays
    (E) Ask about history of asbestosis

239. A 30-year-old African-American female presents to your office with noncaseating granulomas on chest X-ray. She complains of low-grade fevers, weight loss, lymphadenopathy, and joint pain. She is found to have tender nodules on her lower extremities on a physical exam. She is noted to have hypercalcemia and elevated angiotensin-converting enzyme levels during laboratory workup. Which of the following is the most likely diagnosis?

    (A) Pneumonia
    (B) Pulmonary lymphoma
    (C) Sarcoidosis
    (D) Small cell lung cancer
    (E) Amyloidosis

240. Which of the following tests would be the only one found to be positive in a case of latent tuberculosis infection?

    (A) Positive interferon gamma release assay
    (B) Positive sputum culture
    (C) Positive sputum smear
    (D) Cavitary lesions seen on chest X-ray
    (E) Diffuse infiltrates on chest X-ray

241. Which of the following is the recommended outpatient treatment of choice for community-acquired pneumonia in a person with no allergies and no comorbidities?

    (A) Aminoglycoside (e.g., gentamicin)
    (B) Macrolide (e.g., azithromycin)
    (C) Quinolone (e.g., ciprofloxacin)
    (D) Sulfonamide (e.g., sulfadiazine)
    (E) Carbapenem (e.g., Cilastatin)

242. Which of the following landmarks, when obscured on an upright chest X-ray, makes one suspect a pleural effusion is present?

    (A) Apex
    (B) Costophrenic angle
    (C) Heart border
    (D) Mediastinum
    (E) Aortic notch

243. A 30-year-old male presents to your clinic with recurrent pulmonary emboli. The most likely inherited cause is a variant in

    (A) factor V Leiden.
    (B) factor VIII.
    (C) factor X.
    (D) factor XII.
    (E) factor IX.

244. In which of the following infections/diseases is amantadine (Symmetrel) used as treatment?

    (A) Acute bronchitis
    (B) Croup
    (C) Influenza
    (D) Tuberculosis
    (E) COPD

245. A 62-year-old patient with a 45 pack-year history of tobacco use presents to your clinic with a productive cough. He describes the cough as harsher than normal over the past month, with occasional colored or blood-tinged sputum. He was seen in an urgent care center and was given a course of antibiotics that did not improve his symptoms. Of the following choices, what is the next best course of action?

(A) Obtain a CT scan
(B) Obtain sputum cultures
(C) Prescribe a cough suppressant
(D) Prescribe a longer course of antibiotics
(E) Perform a Tb skin test

246. A 55-year-old male presents to your clinic with a temperature of 102.3°F, cough, and purulent sputum. His chest X-ray is shown below. He does NOT live in a nursing home and has NOT been hospitalized recently. He has no other medical problems. Which of the following bacteria is the most likely cause of this person's disorder?

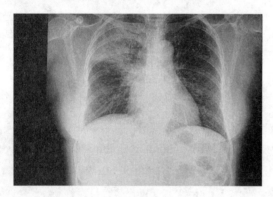

(A) *Mycoplasma* pneumonia
(B) *Pseudomonas aeruginosa*
(C) *Staphylococcus aureus*
(D) *Streptococcus* pneumonia
(E) *Klebsiella pneumoniae*

247. A 36-year-old male presents to your clinic with occasional wheezing for the past 3 weeks. He notes that lately he has experienced more episodes of dyspnea and wheezing, with as many as three episodes per week including nighttime symptoms. He notes this is worse when he walks by someone when they are smoking. His spirometry is normal. Which of the following tests would you order to help determine the etiology of his illness?

(A) Arterial blood gas
(B) Bronchial provocation testing
(C) Chest X-ray
(D) Chest CT
(E) Repeat spirometry

248. What is the most appropriate first-line treatment for moderate obstructive sleep apnea in an adult?

(A) Continuous positive airway pressure
(B) Hypoglossal nerve stimulation
(C) Uvulopalatopharyngoplasty
(D) Pharmacological therapy
(E) Watch for progressive symptoms

249. A 30-year-old non-smoking patient presents to your clinic with complaints of a nagging, non-productive cough and mild wheezing. She is afebrile. Past history is significant for bronchitis. Which of the following options is the best immediate treatment for this person?

(A) Albuterol (a beta2-agonist) and cough suppressant
(B) Azithromycin (a macrolide antibiotic) and cough suppressant
(C) Doxycycline (an antibiotic) and albuterol (a beta2-agonist)
(D) Levaquin (a fluoroquinolone antibiotic), albuterol (a beta2-agonist), and cough suppressant
(E) Flovent (inhaled corticosteroid)

250. In a person with newly diagnosed tuberculosis, which of the following should also be tested for?

    (A) Diabetes
    (B) Histoplasmosis
    (C) HIV
    (D) Lung cancer
    (E) COPD

251. A 56-year-old male with a history of alcoholism is diagnosed with pneumonia. Which of the following organisms is the most likely etiology?

    (A) *Escherichia coli*
    (B) *Klebsiella pneumonia*
    (C) *Mycobacterium tuberculosis*
    (D) *Streptococcus aureus*
    (E) *Staphylococcus aureus*

252. A 66-year-old female presents to your clinic with complaints of progressive dyspnea. On physical examination, you note decreased breath sounds in the lower left lung field and dullness to percussion. Her chest X-ray is shown below. Which of the following is the most likely diagnosis?

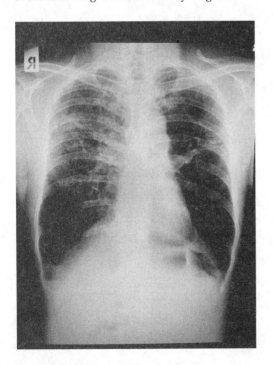

    (A) Atelectasis
    (B) Pneumonia
    (C) Pleural effusion
    (D) Pulmonary embolism
    (E) COPD

253. Which of the following provides the best evidence for small airway disease?

    (A) FEF25–75%
    (B) FEV1
    (C) FEV1/FVC
    (D) Peak flow rate
    (E) FEV > 25%

254. A 65-year-old male with a 55 pack-year history of tobacco use is seen in your clinic with complaints of increasing dyspnea and morning cough. Which of the following PFT results are most consistent with this person?

    (A) FEV1 < 70% normal FVC low FEV1/FVC > 80% predicted
    (B) FEV1 > 80% normal FVC normal FEV1/FVC > 80% predicted
    (C) FEV1 > 80% normal FVC normal FEV1/FVC < 70% predicted
    (D) FEV1 < 70% normal FVC low FEV1/FVC < 70% predicted
    (E) FEV1 < 80% elevated FVC elevated FEV1/FVC < 70% predicted

255. Which of the following treatment options is considered standard first-step therapy for a person with mild, intermittent asthma?

    (A) Inhaled corticosteroid (such as beclomethasone, fluticasone)
    (B) Long-acting beta2-agonist (such as salmeterol)
    (C) Oral prednisone (corticosteroid)
    (D) Long-acting beta-agonist (salmeterol) and muscarinic agent (atropine)
    (E) Short-acting beta2-agonist (such as albuterol) and inhaled corticosteroid

256. A 78-year-old male with an eighty pack-year history of tobacco abuse presents to the emergency department with confusion and muscle weakness. Laboratory values obtained in the ED are noteworthy for a sodium value of 118 mEq/L (normal 136–145). Which of the following is the most likely cause?

   (A) Adenocarcinoma
   (B) Bronchial adenoma
   (C) Small cell carcinoma
   (D) Squamous cell carcinoma
   (E) Melanoma

257. Diagnosis of a pneumothorax includes which of the following chest X-ray findings?

   (A) Air bronchogram
   (B) Elevated hemidiaphragm
   (C) Kerley B lines
   (D) Visceral pleural line
   (E) Depressed hemidiaphragm

258. The most prominent physical finding early in COPD is

   (A) diminished breath sounds and coarse rhonchi.
   (B) jugular venous distension.
   (C) low position of the diaphragm on percussion.
   (D) prolonged expiration.
   (E) hyperresonance of lung field percussion.

259. Which of the following physical examination findings helps differentiate a pleural effusion from pneumonia? What would a pleural effusion have that pneumonia does not?

   (A) Bronchial breath sounds
   (B) Decreased fremitus
   (C) Hyperresonance to percussion
   (D) Increased respiratory rate
   (E) Tympany of left anterior costal margin

260. Which of the following is the most ominous sign of impending doom in a person with an acute exacerbation of asthma?

   (A) $PaCO_2$ 57 mmHg (normal 36–44)
   (B) PaO_2 80 mmHg (normal 80–100)
   (C) Respiratory rate of 26/minute (normal adult 12–20/minute)
   (D) Oxygen saturation 88% (normal > 90%)
   (E) Use of accessory muscles of respiration

261. A 25-year-old graduate student is admitted to the hospital for increasing SOB. He first noticed a decrease in his exercise tolerance and started experiencing incidences of SOB at age 16 years. The incidences of SOB are unrelated to any physical activity, places, or other temporal factors. At age 18 years, a chest X-ray showed hyper-inflated lungs and lower lobe bullae (cystic collections of air within the lung parenchyma). By age 19 years, he required supplemental oxygen. He has had multiple hospital admissions for SOB. He denies use of tobacco and has never had a job. He denies unusual exposures. His family history is significant for an older brother who died at age 26 years from an unknown lung disease. Both sets of parents and grandparents are alive and in good health. Physical examination reveals a thin male in moderate respiratory distress. There is no clubbing or cyanosis noted. Chest examination reveals a marked increase in his AP diameter, hyperresonance to percussion, distant breath sounds with occasional end-expiratory wheezes. Cardiovascular examination is normal. PFTs reveal the following:

	Predicted	Patient Post-bronchodilator
FEV1	3.8	0.6
		0.9
FVC	4.8	1.4
		1.8
FEV1/FVC	⩾70%	44%
		50%
FEF25–75%	4.0	0.4
		0.4

TLC is 129% predicted; FRC is 188% predicted; RV is 318% predicted. Based on this information, which of the following is the correct diagnosis for this person?

(A) Asthma
(B) Emphysema
(C) Idiopathic pulmonary fibrosis
(D) Sarcoidosis
(E) Tuberculosis

262. A 60-year-old male with a history of COPD presents to your clinic with increased cough and increased sputum production. He states he is "getting over a cold" and is feeling sicker than normal. He is short of breath but no more than usual. His vital signs are: temperature 100.4°F, respiratory rate of 22/minute, heart rate 88 bpm, and oxygen saturation 92% on room air. Chest examination reveals an increased AP diameter and diminished breath sounds without wheezes, rhochi, or crackles. Cardiovascular examination reveals distant heart sounds. His ABG is: pH 7.44 (normal 7.36–7.44), PaO_2 75 mmHg (normal 80–100), $PaCO_2$ 40 mmHg (normal 36–44). Which of the following is the most appropriate management of this person at this time?

(A) Admission to the hospital
(B) Brief course of oral theophylline
(C) Oral antibiotics
(D) Oxygen therapy
(E) Short acting bronchodilator

263. In a person with suspected pleural effusion, which of the following standard imaging studies would be best to initially select to visualize the effusion?

(A) Lateral decubitus X-ray
(B) Chest ultrasound
(C) Lateral view X-ray with full inspiration
(D) PA view X-ray with full inspiration
(E) CT scan

264. A 2-year-old child is brought to the emergency department by his mother for altered mental status, cough, and difficulty breathing. On examination, you note a cyanotic, poorly responsive child with audible inspiratory stridor, use of accessory muscles of respiration, and respirations of 55/minute. Pulse oximetry reveals oxygen saturation of 60%. Which of the following is the most appropriate NEXT step to perform in the management of this child?

(A) Immediate intubation
(B) IV antibiotics
(C) Nebulized albuterol
(D) Nebulized racemic epinephrine
(E) Atropine

265. A patient with FEV1/FVC ratio of 0.8 (normal > 0.7 of predicted) in addition to a less than lower limit of normal FVC and less than lower limit of normal total lung capacity most suggests which of the following?

(A) Restrictive pattern
(B) Obstructive pattern
(C) Mixed, obstructive and restrictive
(D) Normal spirometry study
(E) Kussmaul respiration

266. A 66-year-old male presents to the ED for evaluation of altered mental status and seizure. On physical examination, you find Trousseau sign. Which of the following is the most likely diagnosis?

(A) Hypercalcemia
(B) Hyperkalemia
(C) Hypocalcemia
(D) Hypokalemia
(E) Hyponatremia

267. A 21-year-old male presents to student health with severe flank pain, and vomiting since the pain began 5 hours ago. He states that he had blood in his urine this morning. He has severe right-sided CVA tenderness on exams. What is the currently preferred diagnostic test to confirm your suspected diagnosis?

(A) Renal ultrasound
(B) Kidney, ureter, and bladder X-ray (KUB)
(C) Magnetic resonance imaging (MRI)
(D) Non-contrast computed tomography (CT)
(E) Urinalysis

268. Given the picture, which structure best represents the efferent arteriole?

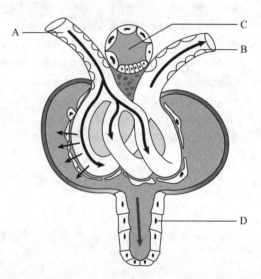

(A) A
(B) B
(C) C
(D) D
(E) E

269. A 46-year-old male presents to the emergency department with a 3-day history of vomiting. He states that he cannot hold anything down and just keeps vomiting. He has become increasingly weak and "just feels bad." His pertinent laboratory data is as follows:

ABG:

pH 7.64

PCO_2 44 mm Hg

HCO_3 50 mEq/L

Which of the following represents his acid-base disorder?

(A) Metabolic acidosis
(B) Respiratory acidosis
(C) Respiratory alkalosis
(D) Metabolic alkalosis
(E) Mixed acidosis

270. A 4-year-old male with a history of allergic rhinitis is brought in for evaluation of facial and leg swelling. The swelling started yesterday according to the mother. There have been no injuries. The urine shows large protein and hyaline casts. What is the most likely diagnosis?

(A) IgA nephropathy
(B) Goodpasture syndrome
(C) Henoch-Schonlein purpura
(D) Minimal change disease
(E) Lupus nephritis

271. Which condition below commonly presents with asymptomatic microscopic hematuria or with recurrent episodes of gross hematuria during or immediately following an upper respiratory infection?

(A) Focal segmental glomerulosclerosis
(B) IgA nephropathy
(C) Nephrotic syndrome
(D) Rapidly progressive glomerulopathy
(E) Polycystic kidney disease

272. A 24-year-old male presents with fever, dysuria, and perineal pain × 4 days. On exam, you note prostate tenderness on rectal examination and a urinalysis reveals pyuria, bacteriuria, and 2+ hematuria. What is the most likely diagnosis?

(A) Acute bacterial prostatitis
(B) Benign prostatic hyperplasia
(C) Prostate cancer
(D) Pyelonephritis
(E) Sigmoid colon tumor

273. Which of the following clinical scenarios meets the definition of chronic kidney disease?

(A) 48-year-old male with hypertension and a GFR of 62 mL/min
(B) 48-year-old female with a 10-year history of smoking and GFR of 65 mL/min
(C) 48-year-old male with pyelonephritis and current GFR of 67 mL/min
(D) 48-year-old female with a congenital solitary kidney and GFR of 70 mL/min
(E) 48-year-old male with diabetes and GFR of 90 mL/min

274. Which of the following scrotal masses presents as a non-tender mass?

(A) Epididymitis
(B) Hydrocele
(C) Orchitis
(D) Testicular torsion
(E) Spermatocele

275. A 28-year-old woman is admitted with tachycardia and a BP of 90/60. She just returned from a trip to South Africa and has had intractable diarrhea. Her chemistry panel shows: Na 145 meq/L, K 3.1 meq/L, Cl 122 meq/L, HCO_3 12 meq/L, glucose 180 mg/dL, BUN 28 mg/dL. ABG: pH 7.32 pCO_2 26 HCO_3 12. What is her disorder?

   (A) Compensated non-anion gap metabolic acidosis
   (B) Uncompensated non-anion gap metabolic acidosis
   (C) Compensated anion gap metabolic acidosis
   (D) Uncompensated anion gap metabolic acidosis
   (E) Uncompensated anion gap respiratory acidosis

276. A signs of lupus includes which of the following?

   (A) Malar rash
   (B) Joint stiffness
   (C) Reduced vision
   (D) Polyuria
   (E) Shortness of breath

277. What is the most common type of glomerulonephritis worldwide?

   (A) Post infectious glomerulonephritis
   (B) IgA nephropathy
   (C) Goodpasture's disease
   (D) Lupus nephritis
   (E) Bright's disease

278. Which of the following is the most common sign for nephroblastoma/Wilms tumor?

   (A) Weight loss
   (B) Abdominal mass
   (C) Fever
   (D) Lymphadenopathy
   (E) Reduced urine output

279. A 75-year-old patient with PMH of constipation presents for evaluation of nausea. An ECG is obtained revealing a prolonged PR interval and tall T-waves. Physical exam shows absent deep tendon reflexes. Which of the following is the most likely underlying electrolyte disorder?

   (A) Hyperphosphatemia
   (B) Hypokalemia
   (C) Hypomagnesemia
   (D) Hypernatremia
   (E) Hypermagnesemia

280. Increased incidence of bacteremia caused by gram negative bacilli is caused by which of the following?

   (A) Anemia
   (B) Lymphopenia
   (C) Hypogammaglobulinemia
   (D) Neutropenia
   (E) Eosinophilia

281. Which of the following can be considered the most common type of kidney stone?

   (A) Calcium oxalate
   (B) Struvite
   (C) Uric acid
   (D) Cystine
   (E) Bilirubin

282. A 30-year-old male presents with scrotal swelling over the past several months after being hit with a softball. He denies associated pain, hematuria, and penile discharge. On exam, he has hemiscrotal swelling that is nontender and transilluminates. There is no discrete palpable mass. Which of the following is the most likely diagnosis?

   (A) Hydrocele
   (B) Orchitis
   (C) Spermatocele
   (D) Varicocele
   (E) Inguinal hernia

283. An 8-month-old male infant is brought into his pediatrician's office for continued evaluation of undescended testes. The parents were previously advised to wait for 4 months but have not noted any change to his exam. Physical exam confirms that one of his testes is still undescended. As the provider, what advice would you give the parents for the next course of action in his management plan?

    (A) Refer to a pediatric urologist for surgery
    (B) Advise the parents to wait another 6 months
    (C) Order an ultrasound
    (D) Attempt to pull the testis down
    (E) Measure urine output

284. A 22-year-old male is diagnosed with testicular cancer. Which of the following aspects of his history is a key risk factor for this condition?

    (A) Multiple STDs
    (B) Tobacco abuse
    (C) Undescended testis
    (D) Uncircumcised penis
    (E) Family history

285. How long must a diaphragm be left in place after intercourse for efficacy?

    (A) 1/2 hour
    (B) 1 hour
    (C) 2 hours
    (D) 4 hours
    (E) 6 hours

286. A 34-year-old patient wants to know what guidelines she should follow for her pap testing. Her last cervical cytology was last year. The results were negative for intraepithelial lesion and co-testing was negative for HPV. When should she get her next pap test?

    (A) In 1 year with HPV screening
    (B) In 2 years without HPV screening
    (C) In 4 years with HPV screening
    (D) In 10 years with HPV screening
    (E) In 4 years without HPV screening

287. A 29-year-old patient at 28 weeks gestation presents for a routine prenatal visit. You review her lab study results and note that her 1-hour GTT (glucose tolerance test) yielded a glucose level of 155 mg/dl. She has no history of diabetes. Which of the following is the most appropriate next step for this patient?

    (A) Repeat 1-hour GTT
    (B) Order a 3-hour GTT
    (C) Initiate a diabetic diet and repeat fasting glucose level in 1 week
    (D) Start patient on oral metformin
    (E) Start patient on insulin therapy

288. A newly pregnant patient presents to the office with bleeding in the first trimester. If the initial beta HcG value is 48 on Monday, what should the value be on Friday?

    (A) 60
    (B) 90
    (C) 192
    (D) 210
    (E) 420

289. You are taking the history of a new obstetrical patient. Her pregnancy is confirmed in your office. She has had two prior spontaneous abortions in the first trimester. She also has two living children, one at 41 weeks and the other at 30. What is her gravitation and parity?

    (A) G4P1-1-2-2
    (B) G5P1-1-2-2
    (C) G4P2-0-2-2
    (D) G5P2-0-2-2
    (E) G5P2-0-1-1

290. You are attempting to deliver an infant to a mother who has been in the 2nd stage of labor for some time. She is exhausted and you are considering an operative delivery. On the next push, the head is delivered and you note the body is trapped. What should you attempt FIRST in order to prevent an adverse outcome?

   (A) Leopold's maneuver
   (B) McRobert's maneuver
   (C) Anterior clavicle fracture
   (D) Vacuum delivery
   (E) Rubin's maneuver

291. A 31-year-old woman is 5 days status post uncomplicated primary c-section for failure to progress. Her mother drives her to the office after the patient complains of shortness of breath, chest pain, and has several coughing fits. Upon arrival, she has a respiratory rate of 28, appears anxious, and has a pulse of 120. Which of the following tests will CONFIRM your diagnosis?

   (A) Chest X-ray
   (B) CTA of the chest (pulmonary angiogram)
   (C) MRA of the chest (magnetic resonance angiogram)
   (D) Echocardiogram
   (E) Sputum stain

292. A patient with necrotic vaginal discharge and a barrel shaped cervix would most likely have which of the following findings on cervical pathology?

   (A) Adenocarcinoma
   (B) Squamous cell
   (C) Carcinosarcoma
   (D) Stromal cell
   (E) Melanoma

293. A 30-year-old G2P1 patient, who is at 32 weeks in her pregnancy, presents with painless bright red vaginal bleeding of sudden onset. She was sitting on the couch at home when the bleeding began. Based on these symptoms, which of the following is the most likely diagnosis?

   (A) Rupture of membranes
   (B) Placental abruption
   (C) Placenta previa
   (D) Uterine rupture
   (E) Vaginal laceration

294. A pregnant patient presents at 12 weeks gestation. Her BP is 160/110. Repeat blood pressure at the end of the visit is the same. She notes a history of elevated blood pressure but never took medication. She has had sporadic health care her whole life. This is her first pregnancy. Which of the following treatment options is recommended?

   (A) Methyldopa (dopamine analog)
   (B) Lasix (loop diuretic)
   (C) Lisinopril (ace inhibitor)
   (D) Hydralazine (vasodilator)
   (E) Nifedipine (calcium channel blocker)

295. A 31-year-old female has been attempting to get pregnant for the last year. She reports menses every 30 days with no complaints of pain or bleeding problems. She has no history of pelvic inflammatory disease or known sexually transmitted infections. She has no issues with her weight. She has two children spontaneously conceived with her last partner. Her partner is 39 and has never fathered any children. Which of the following is the first step in their workup?

   (A) Hysterosalpingogram
   (B) Reassurance
   (C) Ovarian reserve testing
   (D) Semen analysis
   (E) Testicular transillumination

296. A patient presents to the emergency department with profuse vaginal bleeding, left sided abdominal pain, and a bHCG of 2500. She is moderately tender to palpation during the exam, and on the bimanual exam you can palpate an enlarged adnexa on the left. Ultrasound reveals an empty uterus and the left adnexa has a mass of ~3 cm. Color flow doppler indicates a blood collection surrounding this mass. Which of the following is appropriate management for this patient?

    (A) Expectant management
    (B) Methotrexate
    (C) Laparotomy
    (D) D+C
    (E) Hysterectomy

297. A G1 female patient presents at 7 weeks gestation with cramping and vaginal bleeding over the last several hours. She notes the bleeding is getting heavier. On exam, you find that her cervical os is dilated to 2 cm. Transvaginal ultrasound reveals an intrauterine pregnancy with positive fetal heart tones at 140 bpm. Which of the following measures should you take at this time?

    (A) ABO/Rh typing
    (B) Schedule D+C
    (C) Prescribe mifepristone
    (D) Administer methotrexate
    (E) Hysteroscopy

298. A 45-year-old patient presents to the office for complaints of pelvic pressure and dyspareunia. She is found to have a prolapsed uterus stage 4 on pelvic exam and desires definitive treatment. She has no significant medical history. Surgical history is notable for a bilateral tubal ligation 7 years ago. Which of the following would best benefit her?

    (A) Medications
    (B) Pessary
    (C) Pelvic floor physical therapy
    (D) Surgical repair
    (E) Oncology referral

299. A 42-year-old patient comes to the office 2 months after undergoing a total abdominal hysterectomy/bilateral salpingo-oophorectomy for leiomyomas and recurrent benign cysts. She has unrelenting night sweats, hot flashes, and mood changes. Pathology from surgery was benign. Which of the following would be the most appropriate type of medication for her symptoms?

    (A) Combination hormone replacement therapy
    (B) Estrogen-only hormone replacement therapy
    (C) Vaginal estrogen cream therapy
    (D) Progesterone only hormone replacement therapy
    (E) Progest

300. At 38 weeks gestation, a 26-year-old G1P0 presents with the complaint of leaking fluid from her vagina 1 hour ago for 3–4 minutes. Which of the following would be a positive test for rupture of membranes?

    (A) Lecithin-sphingomyelin (L/S) ratio greater than 2
    (B) The presence of "ferning" on glass slide made from fluid
    (C) A low estimate of amniotic fluid volume on ultrasound exam
    (D) Testing with nitrazine paper to show fluid is acidic
    (E) The presence of spinnbarkeit in the cervical mucus

ANSWER KEY
Practice Test 2

PRACTICE TEST 2

1. A	39. B	77. D	115. D	153. E	191. A	229. A	267. D
2. D	40. D	78. D	116. B	154. A	192. B	230. C	268. B
3. C	41. C	79. A	117. C	155. C	193. D	231. A	269. D
4. B	42. A	80. D	118. A	156. C	194. C	232. A	270. D
5. D	43. C	81. C	119. A	157. A	195. B	233. B	271. B
6. A	44. B	82. C	120. B	158. D	196. D	234. B	272. A
7. E	45. B	83. D	121. B	159. D	197. C	235. D	273. D
8. B	46. B	84. A	122. C	160. A	198. D	236. A	274. B
9. D	47. E	85. B	123. B	161. D	199. D	237. B	275. A
10. A	48. C	86. E	124. A	162. A	200. E	238. D	276. A
11. C	49. C	87. D	125. C	163. C	201. C	239. C	277. B
12. B	50. D	88. D	126. A	164. C	202. C	240. A	278. B
13. C	51. C	89. A	127. B	165. C	203. D	241. B	279. E
14. D	52. A	90. D	128. B	166. B	204. A	242. A	280. D
15. A	53. D	91. B	129. A	167. A	205. A	243. A	281. A
16. A	54. C	92. E	130. B	168. A	206. A	244. C	282. A
17. C	55. C	93. B	131. A	169. D	207. B	245. A	283. A
18. C	56. B	94. A	132. D	170. B	208. A	246. D	284. C
19. C	57. A	95. C	133. C	171. A	209. B	247. B	285. E
20. B	58. C	96. C	134. A	172. B	210. C	248. A	286. C
21. A	59. C	97. A	135. A	173. C	211. D	249. A	287. B
22. E	60. A	98. D	136. B	174. C	212. D	250. C	288. C
23. C	61. A	99. C	137. B	175. B	213. A	251. B	289. B
24. C	62. A	100. D	138. A	176. B	214. C	252. C	290. B
25. B	63. B	101. D	139. D	177. B	215. B	253. A	291. B
26. A	64. A	102. A	140. A	178. C	216. D	254. D	292. B
27. A	65. A	103. C	141. A	179. B	217. B	255. E	293. C
28. E	66. C	104. B	142. B	180. B	218. C	256. C	294. A
29. C	67. C	105. C	143. B	181. D	219. C	257. D	295. D
30. A	68. B	106. D	144. C	182. D	220. B	258. D	296. D
31. C	69. A	107. A	145. A	183. C	221. A	259. B	297. B
32. C	70. E	108. B	146. A	184. B	222. A	260. A	298. D
33. B	71. B	109. C	147. B	185. A	223. C	261. B	299. B
34. A	72. D	110. B	148. B	186. B	224. D	262. C	300. B
35. B	73. A	111. C	149. C	187. B	225. E	263. B	
36. A	74. A	112. C	150. D	188. B	226. E	264. A	
37. A	75. B	113. B	151. B	189. C	227. D	265. A	
38. B	76. A	114. E	152. A	190. B	228. B	266. C	

Answer Explanations

1. **(A)** This patient has coarctation of the aorta based on pulse discrepancies stated above. The murmur of coarctation usually is heard in the left back or axilla.

2. **(D)** Troponin is the most sensitive and specific of all the cardiac biomarkers. Troponins I and T are not present in any organ other than the heart. Troponin does not peak or fall quickly. CK & CK-MB can be increased due to muscle injury or disease and renal failure. CK is found in skeletal muscle.

3. **(C)** Patient has right heart failure symptoms and signs. Cough, dyspnea, JVD, and murmur of pulmonic regurgitation. On echo and exam, there is no evidence of left-sided CHF, which eliminates Choices B and D. RVSP is high, indicating pulmonary HTN. The murmur is not consistent with MR.

4. **(B)** This patient has acute pulmonary edema. Evidence is hypoxia, crackles, and pink sputum. Furosemide will improve the pulmonary edema and an ACE is a good choice for heart failure treatment and can be used acutely. He does not need an inotrope, as he is hypertensive and warm. Beta-blockers are not typically used in acute heart failure; they are used in treatment after the acute heart failure resolves. Thiazide diuretics are superior for HTN control, but loop diuretics are better for pulmonary edema.

5. **(D)** ASDs allow for a left to right shunt of blood. This delays closure of the pulmonic valve and would increase pulmonary artery pressure. It is not a part of Tetralogy, and equal pressures in the atria would be bad. Large ASDs are repaired.

6. **(A)** Cocaine can cause vasospasm of the coronary arteries and result in MI.

7. **(E)** Beta-blockers are used in patients who have sustained an MI and have hypertension. This is one of the compelling indications for beta-blocker use.

8. **(B)** The correct conduction pathway begins at the SA node with impulse generation, then spreads through the atria to the AV node. From the AV node, the impulse spreads to the bundle of His and then to the bundle branches before finally reaching the Purkinje fibers.

9. **(D)** The patient has signs of CHF, with dyspnea and orthopnea. Medications are relatively ineffective for stenosis. Balloon valvuloplasty is the best treatment.

10. **(A)** OSA is a cause of pulmonary venous hypertension and can result in right heart failure.

11. **(C)** This patient is suffering from the most feared complication of a MI, which is cardiogenic shock. This patient needs inotropic support. Nitroglycerin, furosemide, and lisinopril will worsen the hypotension. He will need diuresis, but his BP should be elevated first.

12. **(B)** ABI is the best test for screening for peripheral arterial disease. Smoking and hypercholesterolemia are major risk factors. Physical therapy will not improve the claudication. Angiography may be necessary to localize and treat PAD but is not the first diagnostic test.

13. **(C)** This patient has A-fib with RVR. She is alert and oriented and has strong peripheral pulses. She is not hypotensive and is not unstable. The best management for this patient is a calcium channel blocker drip for rate control. You would also begin to anticoagulate the patient to prevent a thrombotic event.

14. **(D)** This patient has sustained ventricular tachycardia and is unstable. The best treatment is synchronized cardioversion.

15. **(A)** Aortic regurgitation is oftentimes best heard by having the patient sit up and lean forward. It is a diastolic murmur best heard at the left sternal border. There are hyperdynamic pulses and a wide pulse pressure.

16. **(A)** S4 is caused by pushing blood in during atrial contraction against a stiff left ventricle, as would be seen in HTN and LVH. Pericarditis may result in a rub; postpartum cardiomyopathy should be dilated and would be associated with an S3. The other choice is unlikely to change the heart sounds.

17. **(C)** AV dissociation is described. Treatment would be a pacemaker as soon as possible. Don't panic. Observation is too conservative; death from poor perfusion from bradycardia could result. Adenosine is for supraventricular tachycardias and does not promote resynchronization.

18. **(C)** Aneurysms have little to do with an HFpEF 65-year-old who has normal EF, but PR is likely causing right heart failure. The child has a description of tamponade, which is distinct from HFpEF.

19. **(C)** This patient is having a STEMI and needs emergent cardiac catheterization. Before going to the cath lab, you need to start an IV nitroglycerin drip, give IV beta-blocker, start an antiplatelet strategy, and start the patient on heparin. If catheterization can happen in 90 minutes, this is the preferred treatment. TPA is contraindicated in this patient due to cerebral aneurysm history. (D) is not the best choice because of the delay in STEMI treatment, waiting for results, and no medications ordered for immediate angina treatment.

20. **(B)** This patient has CAD risk factors with smoking and cholesterol. He has sx of left and right heart failure with dyspnea on exertion, crackles, JVD, and edema. EF not provided.

21. **(A)** Patients will describe a tearing sensation during an aortic dissection. He has the murmur of aortic regurgitation, indicating the dissection involves his aortic valve. Asymmetric pulses in the upper extremities are typical with a dissection.

22. **(E)** This patient has superficial thrombophlebitis from an IV. The best management would be to advise the patient to take an NSAID and apply moist heat to the affected area.

23. **(C)** Pericarditis and myocarditis are associated with recent viral illness, but pericarditis is not associated with high troponin levels and myocarditis is typically not associated with pain. (A) describes pulmonary edema or PE. (B) describes myocarditis (troponin elevated but no blockage). (D) is heartburn or GERD.

24. **(C)** BNP elevation indicates Acute HF. Troponin elevation would indicate MI but is not requisite for the diagnosis of acute heart failure.

25. **(B)** MR should not change S2. LBBB should cause paradoxical split not fixed split. Deep inspiration should cause physiological split.

26. **(A)** Unfractionated heparin is the best choice immediately, as warfarin will not effectively anticoagulate for several days. IVC filters and TPAs are reserved for severe cases, such as hypotension or when anticoagulants cannot be used, like after trauma or brain surgery.

27. **(A)** Right coronary feeds the inferior wall of the left ventricle.

28. **(E)** Critical stenosis is 75%.

29. **(C)** COPD, PE, OSA, or a valve lesion can cause RV failure.

30. **(A)** Heavy drinking is a risk factor of cardiovascular disease, with direct effect on cardiac structure and function.

31. **(C)** Atrial fibrillation is commonly associated with cardiac conditions, but is also associated with non-cardiac conditions. Pericarditis is strongly associated with atrial fibrillation. The follwing are also associated with atrial fibrillation: EtOH abuse, hyperthyroidism, CAD, cardiomyopathy, pericarditis, LVH from HTN, any one of many valve diseases.

32. **(C)** Calcium channel blockers and ACE inhibitors are preferred antihypertensive agents for patients with atherosclerosis, peripheral artery disease, and systolic hypertension. Two or more antihypertensives for blood pressure control are often needed, and it is recommended to combine drugs at low-to-medium doses.

33. **(B)** In choice B, patient has tachycardia as a cause for increased oxygen demand and the troponin pattern is slightly elevated and flat, suggesting Type 2 MI. In (A), (C), and (D) patients have symptoms and clinical data pointing to a blocked coronary artery. When present, the troponin levels indicate a pattern of acute increasing damage. In choice (E), risk factors are present, requiring further evaluation and lab work.

34. **(A)** Patients with unstable angina and NSTEMI should go to cath lab if:

   ▪ Cardiac cath and revascularization is indicated
   ▪ Persistent symptoms despite optimal medical therapy
   ▪ Persistent elevations in troponin
   ▪ Persistent ST segment depression
   ▪ CHF
   ▪ Hemodynamic instability
   ▪ Dysrhythmia
   ▪ Recent coronary intervention (6 months)
   ▪ TIMI risk score (5–7)

35. **(B)** Maintaining a high dose will not give relief from muscle pain. Switching to another class is not likely to reduce risk. Diet and exercise alone is unlikely to maintain a good LDL result.

36. **(A)** Echo is less expensive, less invasive, more reliable, and gives more information on the squeeze (function of the heart). Fluid sampling has low sensitivity and specificity. EKG can suggest, but not detect, effusion, and it cannot really determine the impact of an effusion. MRI is the second best choice here but is expensive.

37. **(A)** TR comes primarily from heart failure, either left causing right or pulmonary HTN causing right failure. Its main sx are JVD, ascites, edema in legs, and murmur increases during inspiration. The other choices represent pulm stenosis, aortic stenosis, and HOCM (obstructive cardiomyopathy).

38. **(B)** Patient has a tachycardia that is regular, narrow QRS, and sinus. An objective is to be able to identify sinus rhythm (P in front of every QRS). The best treatment for sinus tachycardia is to treat the underlying cause. Atropine is for bradycardia; beta-blocker is for other tachycardias but not for sinus tach with a defined cause.

39. **(B)** Diastolic murmur that changes with inspiration narrows the type of murmur down to TR and PS. Only TR causes a wave and large P on EKG. Also, the location of the left 5th intercostal space is the tricuspid location.

40. **(D)** Squamous cell carcinoma usually occurs subsequent to prolonged sun exposure on exposed parts in fair-skinned individuals who sunburn easily.

41. **(C)** A photosensitive drug interaction is an adverse reaction of the skin (erythema, edema, vesicles, and/or bullae) that results from simultaneous exposure to certain drugs (via ingestion, injection, or topical application) and to UVR or visible light.

42. **(A)** Oral antifungal therapy is needed. Topical therapy alone is insufficient. A KOH preparation may help to choose the best oral antifungal agent initially. Fungal cultures are not always available and may take 1 to 2 weeks for results. However, they can confirm the diagnosis and influence the choice of ongoing oral antifungal therapy. In the United States, where *T. tonsurans* is most common, oral terbinafine is the best choice as initial therapy.

43. **(C)** Discontinue the medication and start an antihistamine (H1-Histamine blocker). The rash may persist up to 4 weeks after the drug has stopped.

44. **(B)** Chronic venous insufficiency results from pooling of venous blood in the lower extremities. Anterior shins are affected most, followed by calves, dorsal feet, and ankles. Primary lesions are red-brown to brown hyperpigmented macules and patches, often with pedal edema.

45. **(B)** Vitiligo may be associated with autoimmune disorders, such as autoimmune thyroid disease.

46. **(B)** Treatment is recommended when there is a clinical suspicion of Lyme disease. Standard treatment is doxycycline for 10–14 days.

47. **(E)** Impetigo, a superficial infection of the skin, is caused primarily by GAS and occasionally by other streptococci or *Staphylococcus aureus*. Impetigo is seen most often in young children, tends to occur during warmer months, and is more common in warm climates and among children living under conditions of poor hygiene.

48. **(C)** Patients may benefit from avoidance of potential urticarial precipitants such as aspirin, NSAIDs, opiates, and alcohol.

49. **(C)** Severe or widespread involvement should be managed with systemic corticosteroids. Topical treatment does not work well on vesicular and weepy lesions.

50. **(D)** In pemphigus vulgaris, lesions often appear first on the oral mucous membranes. Pemphigus is characterized by an insidious onset of bullae, crusts, and erosions, which rapidly become erosive.

51. **(C)** Pityriasis rosea is a papulosquamous rash occurring more commonly in the spring and fall. Initially a 2–6 cm annular lesion (the herald patch) develops and is followed in a few days to a few weeks by the appearance of many smaller annular or papular lesions, usually presenting on the trunk. Individual lesions may range in color from red to brown and have a trailing scale. Pityriasis rosea shares many clinical features with the rash of secondary syphilis, but palm and sole lesions are extremely rare in PR and common in secondary syphilis.

52. **(A)** Ticks cause illness by acting as vectors for pathogens or by secreting toxins or venoms. Ticks carry more types of infectious pathogens than any other arthropods, except mosquitoes. The most important pathogens include Borrelia (responsible for Lyme disease and relapsing fever) and Rickettsia/Rocky Mountain spotted fever (RMSF). Clinical presentation and findings are consistent with Rickettsia.

53. **(D)** Rosacea is distinguished from acne by the presence of a neurovascular component and the absence of comedones.

54. **(C)** Syphilis can become the "great imitator" in the secondary and subsequent phases of the disease. Secondary skin manifestations appear 1–3 months after the initial papule. This rash is maculopapular and noted on the palms and soles.

55. **(C)** Monofilament testing is used to determine the loss of pressure sensation. The filament is placed on the test spot on the patient's extremity and pressed until the filament bends. The patient responds whether or not the pressure is felt.

56. **(B)** Initial lab workup to identify catecholamine-secreting tumor (pheochromocytoma) is to measure fractionated metanephrine and catecholamine in 24-hour urine collection.

57. **(A)** Fine needle aspiration should be performed to rule out malignancy.

58. **(C)** ADH is produced in the posterior pituitary.

59. **(C)** Hydrocortisone is a good treatment option for the prevention of adrenal crisis, but longer-acting prednisone may be needed to control androgen excess.

60. **(A)** Metformin toxicity can occur after an overdose or in chronic use in patients with renal impairment. Metformin inhibits gluconeogenesis and glycogen breakdown, decreasing glucose absorption and improving peripheral insulin sensitivity.

61. **(A)** Diabetic ketoacidosis (DKA) is a serious complication of diabetes that can be life-threatening. DKA is most common among people with type 1 diabetes. Patients with type 2 diabetes can also develop DKA.

62. **(A)** Acromegaly is usually caused by the pituitary gland producing excess growth hormone. In most cases, the excess production is due to a benign tumor, known as a pituitary adenoma.

63. **(B)** Proteinuria is an expected finding in a diabetic patient with renal compromise.

64. **(A)** Primary hyperaldosteronism is usually diagnosed when a patient with hypertension has unexplained hypokalemia or when a patient has resistant hypertension.

65. **(A)** The dawn phenomenon is an increase in blood sugar levels (hyperglycemia) that happens in the morning. This typically occurs between 3:00 A.M. and 8:00 A.M.

66. **(C)** Symptoms of hyperosmolar hyperglycemic state include: blood sugar level > 600 milligrams per deciliter (mg/dL) or 33.3 millimoles per liter (mmol/L) or excessive thirst, dry mouth, increased urination, warm and dry skin, fever, lethargy, and confusion.

67. **(C)** Early in the course of Cushing's, patients frequently complain of nonspecific symptoms such as fatigue. Most patients eventually develop central obesity with a plethoric "moon face," "buffalo hump," supraclavicular fat pads, protuberant abdomen, and thin extremities.

68. **(B)** Diabetes mellitus 2 is the condition of decreased insulin secretion and peripheral resistance. Factors contributing to hyperglycemia include reduced insulin secretion, decreased glucose utilization, and increased glucose production.

69. **(A)** Radioiodine causes progressive destruction of thyroid cells and can be used as initial treatment or for relapses after a trial of antithyroid drugs. Hypothyroidism is a consequence.

70. **(E)** The goals of therapy for type 1 or type 2 diabetes mellitus are to eliminate symptoms related to hyperglycemia and reduce or eliminate the long-term microvascular and macrovascular complications of DM. Therefore, (E) is correct. All of the above are important.

71. **(B)** All patients with a pituitary adenoma require testing for pituitary hormone hypersecretion.

72. **(D)** Osteomalacia is characterized by markedly reduced serum phosphorus and renal phosphate wasting, leading to muscle weakness, bone pain, and osteomalacia.

73. **(A)** Patients with Turner's syndrome require a multidisciplinary approach because many different organ systems can be affected. In addition to karyotyping, a thorough cardiac and renal evaluation should be performed at the time of diagnosis.

74. **(A)** Hyperparathyroidism (HPT), characterized by excess production of PTH, is a common cause of hypercalcemia and is usually the result of adenomas or hyperplasia.

75. **(B)** The normal range of intraocular pressure is 10–20 mm Hg. Monitoring for the development of glaucoma is required in optic disk or visual field abnormalities, as a significant proportion of eyes with primary open-angle glaucoma have normal intraocular pressure when it is first measured. Repeated measurements identify the abnormally high pressure.

76. **(A)** In central retinal artery occlusion, patients experience a sudden painless monocular loss of vision, either segmental or complete. Visual acuity may range from finger counting or light perception to complete blindness. Fundal findings may include fundal paleness caused by retinal edema (fovea does not have the edema and appears as a cherry-red spot), narrow and irregular retinal arteries, and a "boxcar" appearance of the retinal veins.

77. **(D)** A hordeolum is a painful infection of the glands of the eyelid that is located on the internal or external eyelid. Internal hordeola that do not completely resolve become cysts called chalazia. External hordeola are commonly known as styes.

78. **(D)** Glaucoma causes progressive painless degeneration of the optic nerve. If left untreated, the optic nerve damage results in irreversible and complete blindness. Intraocular lowering therapy is most effective at early stages of the disease. Screening, early detection, and treatment are important.

79. **(A)** The most common form of blepharitis occurs along with acne rosacea or seborrheic dermatitis. The eyelid margins usually are colonized by staphylococci. Upon close inspection, they appear greasy, ulcerated, and crusted, with scaling debris that clings to the lashes. Treatment consists of strict eyelid hygiene, using warm compresses, and eyelash scrubs with baby shampoo.

80. **(D)** Injury to the anterior chamber that disrupts the vasculature supporting the iris or ciliary body results in a hyphema. Nausea and vomiting suggest a possible rise in intraocular pressure caused by blood cells clogging the trabecular meshwork.

81. **(C)** Many types of bacterial corneal ulcers look alike and vary only in severity. Inflammation and ulcers caused by alpha-hemolytic streptococci, *Staphylococcus aureus*, *Staphylococcus epidermidis*, and *Mycobacterium chelonae* often cause corneal ulcers that tend to spread slowly and superficially.

82. **(C)** Topical antibiotics should be used to treat keratitis of bacterial origin.

83. **(D)** A retinal detachment produces symptoms of floaters, flashing lights, and a scotoma in the peripheral visual field corresponding to the detachment. If the detachment includes the fovea, there is an afferent pupil defect and the visual acuity is reduced. Patients with a history of myopia, trauma, or previous cataract extraction are at highest risk for retinal detachment.

84. **(A)** Acute angle closure glaucoma is noted by a red and painful eye. When the pupil becomes mid-dilated, the iris blocks aqueous outflow via the anterior chamber angle and the intraocular pressure rises abruptly, producing pain, injection, corneal edema, obscurations, and blurred vision. In some patients, ocular symptoms occur with nausea, vomiting, or headache.

85. **(B)** Incision and drainage is the recommended treatment for abscesses because it is a safe and effective way of treating an infection.

86. **(E)** Lips, floor of the mouth, and central and lateral sides of the tongue are the most common sites. The tongue is the most common site in male patients.

87. **(D)** Phenytoin causes gingival hyperplasia. Diagnosis is made by history of gums, which may bleed with minor trauma from eating, brushing, or flossing, and inflamed gingiva that are red and friable.

88. **(D)** Chronic otitis media is characterized by persistent or recurrent purulent otorrhea in the setting of TM perforation. Usually, there is also some degree of conductive hearing loss.

89. **(A)** Croup is a viral respiratory condition characterized by marked swelling of the subglottic region of the larynx. Croup primarily affects children < 6 years old.

90. **(D)** Lateral neck X-rays may be helpful in demonstrating a classic "thumbprint" sign caused by the swollen epiglottis.

91. **(B)** Oral candidiasis is usually painful and looks like creamy-white curd-like patches overlying erythematous mucosa.

92. **(E)** When the tuning fork is placed on the patient's head, sound should lateralize toward the ear with a conductive loss and away from the ear with a sensorineural loss.

93. **(B)** Benign paroxysmal positional vertigo is a common cause of recurrent vertigo. Episodes are brief (< 1 min, usually 15–20 s) and are always initiated by changes in head position.

94. **(A)** This child has croup. Antibiotics are rarely indicated; supportive care is most appropriate. Given the signs of respiratory distress, admission is warranted.

95. **(C)** The typical bleeding site is the Kiesselbach area of the anteromedial septum, an area at risk due to the anastomoses of three arteries.

96. **(C)** Most patients with clinically apparent ascites will require diuretic therapy in addition to dietary sodium restriction. Lactulose should be administered to treat the somnolence.

97. **(A)** The model for end-stage liver disease (MELD) score predicts short term mortality in patients with cirrhosis. The scoring system uses serum bilirubin, creatinine, and prothrombin time to assess hepatic function.

98. **(D)** Vitamins with added triglycerides should be started. Symptoms suggestive of functional gallbladder disorder can resolve spontaneously, so early intervention should be avoided.

99. **(C)** Cholera occurs under conditions of crowding, war, and famine (e.g., in and where sanitation is inadequate).

100. **(D)** Treatment for cholera is primarily by replacement of fluids. In mild or moderate illness, oral rehydration is usually adequate.

101. **(D)** Most patients with IBS have mild symptoms that respond readily to education, reassurance, and dietary interventions. Pharmacotherapy should be reserved for patients with moderate to severe symptoms that do not respond to conservative measures. Treatment targeted at the specific dominant symptom (abdominal pain, constipation, or diarrhea) may be beneficial.

102. **(A)** In most cases, the tumor is located in the head of the pancreas.

103. **(C)** Patients typically complain of intermittent abdominal pain accompanied by diarrhea or constipation or both with long-standing duration. The diarrhea is often accompanied by cramps that are relieved with defecation.

104. **(B)** The choice of therapy varies depending upon the anatomic location of disease, the severity of disease, and whether the treatment goal is to induce remission or maintain remission. Medical therapies that are used for Crohn's disease include: oral 5-aminosalicylates (e.g., sulfasalazine, mesalamine), glucocorticoids (e.g., prednisone), and immunomodulators (e.g., azathioprine, methotrexate).

105. **(C)** Signs and symptoms of *E. coli* infection usually begin 3–4 days after exposure to the bacteria. Signs and symptoms include diarrhea, abdominal cramping, abdominal pain or tenderness, nausea, and vomiting.

106. **(D)** Gallstones are the most common cause of acute pancreatitis, accounting for more than 50 percent of cases. However, only a small percent of patients with gallstones develop pancreatitis.

107. **(A)** Biliary colic usually occurs after meals, when the gallbladder contracts to push bile out into the digestive tract. After a first attack of biliary colic, more than 90% of people will have a repeat attack. Repeated attacks of biliary colic are the most common reason for removing the gallbladder.

108. **(B)** The *H. pylori* stool antigen test can be used to assess the success of treatment.

109. **(C)** A small bowel obstruction can be treated successfully with nonoperative management, such as NG tube decompression in many cases.

110. **(B)** Tubular adenomas may cause obstruction, and the overall risk of malignant degeneration correlates with size. Diagnosis is made by barium enema, sigmoidoscopy, or colonoscopy.

111. **(C)** Blood exposed to gastric acid and digestive enzymes produces a black, sticky (tarry) stool. EGD would be indicated in the primary evaluation of this patient with upper GI bleeding.

112. **(C)** When a mechanical obstruction is suspected, endoscopy is a useful initial diagnostic test. The presence of furrows and multiple rings throughout a narrowed esophagus confirm feline esophagus and should raise suspicion for recurrent dysphagia and food impaction.

113. **(B)** When mechanical obstruction is suspected, endoscopy is a useful initial diagnostic test, since it permits immediate biopsy and/or dilation of strictures, masses, or rings. The presence of linear furrows and multiple corrugated rings throughout a narrowed esophagus (feline esophagus) should raise suspicion for eosinophilic esophagitis, an increasingly recognized cause for recurrent dysphagia and food impaction.

114. **(E)** Primary sclerosing cholangitis is thought to result from an increased immune response to intestinal endotoxins and characterized by diffuse inflammation of the biliary tract leading to fibrosis and strictures of the biliary system. Affected persons are typically male and 20–50 years of age.

115. **(D)** There is increasing evidence that frequent, severe GERD, particularly nocturnal, is a major risk factor for the development of esophageal adenocarcinoma. Anemia supports the diagnosis.

116. **(B)** For unvaccinated persons sustaining an exposure to HBV, postexposure prophylaxis with a combination of HBIG and hepatitis B vaccine (for long-lasting immunity, as well as its apparent efficacy in moderating clinical illness after exposure) is recommended.

117. **(C)** Hepatocellular carcinomas are a common cause of cancer-related deaths. They are associated with hepatitis B.

118. **(A)** **HBsAg:** The appearance of HBsAg in serum is the first evidence of infection, appearing evidence of liver disease and persisting throughout the clinical illness. Persistence of HBsAg more than 6 months after the acute illness signifies chronic hepatitis B.

    Anti-HBs: Anti-HBs appear in most individuals after clearance of HBsAg and after successful vaccination against hepatitis B. Disappearance of HBsAg and the appearance of anti-HBs signal recovery from HBV infection, non-infectivity, and immunity.

    Anti-HBc: IgM anti-HBc appears shortly after HBsAg is detected.

    HBeAg: HBeAg is a secretory form of HBcAg that appears in serum during the incubation period shortly after the detection of HBsAg. HBeAg indicates viral replication and infectivity.

119. **(A)** Serologic pattern in chronic hepatitis B virus (HBV) infection with active viral replication:

    HBsAg

    Anti-HBs

    Anti-HBc

    HBeag

    Anti-HBe

    +

    −

    IgG

    +

    −

    HBsAg: The appearance of HBsAg in serum is the first evidence of infection, appearing evidence of liver disease, and persisting throughout the clinical illness. Persistence of HBsAg more than 6 months after the acute illness signifies chronic hepatitis B.

    Anti-HBs: Anti-HBs appear in most individuals after clearance of HBsAg and after successful vaccination against hepatitis B. Disappearance of HBsAg and the appearance of anti-HBs signal recovery from HBV infection, non-infectivity, and immunity.

    Anti-HBc: IgM anti-HBc appears shortly after HBsAg is detected.

    HBeAg: HBeAg is a secretory form of HBcAg that appears in serum during the incubation period shortly after the detection of HBsAg. HBeAg indicates viral replication and infectivity.

120. **(B)** 24-hour pH monitoring is accepted as the standard with a sensitivity of 85% and specificity of 95%. False positives and false negatives still exist. Endoscopy lacks sensitivity in determining pathologic reflux but can identify complications (e.g., strictures, erosive esophagitis, Barrett's esophagus). Barium radiography has limited usefulness in the diagnosis of GERD.

121. **(B)** *S. aureus* is an important cause of food poisoning and is a common etiology identified in foodborne outbreaks around the world.

122. **(C)** Somatostatin receptor scintigraphy is appropriate for the evaluation of a suspected neuroendocrine tumor, as in this case when Zolliger-Ellison syndrome is suspected. Zollinger-Ellison syndrome is caused by the hypersecretion of gastrin, typically by a duodenal or pancreatic neuroendocrine tumor.

123. **(B)** Due to his family history, this patient should begin his screening at age 40 (10 years prior to first degree relatives diagnosis). In the current USPSTF recommendation, while continuing to recommend colorectal cancer screening in adults aged 50 to 75 years (A recommendation), the USPSTF now recommends screening starting at age 45 years (B recommendation).

124. **(A)** Alkaline phosphatase elevations greater than normal occur primarily in patients with cholestatic liver disorders (i.e., cholecystitis), infiltrative liver diseases, and bone conditions characterized by rapid bone turnover. In liver diseases, the elevation is almost always due to increased amounts of the liver isoenzyme.

125. **(C)** PSA is excellent for assessing response to therapy. PSA is NOT specific for cancer. Although a value of 4.0 ng/mL is used as the level above which the incidence of prostate cancer increases, values below this may still occur in people with prostate cancer. PSA has a higher accuracy rate of detecting prostate cancer than DRE alone.

126. **(A)** This scenario represents stress incontinence, which is one of the types of incontinence that should first be addressed with conservative measures. The first-line therapies for stress incontinence are weight loss, behavioral therapy (avoiding caffeinated beverages and timed voiding), and pelvic floor exercises (Kegel exercises). These should be tried prior to cystoscopy or surgery.

127. **(B)** In glomerulonephritis, dipstick and microscopic evaluation reveal evidence of hematuria and typically proteinuria. There may be cellular elements, such as dysmorphic red cells, red cell casts, and white cells. Red cell casts are specific for glomerulonephritis, and a detailed search on urine microscopy is warranted.

128. **(B)** SIADH is associated with euvolemic hyponatremia. Symptomatic hyponatremia with confusion is best treated with 3% saline; hypertonic saline should be used.

129. **(A)** This is the classic clinical picture and biopsy result of Goodpasture syndrome. Symptoms of Goodpasture syndrome include recurrent episodes of coughing up of blood (hemoptysis), difficulty breathing (dyspnea), fatigue, chest pain, and/or abnormally low levels of circulating red blood cells.

130. **(B)** This patient has BPH. Alpha-blockers are the only choice listed that will be effective in management of BPH.

131. **(A)** Cigarette smoking is an established cause of bladder cancer. Bladder cancer risk for a current smoker is approximately two to three times that of a nonsmoker.

132. **(D)** Underlying vascular disorders are the most likely etiology for ED.

133. **(C)** Excess urinary output may be caused by diuretics, excess fluid intake, metabolic abnormalities (e.g., hyperglycemia, hypercalcemia, diabetes insipidus), or peripheral edema. Appropriate pharmacotherapy is warranted.

134. **(A)** The cornerstone of treatment is bladder training before implementing medication management.

135. **(A)** The principal symptoms of a Bartholin cyst are periodic painful swelling on either side of the introitus and dyspareunia. A fluctuant swelling 1–4 cm in diameter lateral to either labium minus is a sign of occlusion of a Bartholin duct. Tenderness is evidence of active infection.

136. **(B)** The standard treatment for bacterial vaginosis is oral metronidazole 500 mg twice daily for 7 days.

137. **(B)** The most common organism associated with UTIs is *E. coli*, which is implicated in ~80% of UTIs.

138. **(A)** A diet high in fats may cause decreased absorption of Viagra.

139. **(D)** Patients with alpha thalassemia trait (two-gene deletion of chromosome 16) exhibit mild microcytic, hypochromic anemia. The hemoglobin electrophoresis is usually normal. Individuals with one gene deletion usually have a normal hemoglobin and are not microcytic. In iron deficiency anemia, the RDW is typically elevated, and the RBC count would be expected to be decreased. Beta thalassemia major results in more severe anemia and clinical sequelae of ineffective erythropoiesis. The anemia of chronic inflammation is typically normocytic or mildly microcytic and would also be expected to have a decreased RBC count.

140. **(A)** An African American female patient has a microcytic anemia, normal iron studies, positive family history, and normal hemoglobin electrophoresis, which are all consistent with alpha thalassemia. IDA is unlikely given normal iron studies. Lead poisoning is quite rare and would not have a positive family history. She does not have any inflammatory disorders to make anemia of chronic disease the best choice. Hemoglobin electrophoresis is normal in alpha thalassemia.

141. **(A)** Acute ITP commonly follows a viral infection and is characterized by easy bruising, epistaxis, and gingival bleeding.

142. **(B)** The insoluble material derived by centrifuging thawed, previously frozen plasma is cryoprecipitate. It contains von Willebrand's factor, factor VIII, factor XIII, and fibrinogen.

143. **(B)** The INR was developed as a standardization to eliminate the variability caused by obtaining reagents from several sources. Coumadin (warfarin) interferes with vitamin K dependent coagulation factors, and the prothrombin time is commonly used to measure Coumadin therapy.

144. **(C)** This is consistent with tumor lysis syndrome, which can be a life-threatening condition. This is caused by lysis of the large tumor burden, causing release of the intracellular electrolytes into the bloodstream.

145. **(A)** Penicillin-induced type I hypersensitivity reactions can present immediately and result in death. In the classic form, the mediator release occurs when penicillin binds to two antigen-specific IgE immunoglobulins, resulting in cross-linking on previously sensitized basophils and mast cells.

146. **(A)** Ferritin is the earliest and most sensitive indicator of iron deficiency.

147. **(B)** Bence-Jones proteins may be seen in multiple myeloma.

148. **(B)** Apoptosis occurs when both the chromatin and cytoplasm rapidly shrink and eliminate unneeded cells or cells in which potentially pathogenic defects have occurred. It can be difficult to distinguish from mitosis on a slide.

149. **(C)** Contaminated lab draw should be suspected due to other clinical features including recent normal results.

150. **(D)** This patient with hemoglobin SS (sickle cell anemia) should be prescribed hydroxyurea based upon her history of acute chest syndrome and > three sickle cell pain crises per year. Aspirin, multivitamin, vitamin D, and vitamin B12 do not have a role in alleviating the clinical manifestations of the pathophysiology of sickle cell anemia.

151. **(B)** Hereditary hemochromatosis is associated with increased intestinal iron absorption and accumulation of the iron within various sites, including the pancreas, skin, liver, and heart.

152. **(A)** Cytoplasmic granules in basophils contain heparin and histamine. Basophils migrate from the circulation into tissue where they become mast cells, which play a role in hypersensitivity reactions.

153. **(E)** This is remission of AML. She needs consolidation chemotherapy. Maintenance chemotherapy regimens are for ALL.

154. **(A)** Culture remains the most sensitive and specific manner to diagnose TB. Acid-fast smear helps determine infectivity. Quantiferon only suggests exposure and cannot diagnose whether exposure is acute or latent.

155. **(C)** Pandemics are caused by antigenic drift, which is the process described by mixing genomes in a common host. Mutation of surface protein results in epidemics and is called antigenic shift. Plasmid transfer occurs in bacteria, not influenza.

156. **(C)** Picture shows vesicles at vermillion border. Labial vesicles worsened by stress or sunlight suggests HSV-1 infection.

157. **(A)** *Clostridium botulinum* releases a toxin that cleaves the snare protein complex so that neurotransmitter vesicles cannot undergo exocytosis and release acetylcholine.

158. **(D)** AB/AG combo is the best test for diagnosis. Genotype, viral load, and CD4 all assist with determining drug therapy but are not for diagnosis.

159. **(D)** The only major criterion mentioned above is the two blood cultures positive for typical organisms. All the other choices are minor criteria, including the murmur. Major criteria would be a new regurgitant murmur.

160. **(A)** Based on the history, this woman has multiple risk factors for meningitis from Listeria. She ate unpasteurized dairy and has gram positive bacilli on the Gram stain, which confirms the diagnosis. She should be treated with ampicillin.

161. **(D)** Cefepime maintains excellent gram-positive coverage and also has a wide spectrum for gram-negative organisms, including pseudomonas.

162. **(A)** All viruses use host ribosomes for protein production. DNA viruses use HOST polymerase. Viral envelope is mostly from the host cell membrane and viruses can't produce or store energy on their own.

163. **(C)** This patient has malaria as she traveled to Nigeria where it is endemic. She now has jaundice and hemoglobinuria from lysis of the RBCs. AG/AB combo is diagnostic for HIV, AFB for TB, and MRI for bone destruction, indicating osteomyelitis.

164. **(C)** The correct answer is no treatment required, except supportive care. This is most likely hemolytic uremic syndrome caused by enterohemorrhagic *E. coli.* (EHEC is a strain of *E.coli* that produces Shiga toxin.) Antibiotics will increase Shiga toxin production, causing further damage to the intestinal wall.

165. **(C)** This is *C. difficile* colitis, and it is caused by broad-spectrum anaerobic abx use. *C. diff* is transmissible on objects and person to person. Therapy is metronidazole orally for 14 days. Antidiarrheals will worsen the condition by causing retention of toxins.

166. **(B)** Brucellosis—risk is hunter with typical febrile illness. Lyme is incorrect as it is not typically seen in Montana. Schistosomiasis is a parasite and not treated with doxy.

167. **(A)** Pasteurella is most likely. Beta lactamase-resistant penicillin is best.

168. **(A)** The patient is not responding to the best antibiotic therapy. This is an indication for surgery. Swabbing a foot ulcer is not recommended, as it is unlikely to reveal true pathogens. Propose surgical and antibiotic treatment/management of osteomyelitis.

169. **(D)** Beta-lactams are superior to vancomycin when bacteria is susceptible. Bactericidal antibiotics are preferred.

170. **(B)** The type of bacteria seen in this photo shows impetigo or *streptococcus.*

171. **(A)** DNA probe is the most common mode of diagnosis. It is hard to differentiate causes of urethritis on exam alone. Macrolide is a common treatment for NGU and GU but may not be the best. NG is transmittable via sexual intercourse.

172. **(B)** This pain is often described as having a burning quality. The pain typically begins after a delay of hours to days or even weeks and is accompanied by swelling of the extremity.

173. **(C)** Presentation and MOI are most consistent with injury of the left medial meniscus. MRI is the most appropriate test.

174. **(C)** The anterior talofibular ligament is affected because of an ankle sprain injury.

175. **(B)** Legg-Calvé-Perthes disease is an avascular necrosis of the femoral head due to disruption of blood flow. It typically occurs in children aged 4 to 10 years and is more common in males. Patients typically present with hip pain and a limp, which is exacerbated by activity. X-rays may show widening of the cartilage space or a subchondral stress fracture.

176. **(B)** Components of the musculoskeletal examination—

Grading muscle strength (Oxford scale)

- Grade 0—No muscle movement
- Grade 1—Muscle movement without joint motion
- Grade 2—Moves with gravity eliminated
- Grade 3—Moves against gravity but not resistance
- Grade 4—Moves against gravity and light resistance
- Grade 5—Normal strength

177. **(B)** The classic presentation of a herniated nucleus pulposus is moderate to severe pain radiating from the back down the buttock and leg, usually to the foot or ankle, with associated numbness or paresthesias and exacerbated by coughing, sneezing, or straining.

178. **(C)** The chief complaint of plantar fasciitis is sharp and stabbing heel pain that is most severe in the morning or standing after rest. The pain usually improves with ambulation but may worsen after activity or at the end of the day. On physical examination, there is localized tenderness on palpation of the medial calcaneus. Passive dorsiflexion may cause pain or discomfort in the plantar fascia. Evaluation of the ankle joint may reveal decreased dorsiflexion, indicating a tight Achilles tendon.

179. **(B)** The short-arm ulnar gutter is useful for fracture of the proximal phalanx of the ring or little finger or for fracture of the fourth or fifth metacarpal, including the common "boxer's fracture."

180. **(B)** Cauda equina syndrome should be considered when bowel and bladder dysfunction coincide with back pain. It is a surgical emergency because neurologic results are affected by the time of decompression.

181. **(D)** Anterior shoulder instability is evaluated by the apprehension test. A positive test represents a shoulder dislocation.

182. **(D)** Knee dislocations are high energy traumatic injuries characterized by a high rate of neurovascular injury.

183. **(C)** Spine—anatomic structures of the entire vertebral column and normal curvatures. The cervical spine curves slightly inward, sometimes described as a backward C-shape, or lordotic curve.

184. **(B)** Gamekeeper's thumb is an ulnar collateral ligament rupture of the thumb metacarpal that occurs after a forceful dislocation of the proximal phalanx of the thumb radially with spontaneous relocation that results in rupture of the ulnar collateral ligament.

185. **(A)** Components of the musculoskeletal examination

Grading muscle strength (Oxford scale)

- Grade 0—No muscle movement
- Grade 1—Muscle movement without joint motion
- Grade 2—Moves with gravity eliminated
- Grade 3—Moves against gravity but not resistance
- Grade 4—Moves against gravity and light resistance
- Grade 5—Normal strength

186. **(B)** Finkelstein test is positive if the patient reports pain aggravation at the tip of the radial styloid process consistent with De Quervain tendonitis.

187. **(B)** The most likely diagnosis is radial head subluxation (nursemaid's elbow).

188. **(B)** Anterior and posterior hip dislocations can often be reduced by manipulation. If the imaging reveals fractures or significant damage to soft tissues, blood vessels, or nerves, orthopedic surgery may be required.

189. **(C)** The pediatric musculoskeletal system reflects the active growth and development that occurs during childhood. Fracture classification, treatment approach, and types of complications are directly related to this unique anatomy. A posterior rib fracture is not related to normal growth and development.

190. **(B)** Tension or stress of the tendon near the attachment on the humerus is the primary cause of epicondylitis. It occurs often in repetitive upper extremity activities, such as computer use, heavy lifting, forceful forearm pronation, and supination.

191. **(A)** Passive stretching to straighten the head, causing the sternal head of one muscle to tense more than the other, is an effective initial treatment.

192. **(B)** The fifth metatarsal is the most commonly fractured metatarsal. Distal fifth metatarsal fractures involve the distal shaft, head, and neck region. Fractures of the base of the fifth metatarsal are more common than distal fractures.

193. **(D)** Exam of the wrist in ulnar deviation exposes more of the scaphoid to palpation within the snuffbox. Eliciting pain in this area when the patient resists supination or pronation of the hand, or pain with pressure along the thumb's metacarpal, is also suggestive of injury.

194. **(C)** The lumbar spine has a lordotic curve. Pain of spine origin may be located in the back or referred to the buttocks or legs. Diseases affecting the upper lumbar spine tend to refer pain to the lumbar region, groin, or anterior thighs. Diseases affecting the lower lumbar spine tend to produce pain referred to the buttocks, posterior thighs, calves, or feet.

195. **(B)** Patients with Broca's aphasia have labored speech, which is interrupted by many word-finding pauses.

196. **(D)** Lesions of the upper motor neurons produce weakness through decreased activation of lower motor neurons. In general, distal muscle groups are affected more severely than proximal ones and axial movements are spared, unless the lesion is severe and bilateral. Spasticity is typical but may not be present acutely.

197. **(C)** Guillain-Barré syndrome is characterized by acute or subacute progressive neuropathy. Weakness is more severe than sensory disturbances.

198. **(D)** Parkinson's disease is characterized by a resting tremor, rigidity/stiffness, bradykinesia, and gait instability.

199. **(D)** Symptoms consist of headache, diplopia, and other visual disturbances due to papilledema and abducens nerve dysfunction.

200. **(E)** Occlusion of the proximal middle cerebral artery (MCA), or one of its major branches, is most often due to an embolus and can cause these clinical findings.

201. **(C)** Patients most often present with an insidious loss of episodic memory followed by a slowly progressive dementia. The cognitive changes of Alzheimer's disease tend to follow a characteristic pattern, beginning with memory impairment and progressing to language and visuospatial deficits, followed by executive dysfunction.

202. **(C)** Babinski sign is a pathologic response to stimuli in or to the S1 dermatome resulting from loss of central spinal cord inhibition. It is characterized by great toe dorsiflexion and fanning of other toes.

203. **(D)** Proximal muscle involvement becomes evident in Duchenne muscular dystrophy very early. Boys with DMD have difficulty with gait. As the disease progresses, weakness becomes more generalized. Hypertrophy of muscles, particularly in the calves, is an early and prominent finding. Cardiac involvement is common and may result in heart failure.

204. **(A)** Absence seizures are characterized by sudden, brief lapses of consciousness without loss of postural control. The seizure usually lasts for only seconds, consciousness returns quickly, and there is no postictal confusion.

205. **(A)** In cluster headaches, the pain is usually retro orbital and is often excruciating. At least one of the daily attacks of pain recurs at about the same hour each day for the duration of a cluster period. Cluster headache is associated with conjunctival injection or lacrimation, aural fullness, rhinorrhea, nasal congestion, or ptosis.

206. **(A)** Symptoms and ESR suggest temporal arteritis, and prednisone is the treatment of choice.

207. **(B)** With CN IV palsy, double vision occurs when the head is tilted toward the affected side, since that eye cannot rotate inward to maintain fixation.

208. **(A)** (Uncal) brain herniation leads to compression of parasympathetic fibers of the third cranial nerve, causing an ipsilateral fixed and dilated pupil due to unopposed sympathetic tone.

209. **(B)** Carpal tunnel syndrome initial treatment includes splinting of the affected wrist in the neutral position for up to 3 months.

210. **(C)** Bell's palsy is associated with preauricular pain and hyperacusis.

211. **(D)** Trigeminal neuralgia is characterized by episodes of pain in the lips, gums, cheek, or chin and sometimes in the distribution of the ophthalmic division of the fifth nerve. The pain lasts intensely for a few seconds, occurs individually or in clusters, and tends to recur frequently in the day and/or night for several weeks at a time. They may occur spontaneously or with movements of the affected area.

212. **(D)** Presentation is consistent with cluster HA; verapamil is appropriate preventative treatment. Sumatriptan can be used for acute treatment.

213. **(A)** Migraine headaches are usually episodic headaches associated with certain features such as sensitivity to light, sound, or movement. Gastrointestinal symptoms including nausea and vomiting often accompany the headache.

214. **(C)** MRI is the best modality for evaluating change in chronic HAs. CT is the best modality to evaluate for acute bleeding.

215. **(B)** The cognitive changes of AD tend to follow a characteristic pattern, beginning with memory impairment and progressing to language and visuospatial deficits, followed by diminishing executive functioning.

216. **(D)** Epilepsy describes a condition in which a person has a risk of recurrent seizures due to a chronic, underlying process. Epilepsy is defined as two or more unprovoked seizures occurring 24 hours apart.

217. **(B)** Patients with borderline personality disorder display instability in their self-image, affect, and relationships with others. They are often impulsive and may engage in self-destructive behaviors, such as substance abuse, self-mutilation, and suicide attempts.

218. **(C)** SSRIs are considered first-line treatment in PTSD (in fact, sertraline and paroxetine are FDA approved for PTSD). SNRIs are not currently FDA approved for PTSD, though in some cases they may be considered second-line.

219. **(C)** Patients with paranoid personality disorder have distrust and a suspicious approach to others. They are often reluctant to confide in others and can be overwhelmed with unwarranted feelings about the loyalty or trustworthiness of friends and coworkers.

220. **(B)** Conversion disorder, also known as functional neurological symptom disorder, describes individuals whose somatic complaints involve one or more symptoms of altered motor or sensory function that cannot be medically explained. Significant distress and impairment often requires medical evaluation.

221. **(A)** MDD with suicidality and/or refusal to eat is an indication for ECT. Addition of medications (SSRI) may be concurrent, but the best initial treatment is ECT.

222. **(A)** This patient has anorexia nervosa. DSM criteria for diagnosis of anorexia nervosa includes all of the following: refusal to maintain normal body weight, intense fear of becoming fat, disturbance in the way one experiences his or her weight (or denial of the seriousness of low body weight).

223. **(C)** Paranoid schizophrenia is still one of the most common types of schizophrenia. The mean age of onset is in the early forties, much later than that of the preceding types (Winokur). The central feature is the preoccupation with one or more delusions related to a single or a limited number of topics, accompanied by auditory hallucinations.

224. **(D)** This patient is in opioid withdrawal. He has muscle cramps/abdominal pain, vomiting, dilated pupils, elevated BP, and tachycardia. Opioid overdose results in drowsiness, slurred speech, and impaired memory and attention. Additionally patients will have pupillary constriction. (Pupillary dilation can occur in the most severe form of opioid overdose; the dilation will only occur after the patient has been anoxic.)

Benzodiazepine overdose is associated with a large margin of safety, and patients that take large amounts may have drowsiness, lethargy, ataxia, and confusion. Benzo withdrawal has no specific papillary or pain findings; patients often have vomiting instead of diarrhea and will also frequently have tremors and/or seizures.

225. **(E)** Individuals with schizoid personality disorder are withdrawn from social relationships and have a limited range of emotional expression in their interactions with others, sometimes appearing cold or distant. Patients with this disorder are threatened by experiencing emotions, intimacy, and interpersonal conflict. As a result, they tend to isolate themselves and avoid close relationships. Avoidant PD is associated with social isolation due to fear of rejection and criticism rather than lack of interest or indifference in interacting with others.

226. **(E)** Approximately half of patients presenting with agoraphobia report having panic attacks before the onset of the disorder.

227. **(D)** All others are more broad indicators of possible dx alcohol use disorder but do not necessarily define tolerance.

228. **(B)** Delusions are distorted and highly illogical misinterpretations of actual events or experiences.

229. **(A)** Behavior therapy is the most effective treatment for phobias; exposure therapy is best for specific phobias. Beta-blockers and benzodiazepines may be used in association with exposure therapy, particularly in a patient's phobia is associated with panic attacks.

230. **(C)** Thyroid dysfunction should be considered as a medical reason for depressive symptoms. A TSH can assist in ruling this out. While all other tests can be helpful, they are not likely to yield a diagnosis or rule out anything from the differential that can cause both depressed mood and increased sleepiness.

231. **(A)** Bipolar depression, refractory MDD, and MDD with psychotic features are all potential indications for ECT. Severe COPD, MI within 3 months, and uncontrolled HTN are relative contraindications (conditions that increase risk) with ECT. Panic disorder is not an indication for ECT. TMS can help with panic disorder.

232. **(A)** Schizoaffective dx is made when psychotic sx meet criterion A for schizoaffective but the patient is also experiencing mood (depression or manic) episodes. Psychotic symptoms must be present in the absence of mood sx for at least 2 weeks. Psychotic features may occur in MDD but in the presence of depression.

233. **(B)** The MSE is the assessment in question.

234. **(B)** Buprenorphine, naltrexone, and methadone are approved agents for MAT in opioid dependence. Clonidine is used to assist with symptoms in the setting of opioid withdrawal.

235. **(D)** The symptoms of classic whooping cough (pertussis) last about 6 weeks and are divided into three stages. The initial stage is characterized by its insidious onset, with lacrimation, sneezing and coryza, anorexia and malaise, and a hacking night cough. The paroxysmal second stage is characterized by bursts of rapid, consecutive coughs followed by a deep, high-pitched inspiration. The convalescent stage begins 4 weeks after onset of the illness, with a decrease in the frequency and severity of paroxysms of cough. Azithromycin is the treatment of choice. Treatment shortens the duration of illness and may diminish the severity of coughing paroxysms.

236. **(A)** Blunting of costophrenic angles is seen in pleural effusions. Coin lesions are seen in solitary pulmonary nodules. Hilar lymphadenopathy is seen in inflammatory conditions.

237. **(B)** In a person without hemodynamic compromise, heparin is the immediate therapy. With hemodynamic compromise, of the options listed, surgery might be the treatment of choice. Prednisone has no role in the management of PE. Coumadin is not an initial option but rather a potential long-term anticoagulation option.

238. **(D)** CT, MRI, and PET scans may be used to further characterize solitary pulmonary nodules, but the first choice is to examine old chest X-rays to see the rate of increase in size of the lesion.

239. **(C)** The presence of hypercalcemia and elevated ACE levels are characteristic of sarcoidosis. Hypercalcemia might occur in small cell lung cancer but should have no effect on serum ACE levels. The presentation is inconsistent with pneumonia or pulmonary lymphoma.

240. **(A)** A positive sputum culture, positive sputum smear, and cavitary lesions on chest X-ray are characteristics of active TB. TST or IGRA would be positive in latent TB.

241. **(B)** In a person with no allergies and no comorbidities, a macrolide, such as azithromycin, is the medication of choice for CAP.

242. **(B)** Fluid will collect in the costophrenic angles, with pulmonary effusion when the person is standing upright. If there is enough fluid, it will obscure the angle. In an upright chest X-ray, a pleural effusion should have no effect on visualizing the apex, heart border, or mediastinum.

243. **(A)** Factor V Leiden deficiency will increase coagulation, possibly leading to pulmonary embolisms.

244. **(C)** Amantadine is indicated for influenza A only.

245. **(A)** This person, due to their smoking history, is at risk for lung cancer. His repeated use of antibiotics with recurrent symptoms makes CT scan necessary. Sputum cultures, cough suppressant, and a longer course of antibiotics wouldn't help in this case.

246. **(D)** The most common cause of CAP is *Strep* pneumonia. He has no listed risk factors for *Pseudomonas* or *Staph* and is of the wrong age group normally seen with *Mycoplasma* infection.

247. **(B)** The case presentation is highly suggestive of asthma. His normal spirometry results may be due to him not experiencing symptoms at the present time. Bronchial provocation with methacholine or histamine would aid in the diagnosis of asthma. ABGs, chest X-ray, and chest CT would not be helpful in this case.

248. **(A)** Oral appliances have modest efficacy. Surgical intervention is significantly more invasive. There is no effective pharm therapy for sleep apnea at this time.

249. **(A)** Albuterol is a standard short-acting bronchodilator.

250. **(C)** HIV increases a person's risk for TB. Diabetes, histoplasmosis infection, and lung cancer does not increase a person's risk for TB.

251. **(B)** *Klebsiella* is commonly associated with pneumonia in alcoholics.

252. **(C)** The blunting of the left costophrenic angle is a classic finding in a patient with a pleural effusion. Findings of an obscured left heart border might be seen in left lower lobe pneumonia.

253. **(A)** In some cases, a decreased FEF25–75% may be the only finding in PFTs indicating airway.

254. **(D)** The history of smoking, dyspnea, and morning cough should make COPD a strong consideration. PFTs for an obstructive pattern would reveal decreased FEV1, FVC, and FEV1/FVC ratio values.

255. **(E)** A person with intermittent asthma has the lowest severity level and is treated with short-acting beta2-agonists as needed to relieve symptoms. The other choices would be for asthma that is mild, moderate, or severe persistent in nature.

256. **(C)** Hyponatremia from SIADH is one of the paraneoplastic syndromes seen in small cell lung cancer. Paraneoplastic syndromes are not seen in adenocarcinoma, bronchial adenoma, or squamous cell carcinoma.

257. **(D)** A visceral pleural line is the hallmark of a pneumothorax. Kerley B lines are associated with congestive heart failure. Air bronchograms are seen in pneumonia. An elevated hemidiaphragm is generally not seen in a pneumothorax.

258. **(D)** Prolonged expiration is the earliest finding in COPD, due to the collapse of airways during exhalation. Diminished breath sounds, coarse rhonchi, a low position of the diaphragm during percussion (due to air trapping), and jugular venous distension (from right heart failure/cor pulmonale) are late findings in the disease.

259. **(B)** Bronchial breath sounds are noted in pneumonia. Increased respiratory rates are seen in both pneumonia and a pleural effusion (if the effusion is large enough). Decreased fremitus is found in a pleural effusion due to the buffering of the vibrations by the effusion in the pleural cavity; the consolidation of pneumonia will give increased fremitus. Hyperresonance to percussion is noted in a pneumothorax.

260. **(A)** When a person has an asthma attack (or anything that causes shortness of breath), the first response is to increase respiratory rate. This results in a decrease in $PaCO_2$, which will increase pH. Early findings in an asthma exacerbation include an increased respiratory rate and a respiratory alkalosis. As the exacerbation continues, shortness of breath becomes worse and the person starts to use accessory muscles of respiration due to fatigue setting in. Near the point of respiratory failure, the person can't breath fast enough to eliminate the CO_2 in their system, leading to increased $PaCO_2$ and respiratory acidosis. The finding of a respiratory acidosis in an acute exacerbation of asthma is an ominous finding.

261. **(B)** This person has all the signs and symptoms of COPD, along with PFTs revealing obstructive airway disease. He is young and has never smoked and denies unusual exposures. The death of an older brother from lung disease should make a person think that there is a genetic component to his disease. He has emphysema from alpha-1 antitrypsin deficiency. Asthma is in the differential diagnosis but would show reversibility with bronchodilator challenge. Idiopathic pulmonary fibrosis and sarcoidosis would show a restrictive pattern on PFTs.

262. **(C)** This individual is experiencing an exacerbation of his COPD, and antibiotics are indicated. His ABG is consistent with long-standing COPD, and he has good oxygen saturation levels, which indicates hospital admission is unnecessary at this time.

263. **(B)** Patients suspected of having a pleural effusion should undergo chest imaging to diagnose its extent. Chest ultrasound has replaced the lateral decubitus X-ray in the evaluation of suspected pleural effusions and as a guide to thoracentesis.

264. **(A)** Absolute indications for intubation in an asthma exacerbation are coma and respiratory arrest. Worsening ventilatory status despite maximized treatment is a relative indication.

265. **(A)** A restrictive deficit is typified by a reduced total lung capacity (TLC), and symmetrically reduced measures of forced expiratory volume in 1 s (FEV1) and forced vital capacity (FVC).

266. **(C)** Neurologic signs predominate in hypocalcemia, including seizure and confusion. Classic physical findings include Chvostek sign (contraction of the facial muscle in response to tapping the facial nerve) and Trousseau sign (carpal spasm occurring with occlusion of the brachial artery by a blood pressure cuff).

267. **(D)** Non-contrast CT is the most accurate imaging modality for evaluating flank pain given its increased sensitivity and specificity. Identified in lecture as "gold standard" for urinary lithiasis imaging.

268. **(B)** Blood reaches each nephron through the afferent arteriole, leading into a glomerular capillary with large amounts of fluid and solutes. The distal ends of the glomerular capillaries coalesce to form an efferent arteriole, leading to the first segment of a second capillary network surrounding the tubules.

269. **(D)** The hallmark of metabolic acidosis is decreased HCO_3.

270. **(D)** This child has minimal change disease. Remaining choices represent nephritic syndromes.

271. **(B)** In IgA nephropathy, an episode of gross hematuria is the most common presenting symptom. Frequently, this is associated with an upper respiratory infection.

272. **(A)** Perineal, sacral, or suprapubic pain, fever, and irritative voiding complaints are common. High fevers and a warm and often exquisitely tender prostate are detected on examination.

273. **(D)** Patients with markers of kidney damage, including structural abnormality or decreased GFR that persist for > 3 months, have CKD.

274. **(B)** Of those listed, hydrocele is the only choice that is non-tender. Epididymitis, orchitis, and testicular torsion are painful.

275. **(A)** Non-anion gap metabolic acidosis develops from decreased serum bicarbonate levels via renal loss, GI loss, dilutional effect, impaired excretion of acid by the kidneys, or increased acid intake.

276. **(A)** Clinical features include fever, anorexia, malaise, and weight loss. Most patients have skin lesions at some time. The characteristic "butterfly" (malar) rash affects less than half of patients. Several forms of glomerulonephritis may occur as a result of lupus.

277. **(B)** IgA is the most common glomerulonephritis worldwide.

278. **(B)** While all choices may possibly be present, the most common sign is abdominal mass.

279. **(E)** ECG changes of prolonged PR and tall T-waves, along with absent deep tendon reflexes, are seen in hypermagnesemia. Patient has a history of constipation, and laxatives can contain magnesium.

280. **(D)** Neutropenia, or neutrophilia, often with increased numbers of immature forms of polymorphonuclear leukocytes, is the most common laboratory abnormality in septic patients. Other conditions of lower frequency include: thrombocytopenia, laboratory evidence of coagulation abnormalities , and overt disseminated intravascular coagulation.

281. **(A)** The majority of calcium oxalate stones grow on calcium phosphate. Tubular plugs of calcium phosphate may be the initiating event in calcium phosphate stone development, and the process of stone formation may begin years before a clinically detectable stone is identified.

282. **(A)** A hydrocele and spermatocele transilluminate. A spermatocele is cystic and palpable. A hydrocele is most consistent with the description provided.

283. **(A)** Cryptorchidism is associated with increased risk of malignancy, infertility, inguinal hernia, and torsion. Unilateral cryptorchidism, even when corrected before puberty, is associated with decreased sperm count, possibly reflecting unrecognized damage to the fully descended testis or other genetic factors. Referral is appropriate if testes don't descend in the first few weeks of life.

284. **(C)** Cryptorchidism is a risk factor for testicular germ cell tumor.

285. **(E)** The diaphragm can be inserted up to 6 hours before intercourse and should be left in place for at least 6–24 hours after intercourse.

286. **(C)** Women aged 21 to 29 years should be tested with cervical cytology alone, and screening should be performed every 3 years. Human papillomavirus testing should not be performed in women younger than 30 years. For women aged 30 to 65 years, co-testing with cytology and HPV testing every 5 years is advised.

287. **(B)** A 1-hour result of < 135 is considered normal. A 1-hour GTT of 135–200 mg/dL indicates a 3-hour GTT is needed for further evaluation.

288. **(C)** In normal pregnancies, hCG doubles every 1.5 to 2 days for the first 8 weeks.

289. **(B)** Gravity refers to the number of pregnancies, while parity is defined as the number of deliveries over 20 weeks gestation. A convenient symbol for recording the reproductive history is a nomenclature denoting the number of term pregnancies, premature deliveries, abortions, and living children.

290. **(B)** The McRobert's maneuver is an obstetrical maneuver used to assist in childbirth. It is used in case of shoulder dystocia during childbirth and involves hyperflexing the mother's legs tightly to her abdomen.

291. **(B)** A CT pulmonary angiogram is used to diagnose a blood clot in the lung.

292. **(B)** The most common finding of squamous cell carcinoma on physical examination is a visible tumor on the cervix. Larger tumors may be identified by inspection and biopsied directly. Staging of cervical cancer is performed by clinical examination. Stage I cervical tumors are confined to the cervix.

293. **(C)** Placenta previa accounts for bleeding during late pregnancy and is most common during the third trimester. Placenta previa is abnormal implantation of the placenta over or near the internal cervical os. It results from various risk factors. Bleeding may be spontaneous or triggered by digital examination or by onset of labor.

294. **(A)** The development of elevated blood pressure after 20 weeks of pregnancy, or in the first 24 hours postpartum, in the absence of preexisting chronic hypertension or proteinuria, is

referred to as gestational hypertension. Chronic hypertension in pregnancy can be treated with Aldomet (methyldopa). Nifedipine and labetalol are also acceptable when initiating therapy in pregnancy.

295. **(D)** Identifying the cause of infertility encompasses a thorough evaluation of both female and male factors.

296. **(D)** Obtain gynecologic consultation for dilatation and curettage in all cases. Close monitoring of serum hCG levels is required to rule out the presence of malignant gestational trophoblastic disease.

297. **(B)** Prompt removal of any products of conception remaining within the uterus is required to stop bleeding and prevent infection. Analgesia and a paracervical block are useful, followed by uterine exploration with ovum forceps or uterine aspiration.

298. **(D)** The most common surgical procedure is vaginal or abdominal hysterectomy with additional attention to restoring support after the uterus is removed.

299. **(B)** The first-line of treatment could be with an estrogen-only HRT to treat symptoms for a limited duration.

300. **(B)** Pre-labor rupture of membranes is leakage of amniotic fluid before onset of labor. Diagnosis is clinical. Delivery is recommended when gestational age is $\geq$ 34 weeks and is generally indicated for infection or fetal compromise regardless of gestational age.

Appendix

References and Resources

Al-Ani M, Forkins AS, Townend JN, Coote JH. Respiratory sinus arrhythmia and central respiratory drive in humans. *Clin Sci* (Lond) 1996; 90: 235.

Ashley EA, Niebauer J. *Cardiology Explained.* London: Remedica; 2004. Chapter 8, Arrhythmia. Available from: https://www.ncbi.nlm.nih.gov/books/NBK2219/

Jameson J, Fauci A, Kasper D, Hauser S, Longo D, Loscalzo J. *Harrison's Principles of Internal Medicine*, 20e. McGraw-Hill, 2018.

January CT, Wann LS, Alpert JS, Calkins H, Cigarroa JE, Cleveland JC, Conti JB, Ellinor PT, Ezekowitz MD, Field ME, Murray KT, Sacco RL, Stevenson WG, Tchou PJ, Tracy CM, Yancy CW. 2014 AHA/ACC/HRS guideline for the management of patients with atrial fibrillation: A report of the American College of Cardiology/American Heart Association Task Force on Practice Guidelines and the Heart Rhythm Society. *Circulation* 2014; 130: e199–e247.

Hypertension Guideline Resources. www.heart.org. https://www.heart.org/en/health-topics/high-blood-pressure/high-blood-pressure-toolkit-resources. Accessed February 7, 2021.

Mitchell, LB. *Merck Manual Professional Version*. 2019. Atrial Fibrillation, Atrial Flutter. Available from: https://www.merckmanuals.com/professional/cardiovascular-disorders/arrhythmias-and-conduction-disorders/

National Clinical Guideline Centre (UK). Atrial Fibrillation: The Management of Atrial Fibrillation. London: National Institute for Health and Care Excellence (UK); 2014 Jun. (NICE Clinical Guidelines, No. 180.) Available from: https://www-ncbi-nlm-nih-gov.lp.hscl.ufl.edu/books/NBK248059/

Sudlow M, Rodgers H, Kenny RA, Thomson R. Identification of patients with atrial fibrillation in general practice: a study of screening methods. *BMJ* 1998; 317 (7154): 327–328.

Knoop KJ, Stack LB, Storrow AB, Thurman R. (Eds.). *The Atlas of Emergency Medicine,* 5e. McGraw-Hill; Accessed February 03, 2021. https://accessmedicine.mhmedical.com/content.aspx?bookid=2969&sectionid=250463078

Mitchell, LB. *Merck Manual Professional Version*. 2019. Atrioventricular Block. Available from: https://www.merckmanuals.com/professional/cardiovascular-disorders/arrhythmias-and-conduction-disorders/

Badheka AO, Singh V, Patel NJ, et al. QRS duration on electrocardiography and cardiovascular mortality (from the National Health and Nutrition Examination Survey-III). *Am J Cardiology* 2013; 112:671.

Bussink BE, Holst AG, Jespersen L, et al. Right bundle branch block: prevalence, risk factors, and outcome in the general population: results from the Copenhagen City Heart Study. *Eur Heart J* 2013; 24:138.

Mitchell, LB. *Merck Manual Professional Version*. 2019. Bundle Branch Block and Fascicular Block. Available from: https://www.merckmanuals.com/professional/cardiovascular-disorders/arrhythmias-and-conduction-disorders/

Rasmussen PV, Skov MW, Ghouse J, et al. Clinical implications of electrocardiographic bundle branch block in primary care. *Heart* 2019; 105:1160.

Tan NY, Witt CM. Future Perspectives. *Circ Arrhythm Electrophysiol* 2020: 13:e008239.

Xiong Y, Wang L, Liu W, et al. The prognostic significance of right bundle branch block: a meta-analysis of prospective cohort studies. *Clin Cardiol* 2015; 28:604.

Buckley II C, Garcia B. Cardiac Arrhythmias. In: Stone C, Humphries RL, eds. *Current Diagnosis & Treatment: Emergency Medicine*, 8e. McGraw-Hill; Accessed January 07, 2021. https://accessmedicine.mhmedical.com/content.aspx?bookid=2172&sectionid=165064676

Ganz LI, Friedman PL. Supraventricular tachycardia. *N Engl J Med* 1995; 332:162.

Katritsis DG, Josephson ME. Differential diagnosis of regular, narrow = QRS tachycardias. *Heart Rhythm* 2015; 12:1667.

Chong BH, Pong V, Lam KF, et al. Frequent premature atrial complexes predict new occurrence of atrial fibrillation and adverse cardiovascular events. *Europace* 2012; 14:942.

Dewland TA, Vittinghoff E, Mandyam MC, et al. Atrial ectopy as a predictor of incident atrial fibrillation: a cohort study. *Ann Intern Med* 2013; 159:721.

Inohara T, Kohsaka S, Okamura T, et al. Long-term outcome of healthy participants with atrial premature complex: a 15-year follow-up of the NIPPON DATA 90 cohort. *PLoS One* 2013; 8:380853.

Marcus GM. Evaluation and management of premature ventricular complexes. *Circulation* 2020; 141:1404.

Mitchell, LB. *Merck Manual Professional Version*. 2019. Ectopic Supraventricular Rhythms. Available from: https://www.merckmanuals.com/professional/cardiovascular-disorders/arrhythmias-and-conduction-disorders/

Josephson, ME. Sinus Node Function. In: *Clinical Cardiac Electrophysiology: Techniques and Interpretations*, 4th ed., Lippincott, Williams, & Wilkins, Philadelphia 2008, p. 69–9.

Kusumoto FM, Schoenfeld MH, Barrett C, et al. 2018 ACC/AHA/HRS Guideline on the Evaluation and Management of Patients With Bradycardia and Cardiac Conduction Delay: A Report of the American College of Cardiology/American Heart Association Task Force on Clinical Practice Guidelines and the Heart Rhythm Society. *J Am Coll Cardiol* 2019; 74:e51.

Mitchell, LB. *Merck Manual Professional Version*. 2019. Sinus Node Dysfunction. Available from: https://www.merckmanuals.com/professional/cardiovascular-disorders/arrhythmias-and-conduction-disorders/

Cohagan B, Brandis D. Torsade de Pointes. [Updated 2020 Aug 10.] In: StatPearls [Internet]. Treasure Island (FL): StatPearls Publishing; 2020 Jan. Available from: https://www.ncbi.nlm.nih.gov/books/NBK459388/

Heemskerk CPM, Pereboom M, van Stralen K, Berger FA, van den Bemt PMLA, Kuijper AFM, van der Hoeven RTM, Mantel-Teeuwisse AK, Becker ML. Risk factors for QTc interval prolongation. *Eur J Clin Pharmacol* 2018 Feb;74(2):183–191.

Ludhwani D, Goyal A, Jagtap M. Ventricular Fibrillation. [Updated 2020 Aug 10.] In: StatPearls [Internet]. Treasure Island (FL): StatPearls Publishing; 2020 Jan. Available from: https://www.ncbi.nlm.nih.gov/books/NBK537120/

Kang S, Amagai M, Bruckner AL, et al. *Fitzpatrick's Dermatology*, 9th ed. New Stevens-Johnson syndrome. McGraw-Hill Education, 2019.

Papadakis MA, McPhee SJ, Rabow MW. *Current Medical Diagnosis & Treatment 2021*. New York: McGraw-Hill Education; 2021.

Fitzgerald PA. Hypothyroidism & Myxedema. In: Papadakis MA, McPhee SJ, Rabow MW. eds. *Current Medical Diagnosis & Treatment 2021*. McGraw-Hill; Accessed February 10, 2021. https://accessmedicine.mhmedical.com/content.aspx?bookid=2957&sectionid=249376214

Fitzgerald PA. Thyroiditis. In: Papadakis MA, McPhee SJ, Rabow MW. eds. *Current Medical Diagnosis & Treatment 2021*. McGraw-Hill; Accessed February 10, 2021. https://accessmedicine.mhmedical.com/content.aspx?bookid=2957&sectionid=249376160

Jameson J, Mandel SJ, Weetman AP. Hypothyroidism. In: Jameson J, Fauci AS, Kasper DL, Hauser SL, Longo DL, Loscalzo J. eds. *Harrison's Principles of Internal Medicine*, 20e. McGraw-Hill; Accessed February 10, 2021. https://accessmedicine.mhmedical.com/content.aspx?bookid=2129&sectionid=179924583

Jameson J, Mandel SJ, Weetman AP. Hyperthyroidism. In: Jameson J, Fauci AS, Kasper DL, Hauser SL, Longo DL, Loscalzo J. eds. *Harrison's Principles of Internal Medicine*, 20e. McGraw-Hill; Accessed February 10, 2021. https://accessmedicine.mhmedical.com/content.aspx?bookid=2129&sectionid=179924631

Masharani U. Diabetes Mellitus. In: Papadakis MA, McPhee SJ, Rabow MW. eds. *Current Medical Diagnosis & Treatment 2021*. McGraw-Hill; Accessed February 12, 2021. https://accessmedicine.mhmedical.com/content.aspx?bookid=2957&sectionid=249377601

Powers AC, Niswender KD, Evans-Molina C. Diabetes Mellitus: Diagnosis, Classification, and Pathophysiology. In: Jameson J, Fauci AS, Kasper DL, Hauser SL, Longo DL, Loscalzo J, eds. *Harrison's Principles of Internal Medicine*, 20e. McGraw-Hill; Accessed February 12, 2021. https://accessmedicine.mhmedical.com/content.aspx?bookid=2129&sectionid=1922883228.Standards of Medical Care in Diabetes—2021 Abridged for Primary Care Providers

American Diabetes Association. Clinical Diabetes 2021 Jan; 39(1):14–43. https://doi.org/10.2337/cd21-as01

Ellison DH, Berl T. The syndrome of inappropriate antidiuresis. *N Engl J Med* 2007;356:2064–72.

Robertson GL. Regulation of arginine vasopressin in the syndrome of inappropriate antidiuresis. *Am J Med* 2006 Jul;119(7 Suppl 1):S36–42.

Halperin ML, Skorecki KL. Interpretation of the urine electrolytes and osmolality in the regulation of body fluid tonicity. *Am J Nephrol* 1986;6:241–245.

Vitting KE, Gardenswartz MH, Zabetakis PM, Tapper ML, Gleim GW, Agrawal M, Michelis MF. Frequency of hyponatremia and nonosmolar vasopressin release in the acquired immunodeficiency syndrome. *JAMA* 1990 Feb 16;263(7):973–8.

Hew-Butler T, Almond C, Ayus JC, Dugas J, Meeuwisse W, Noakes T, Reid S, Siegel A, Speedy D, Stuempfle K, Verbalis J, Weschler L; Exercise-Associated Hyponatremia (EAH) Consensus Panel: Consensus statement of the 1st International Exercise-Associated Hyponatremia Consensus Development Conference, Cape Town, South Africa 2005. *Clin J Sport Med* 15:208–213,2005.

Silveira MAD, Seguro AC, da Silva JB, Arantes de Oliveira MF, Seabra VF, Reichert BV, Rodrigues CE, Andrade L. Chronic hyponatremia due to the syndrome of inappropriate antidiuresis (SIAD) in an adult woman with corpus callosum agenesis (CCA). *Am J Case Rep* 2018 Nov 12;19:1345–1349.

Van Amelsvoort T, Bakshi R, Devaux CB, Schwabe S. Hyponatremia associated with carbamazepine and oxcarbazepine therapy: a review. *Epilepsia* 1994 Jan-Feb;35(1):181–8.

Berardi R, Antonuzzo A, Blasi L, Buosi R, Lorusso V, Migliorino MR, Montesarchio V, Zilembo N, Sabbatini R, Peri A. Practical issues for the management of hyponatremia in oncology. *Endocrine* 2018 Jul;61(1):158–164.

Liamis G, Milionis H, Elisaf M. A review of drug-induced hyponatremia. *Am J Kidney Dis* 2008 Jul;52(1):144–53.

Katz MA. Hyperglycemia-induced hyponatremia—calculation of expected serum sodium depression. *N Engl J Med* 1973;289:843–844.

Hillier TA, Abbott RD, Barrett EJ. Hyponatremia: evaluating the correction factor for hyperglycemia. *Am J Med* 1999;106:399–403.

Tageja N, Darden J, Brown L. Cervical spinal epidural abscess complicated with cerebral salt wasting. *South Med J* 2009 Dec;102(12):1279–80. doi: 10.1097/SMJ.0b013e3181bfdaf7. PMID: 20016444.

Gross P. Clinical management of SIADH. *Ther Adv Endocrinol Metab* 2012 Apr;3(2):61–73.

Rondon-Berrios H, Tandukar S, Mor MK, Ray EC, Bender FH, Kleyman TR, Weisbord SD. Urea for the treatment of hyponatremia. *Clin J Am Soc Nephrol* 2018 Nov 07;13(11):1627–1632.

Fassnacht M, et al. Management of adrenal incidentalomas: European Society of Endocrinology clinical practice guideline in collaboration with the European Network for the Study of Adrenal Tumors. *Eur J Endocrinol* 2017. 175(2):G1–G34.

Young, WF et al. Screening for endocrine hypertension: An Endocrine Society scientific statement. *Endocr Rev* 2017;38(2):103–122

Nieman LK et al. The diagnosis of Cushing's syndrome: An Endocrine Society clinical practice guideline. *J Clin Endocrinol Metab* 93: 1526–1540, 2008.

Nieman LK et al. Treatment of Cushing's syndrome: An Endocrine Society clinical practice guideline. *J Clin Endocrinol Metab* 2015 Aug;100(8):2807–31.

Tritos NA. Adrenally Directed Medical Therapies for Cushing Syndrome. *J Clin Endocrinol Metab* 2021 Jan 1;106(1):16–25.

Cacciola I, et al. Evaluation of liver enzyme levels and identification of asymptomatic liver disease patients in primary care. *Intern Emerg Med* 2017 Mar;12(2): 181–86.

Agrawal S, et al. Evaluation of abnormal liver function tests. *Postgrad Med J* 2016 Apr;92(1086): 223–34.

Rahmi R and DC Rockey. Complications of cirrhosis. *Curr Opin Gastroenterol* 2012 May; 28(3): 223–9.

Rubin, David T. MD, FACG1; Ananthakrishnan, Ashwin N. MD, MPH2; Siegel, Corey A. MD, MS3; Sauer, Bryan G. MD, MSc (Clin Res), FACG (GRADE Methodologist)4; Long, Millie D. MD, MPH, FACG5 ACG Clinical Guideline: Ulcerative Colitis in Adults, *The American Journal of Gastroenterology*: March 2019-Volume 114-Issue 3-p 384–413 doi: 10.14309/ajg.0000000000000152

Lichtenstein, Gary R MD, FACG1; Loftus, Edward V MD, FACG2; Isaacs, Kim L MD, PhD, FACG3; Regueiro, Miguel D MD, FACG4; Gerson, Lauren B MD, MSc, MACG (GRADE Methodologist)5,â€ ; Sands, Bruce E MD, MS, FACG6 ACG Clinical Guideline: Management of Crohn's Disease in Adults, American Journal of Gastroenterology: April 2018-Volume 113-Issue 4-p 481–517 doi: 10.1038/ajg.2018.27

Papadakis MA, Rabow MW, McPhee SJ. *Current Medical Diagnosis and Treatment 2016*. McGraw-Hill Education/Medical; 2015.

Williams DA. Pance *Prep Pearls*. 2nd ed. Lexington, KY: CreateSpace; 2017.

Lacy, Brian E. PhD, MD, FACG1; Pimentel, Mark MD, FACG2; Brenner, Darren M. MD, FACG3; Chey, William D. MD, FACG4; Keefer, Laurie A. PhD5; Long, Millie D. MDMPH, FACG (GRADE Methodologist)6; Moshiree, Baha MD, MSc, FACG7 ACG Clinical Guideline: Management of Irritable Bowel Syndrome, *The American Journal of Gastroenterology*: January 2021-Volume 116-Issue 1-p 17–44 doi: 10.14309/ajg.0000000000001036

Anand S. Epispadias. StatPearls [Internet]. https://www.ncbi.nlm.nih.gov/books/NBK563180/. Published December 1, 2020. Accessed February 11, 2021.

McAninch JW, Lue TF. *Smith & Tanagho's General Urology*. New York: McGraw-Hill Education; 2020.

Papadakis MA, McPhee SJ, Rabow MW. *Current Medical Diagnosis & Treatment 2021*. New York: McGraw-Hill Education; 2021.

Jacobson CA, Longo DL. Non-Hodgkin's Lymphoma. In: Jameson J, Fauci AS, Kasper DL, Hauser SL, Longo DL, Loscalzo J. eds. *Harrison's Principles of Internal Medicine*, 20e. McGraw-Hill; Accessed February 15, 2021. https://accessmedicine-mhmedical-com/content.aspx?bookid=2129&sectionid=192018038

Jacobson CA, Longo DL. Hodgkin's Lymphoma. In: Jameson J, Fauci AS, Kasper DL, Hauser SL, Longo DL, Loscalzo J. eds. *Harrison's Principles of Internal Medicine*, 20e. McGraw-Hill; Accessed February 15, 2021. https://accessmedicine-mhmedical-com/content.aspx?bookid=2129&sectionid=192018130

Cancer Facts & Figures 2021. https://www.cancer.org/content/dam/cancer-org/research/cancer-facts-and-statistics/annual-cancer-facts-and-figures/2021/cancer-facts-and-figures-2021.pdf. Published 2021. Accessed February 15, 2021.

Hoelzer D. Acute Lymphoid Leukemia. In: Jameson J, Fauci AS, Kasper DL, Hauser SL, Longo DL, Loscalzo J. eds. *Harrison's Principles of Internal Medicine*, 20e. McGraw-Hill; Accessed February 15, 2021. https://accessmedicine-mhmedical-com/content.aspx?bookid=2129&sectionid=192017841

Young NS. Bone Marrow Failure Syndromes Including Aplastic Anemia and Myelodysplasia. In: Jameson J, Fauci AS, Kasper DL, Hauser SL, Longo DL, Loscalzo J. eds. *Harrison's Principles of Internal Medicine*, 20e. McGraw-Hill; Accessed February 15, 2021. https://accessmedicine-mhmedical-com/content.aspx?bookid=2129&sectionid=192017558

Blum W, Bloomfield CD. Acute Myeloid Leukemia. In: Jameson J, Fauci AS, Kasper DL, Hauser SL, Longo DL, Loscalzo J. eds. *Harrison's Principles of Internal Medicine*, 20e. McGraw-Hill; Accessed February 15, 2021. https://accessmedicine-mhmedical-com/content.aspx?bookid=2129&sectionid=192017732

AMA. https://owl.purdue.edu/owl/research_and_citation/ama_style/index.html

AMA. Munshi NC, Longo DL, Anderson KC. Plasma Cell Disorders. In: Jameson J, Fauci AS, Kasper DL, Hauser SL, Longo DL, Loscalzo J. eds. *Harrison's Principles of Internal Medicine*, 20e. McGraw-Hill; Accessed February 15, 2021. https://accessmedicine-mhmedical-com/content.aspx?bookid=2129&sectionid=19201829

AMA. Kantarjian H, Cortes J. Chronic Myeloid Leukemia. In: Jameson J, Fauci AS, Kasper DL, Hauser SL, Longo DL, Loscalzo J. eds. *Harrison's Principles of Internal Medicine*, 20e. McGraw-Hill; Accessed February 15, 2021. https://accessmedicine-mhmedical-com/content.aspx?bookid=2129&sectionid=192017792

Brown KE. Parvovirus Infections. In: Jameson J, Fauci AS, Kasper DL, Hauser SL, Longo DL, Loscalzo J. eds. *Harrison's Principles of Internal Medicine*, 20e. McGraw-Hill; Accessed February 15, 2021. https://accessmedicine.mhmedical.com/content.aspx?bookid=2129&section id=192024899

Clark E, Shandera WX. Major Vaccine-Preventable Viral Infections. In: Papadakis MA, McPhee SJ, Rabow MW. eds. *Current Medical Diagnosis & Treatment 2021*. McGraw-Hill; Accessed February 15, 2021. https://accessmedicine.mhmedical.com/content.aspx?bookid=2957&section id=249387905

Olson D, Levin MJ, Asturias EJ. Infections: Viral & Rickettsial. In: Hay Jr. WW, Levin MJ, Abzug MJ, Bunik M. eds. *Current Diagnosis & Treatment: Pediatrics*, 25e. McGraw-Hill; Accessed February 15, 2021. https://accessmedicine.mhmedical.com/content.aspx?bookid=2815&section id=244268424

Rainwater-Lovett K, Moss WJ. Measles (Rubeola). In: Jameson J, Fauci AS, Kasper DL, Hauser SL, Longo DL, Loscalzo J. eds. *Harrison's Principles of Internal Medicine*, 20e. McGraw-Hill; Accessed February 15, 2021. https://accessmedicine.mhmedical.com/content.aspx?bookid=2129&section id=192025856

American Psychiatric Association. *Diagnostic and Statistical Manual of Mental Disorders*. 5th ed. Washington D.C.: 2013; 143–149.

Johnson DC, Krystal JH, Southwick SM. Posttraumatic Stress Disorder and Acute Stress Disorder. In: Ebert MH, Leckman JF, Petrakis IL. eds. *Current Diagnosis & Treatment: Psychiatry*, 3e. McGraw-Hill; Accessed January 07, 2021. https://accessmedicine.mhmedical.com/content.aspx?bookid=2509&sectionid=200980381

Raj KS, Williams N, DeBattista C. Psychiatric Trauma & Stressor-Related Disorders. In: Papadakis MA, McPhee SJ, Rabow MW. eds. *Current Medical Diagnosis & Treatment 2021*. McGraw-Hill; Accessed January 05, 2021. https://accessmedicine.mhmedical.com/content.aspx?bookid=2957&sectionid=249375205

Salomon RM. Adjustment Disorders. In: Ebert MH, Leckman JF, Petrakis IL. eds. *Current Diagnosis & Treatment: Psychiatry*, 3e. McGraw-Hill; Accessed January 12, 2021. https://access-medicine.mhmedical.com/content.aspx?bookid=2509&sectionid=200806502

Shelton RC. Anxiety Disorders. In: Ebert MH, Leckman JF, Petrakis IL. eds. *Current Diagnosis & Treatment: Psychiatry*, 3e. McGraw-Hill; Accessed January 20, 2021. https://accessmedicine.mhmedical.com/content.aspx?bookid=2509&sectionid=200804771

Rali P, Gandhi V, Malik K. Pulmonary embolism. *Crit Care Nurs Q* 2016;39(2):131-138. doi:10.1097/CNQ.0000000000000106

Girard P, Decousus M, Laporte S, et al. Diagnosis of pulmonary embolism in patients with proximal deep vein thrombosis: Specificity of symptoms and perfusion defects at baseline and during anticoagulant therapy. *Am J Respir Crit Care Med* 2001;164(6):1033–1037. doi:10.1164/ajrccm.164.6.2101045

Mahan CE, Borrego ME, Woersching AL, et al. Venous thromboembolism: Annualised United States models for total, hospital-acquired and preventable costs utilising long-term attack rates. *Thromb Haemost* 2012;108(2):291–302. doi:10.1160/TH12-03-0162

Cheuk BLY, Cheung GCY, Cheng SWK. Epidemiology of venous thromboembolism in a Chinese population. *Br J Surg* 2004;91(4):424–428. doi:10.1002/bjs.4454

Horlander KT, Mannino DM, Leeper KV. Pulmonary embolism mortality in the United States, 1979-1998: An analysis using multiple-cause mortality data. *Arch Intern Med* 2003;163(14):1711–1717. doi:10.1001/archinte.163.14.1711

Tapson VF. Acute pulmonary embolism. *N Engl J Med* 2008;358(10):1037–1052. doi:10.1056/NEJMra072753

Jiménez D, De Miguel-Díez J, Guijarro R, et al. Trends in the management and outcomes of acute pulmonary embolism analysis from the RIETE registry. *J Am Coll Cardiol* 2016;67(2):162–170. doi:10.1016/j.jacc.2015.10.060

Lehnert P, Lange T, Møller CH, Olsen PS, Carlsen J. Acute pulmonary embolism in a national Danish cohort: Increasing incidence and decreasing mortality. *Thromb Haemost* 2018;118(3):539–546. doi:10.1160/TH17-08-0531

Dentali F, Ageno W, Pomero F, Fenoglio L, Squizzato A, Bonzini M. Time trends and case fatality rate of in-hospital treated pulmonary embolism during 11 years of observation in Northwestern Italy. *Thromb Haemost* 2016;115(2):399–405. doi:10.1160/TH15-02-0172

Alotaibi GS, Wu C, Senthilselvan A, McMurtry MS. Secular trends in incidence and mortality of acute venous thromboembolism: The AB-VTE population-based study. *Am J Med* 2016;129(8):879.e19–879.e25. doi:10.1016/j.amjmed.2016.01.041

Spencer FA, Emery C, Lessard D, et al. The Worcester venous thromboembolism study: A population-based study of the clinical epidemiology of venous thromboembolism. *J Gen Intern Med* 2006;21(7):722–727. doi:10.1111/j.1525-1497.2006.00458.x

Rogers MAM, Levine DA, Blumberg N, Flanders SA, Chopra V, Langa KM. Triggers of hospitalization for venous thromboembolism. *Circulation* 2012;125(17):2092–2099. doi:10.1161/CIRCULATIONAHA.111.084467

Gohil R, Peck G, Sharma P. The genetics of venous thromboembolism: A meta-analysis involving ~120,000 cases and 180,000 controls. *Thromb Haemost* 2009;102(2):360–370. doi:10.1160/TH09-01-0013

Stein PD, Terrin ML, Hales CA, et al. Clinical, laboratory, roentgenographic, and electrocardiographic findings in patients with acute pulmonary embolism and no pre-existing cardiac or pulmonary disease. *Chest* 1991;100(3):598–603. doi:10.1378/chest.100.3.598

Stein PD, Beemath A, Matta F, et al. Clinical Characteristics of patients with acute pulmonary embolism: Data from PIOPED II. *Am J Med* 2007;120(10):871–879. doi:10.1016/j.amjmed.2007.03.024

Stein PD, Fowler SE, Goodman LR, et al. Multidetector computed tomography for acute pulmonary embolism. *N Engl J Med* 2006;354(22):2317–2327. doi:10.1056/nejmoa052367

Lankeit M, Jiménez D, Kostrubiec M, et al. Predictive value of the high-sensitivity troponin T assay and the simplified pulmonary embolism severity index in hemodynamically stable patients with acute pulmonary embolism: A prospective validation study. *Circulation* 2011;124(24):2716–2724. doi:10.1161/CIRCULATIONAHA.111.051177

Klok FA, Mos ICM, Huisman M V. Brain-type natriuretic peptide levels in the prediction of adverse outcome in patients with pulmonary embolism: A systematic review and meta-analysis. *Am J Respir Crit Care Med* 2008;178(4):425–430. doi:10.1164/rccm.200803-459OC

Le Gal G, Righini M, Roy PM, et al. Value of D-dimer testing for the exclusion of pulmonary embolism in patients with previous venous thromboembolism. *Arch Intern Med* 2006;166(2):176–180. doi:10.1001/archinte.166.2.176

Den Exter PL, Van Es J, Erkens PMG, et al. Impact of delay in clinical presentation on the diagnostic management and prognosis of patients with suspected pulmonary embolism. *Am J Respir Crit Care Med* 2013;187(12):1369–1373. doi:10.1164/rccm.201212-2219OC

Konstantinides S V., Meyer G, Galié N, et al. 2019 ESC Guidelines for the diagnosis and management of acute pulmonary embolism developed in collaboration with the European Respiratory Society (ERS). *Eur Respir J* 2019;54(3). doi:10.1183/13993003.01647-2019

Agnelli G, Buller HR, Cohen A, et al. Oral apixaban for the treatment of acute venous thromboembolism. *New England Journal of Medicine* 2013; 369 (9): 799–808.

Schulman S, Kearon C, Kakkar AK, et al. Dabigatran versus warfarin in the treatment of acute venous thromboembolism. *N Engl J Med* 2009;361(24):2342–2352. doi:10.1056/nejmoa0906598

García-Bragado Dalmau F. Rivaroxaban oral para el tratamiento de la embolia pulmonar sintomatica. *Rev Clin Esp* 2013;213(5):256–257. doi:10.1016/j.rce.2013.02.004

Bikdeli B, Chatterjee S, Desai NR, et al. Inferior vena cava filters to prevent pulmonary embolism: Systematic review and meta-analysis. *J Am Coll Cardiol* 2017;70(13):1587–1597. doi:10.1016/j.jacc.2017.07.775

Pengo V, Lensing AWA, Prins MH, et al. Incidence of chronic thromboembolic pulmonary hypertension after pulmonary embolism. *N Engl J Med* 2004;350(22):2257–2264. doi:10.1056/nejmoa032274

Wong E, Done N, Zhao M, Woolley A, Prentice J, Mull H. Comparing Total Medical Costs between Patients Receiving Direct Oral Anticoagulants Versus Warfarin for the Treatment of Atrial Fibrillation: Evidence from the VA. Health Serv Res. 2020;55(S1):79–80. doi:10.1111/1475-6773.13440

Chen A, Stecker E, A Warden B. Direct oral anticoagulant use: a practical guide to common clinical challenges. *J Am Heart Assoc* 2020;9(13):e017559. doi:10.1161/JAHA.120.017559

United States Renal Data System. 2020 USRDS Annual Data Report: Epidemiology of kidney disease in the United States. National Institutes of Health, National Institute of Diabetes and Digestive and Kidney Diseases, Bethesda, MD, 2020.

Hart A, Smith JM, Skeans MA, Gustafson SK, Wilk AR, Castro S, Foutz J, Wainright JL, Snyder JJ, Kasiske BL & Israni AK OPTN/SRTR 2018 Annual data report: Kidney. *Am J Transplant* 2019; 20 (Suppl 1): 20–130. doi: 10.1111/ajt.15672

Drüeke TB, Parfrey PS. Summary of the KDIGO guideline on anemia and comment: reading between the (guide)line(s). *Kidney Int* 2012 Nov;82(9):952–60. doi: 10.1038/ki.2012.270. Epub 2012 Aug 1. PMID: 22854645.

Kidney Disease: Improving Global Outcomes (KDIGO) CKD-MBD Update Work Group. KDIGO 2017 Clinical Practice Guideline Update for the Diagnosis, Evaluation, Prevention, and Treatment of Chronic Kidney Disease-Mineral and Bone Disorder (CKD-MBD). *Kidney Int Suppl* (2011). 2017 Jul;7(1):1–59. doi: 10.1016/j.kisu.2017.04.001. Epub 2017 Jun 21. Erratum in: *Kidney Int Suppl* (2011). 2017 Dec;7(3):e1. PMID: 30675420; PMCID: PMC6340919.

A Hoffman BL, Schorge JO, Halvorson LM, Hamid C, Corton M, Schaffer JI. *Williams Gynecology*. New York: McGraw-Hill; 2020.

B De La Cruz M, and Buchanan E. Uterine fibroids and treatment. *Am Fam Physician* 2017 Jan 15;95(2):100–107

Cyr S, Barbee L, Workowski K, et al. Update to CDC's Treatment Guidelines for Gonococcal Infection, 2020. Centers for Disease Control and Prevention. https://www.cdc.gov/mmwr/volumes/69/wr/mm6950a6.htm. Published December 17, 2020. Accessed February 9, 2021.

ASCCP Interim Guidelines. ASCCP. https://www.asccp.org, Accessed February 9, 2021.

Current Medical Diagnosis & Treatment 2022 Eds. Maxine A. Papadakis, et al. McGraw Hill, 2022, https://accessmedicine.mhmedical.com/content.aspx?bookid=3081&sectionid=258579240

Harrison's Principles of Internal Medicine 21e Eds. Joseph Loscalzo, et al. McGraw Hill, 2022, https://accessmedicine.mhmedical.com/content.aspx?bookid=3095&sectionid=259856983.

Index